Doing psychiatry in post-war Europe

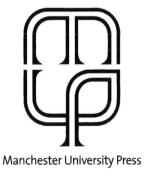

Manchester University Press

SOCIAL HISTORIES OF MEDICINE

Series editors: David Cantor, Anne Hanley and Elaine Leong

Social Histories of Medicine is concerned with all aspects of health, illness and medicine, from prehistory to the present, in every part of the world. The series covers the circumstances that promote health or illness, the ways in which people experience and explain such conditions, and what, practically, they do about them. Practitioners of all approaches to health and healing come within its scope, as do their ideas, beliefs, and practices, and the social, economic and cultural contexts in which they operate. Methodologically, the series welcomes relevant studies in social, economic, cultural, and intellectual history, as well as approaches derived from other disciplines in the arts, sciences, social sciences and humanities. The series is a collaboration between Manchester University Press and the Society for the Social History of Medicine.

To buy or to find out more about the books currently available in this series, please go to: https://manchesteruniversitypress.co.uk/series/social-histories-of-medicine/

Doing psychiatry in postwar Europe

Practices, routines and experiences

Edited by

Gundula Gahlen, Volker Hess,
Marianna Scarfone and Henriette Voelker

MANCHESTER UNIVERSITY PRESS

The publication of this work was supported by the ANR (Agence Nationale de la Recherche), the IUF (Institut Universitaire de France) and by the Open Access Publication Fund of the Humboldt-Universität zu Berlin

The research was funded by the ANR (ANR-18-FRAL-0004) and the DFG (411115568).

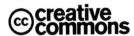

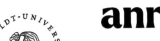

Published by Manchester University Press
Oxford Road, Manchester M13 9PL

www.manchesteruniversitypress.co.uk

British Library Cataloguing-in-Publication Data
A catalogue record for this book is available from the British Library

ISBN   978 1 5261 7346 1   hardback

First published 2024

Typeset
by New Best-set Typesetters Ltd

Contents

Part III – Reflections

Part IV – Crossing institutional boundaries

Figures

Contributors

Monika Ankele is a postdoctoral researcher at the Medical University of Vienna. She works on the history of psychiatry and its institutional cultures in the nineteenth and twentieth century, material cultures and medical humanities. Among her publications are: Monika Ankele and Benoît Majerus (eds), *Material Cultures of Psychiatry* (Bielefeld: Transcript, 2020); Monika Ankele, 'From a patient's view: A sensual-perceptual approach to bed rest', in Bettina Hitzer and Rob Boddice (eds), *Feeling Dis/Ease: Experiencing Medicine and Illness in Modern History* (London: Bloomsbury, 2022), pp. 237–54; Monika Ankele, Sophie Ledebur and Céline Kaiser (eds), *Aufführen, Aufzeichnen, Anordnen: Wissenspraktiken in Psychiatrie und Psychotherapie* (Wiesbaden: Springer Verlag, 2018).

Gábor Csikós is a senior lecturer at the András Pető Faculty of Semmelweis University and research fellow at the Institute of History of the ELKH Research Centre for the Humanities in Budapest. He is interested in rural history, socialist modernisation and the history of psychiatry. Among his publications are: Gábor Csikós, Gergely Krisztián Horváth and József Ö. Kovács (eds), *The Sovietization of Rural Hungary, 1945–1980: Subjugation in the Name of Equality* (London: Routledge, 2023); Gábor Csikós (ed.), *Forrásvidékek: Visszaemlékezések a 20. századra* (Budapest: ELKH – NEB, 2022).

Gundula Gahlen is a research associate at the Ludwig-Maximilians-University Munich. She works on the military history of the eighteenth to twentieth century, the history of psychiatry and cultural history. Among her publications are: Gundula Gahlen, *Nerven, Krieg und militärische Führung: Psychisch erkrankte Offiziere in Deutschland (1890–1939)* (Frankfurt: Campus, 2022); Nikolas Funke, Gundula Gahlen and Ulrike Ludwig (eds), *Krank vom Krieg: Umgangsweisen und kulturelle Deutungsmuster von der Antike bis in die Moderne* (Frankfurt: Campus, 2020); Gundula Gahlen, *Das bayerische Offizierskorps 1815–1866* (Paderborn: Schöningh, 2011).

Volker Hess is Chair of the Institute for the History of Medicine and Ethics in Medicine at the Charité Medical School in Berlin and affiliated professor in the History Department of the Humboldt University. He works on the history of medicine, on the cultural history of psychiatry and madness, and on paper technologies and *Aufschreibesysteme*. Volker has been involved in various collaborative projects in recent years, including the DFG research group 'Cultures of madness' as well as the DFG research group 'Normal#Verrückt'. In 2011 he was awarded an ERC Advanced Grant as principal investigator of 'How physicians know', and in 2019 an ERC Synergy Grant for 'Taming the European Leviathan'. His publications include Volker Hess, 'Bookkeeping madness: Archives and filing between court and ward', *Rethinking History*, 22:3 (2018), 302–35; Volker Hess, 'A paper machine of clinical research in the early 20th century', *ISIS*, 109:3 (2018), 473–93; Volker Hess and J. Andrew Mendelsohn, 'Case and series: Medical knowledge and paper technology, 1600–1900', *History of Science*, 48:3–4 (2010), 287–314.

Despo Kritsotaki is a researcher at the Modern Greek History Research Centre of the Academy of Athens. Her research focuses are the history of mental health and the mental health sciences, history of childhood and the family, and history of sexuality in the twentieth century. Among her publications are: Despo Kritsotaki, *Mental Hygiene, Social Welfare and Psychiatric Reform in Post-War Greece: The Centre for Mental Health and Research, 1956–1978* (Athens: Pedio, 2016) (in Greek); Despo Kritsotaki, Vicky Long and Matthew Smith, *Deinstitutionalisation and After: Post-War Psychiatry in the Western World* (Basingstoke: Palgrave MacMillan, 2016); Despo Kritsotaki, 'Changing psychiatry or changing society? The Motion for the Rights of the "Mentally Ill" in Greece, 1980–1990', *Journal for the History of Medicine and Allied Sciences*, 76:4 (2021), 440–61.

Benoît Majerus is professor of European history at the Centre for Contemporary and Digital History at the University Luxembourg.

He mainly publishes on the history of World War I and II and on the history of psychiatry in the twentieth century. Among his recent publications are: Nicolas Henckes and Benoît Majerus, *Maladies mentales et société (XIXᵉ–XXIᵉ siècles)* (Paris: La Découverte, 2022); Joris Vandendriessche and Benoît Majerus (eds), *Medical Histories of Belgium: New Narratives on Health, Care and Citizenship in the Nineteenth and Twentieth Centuries* (Manchester: Manchester University Press, 2021); Monika Ankele and Benoît Majerus (eds), *Material Cultures of Psychiatry* (Bielefeld: Transcript, 2020).

Christina Malathouni is a senior lecturer at the University of Liverpool School of Architecture. Her main research areas are twentieth-century mental health architecture and twentieth-century architectural heritage. Among her publications are: Christina Malathouni, 'In line with the modern conception of much mental illness: Architectural design contributions to psychiatric reforms in post-war Britain', *Architecture_MPS*, 24:1 (2023), 1–21; Christina Malathouni, 'Beyond the asylum and before the "care in the community" model: Exploring an overlooked early NHS mental health facility', *History of Psychiatry*, 31:4 (2020), 455–69.

Marietta Meier is a full professor and research associate at the University of Zurich. Her research focuses on the history of psychiatry, history of knowledge and history of emotions. Among her publications are: Marietta Meier, 'Third person: Narrating dis-ease and knowledge in psychiatric case histories', in Rob Boddice and Bettina Hitzer (eds), *Feeling Dis-Ease: Experiencing Medicine and Illness in Modern History* (London: Bloomsbury Academic, 2022), pp. 103–20; Marietta Meier, Mario König and Magaly Tornay, *Testfall Münsterlingen: Klinische Versuche in der Psychiatrie, 1940–1980* (Zurich: Chronos, 2019); Marietta Meier, *Spannungsherde: Psychochirurgie nach dem Zweiten Weltkrieg* (Göttingen: Wallstein, 2015).

David Niget is an associate professor in the Department of History at the University of Angers. His primary research topic is juvenile delinquency and youth culture from a gender perspective, expertise and child guidance, moral panics and risk. Among his publications are: David Niget, 'Gender, agency, and sex: Postwar European youth and the generation gap', in J. Marten (ed.), *The Oxford Handbook of the History of Youth Culture* (Oxford: Oxford University Press, 2023); David Niget, 'Sciences du psychisme et citoyenneté dans les institutions de rééducation pour jeunes filles délinquantes en France et en Belgique au XXe siècle', in M. Petitclerc, L. Bienvenue, D. Niget, M. Robert and C. Verbauwhede (eds), *Question sociale et citoyenneté: La dimension politique des régulations sociales (XIXe–XXIe siècles)* (Québec: Presses de l'Université du Québec, 2021); David Niget, 'From criminal justice to the social clinic: The role of magistrates in the circulation of transnational models in the twentieth century', in W. S. Bush and D. S. Tanenhaus (eds), *Ages of Anxiety: Historical and Transnational Perspectives on Juvenile Justice* (New York: New York University Press, 2018), pp. 15–38.

Katariina Parhi is a postdoctoral research fellow at the Academy of Finland Centre of Excellence in the History of Experiences at Tampere University. Her research areas are the social history of medicine, history of psychiatry, historical criminology and history of social control. Among her publications are: Heini Hakosalo, Katariina Parhi and Annukka Sailo (eds), *Historical Explorations of Modern Epidemiology: Patterns, Populations and Pathologies* (London: Palgrave Macmillan, 2023); Katariina Parhi, 'No coming back to sick society: The emergence of new drug user segment in the Järvenpää Social Hospital in Finland, 1965–1975', *Journal of the History of Medicine and Allied Sciences*, 76:4 (2021), 417–39.

Marianna Scarfone is an associate professor at the Department for the History of Medicine at Strasbourg University and a member of the Institut Universitaire de France. Her research focuses on the history of Italian and French psychiatry, and their colonial developments, as well as the mental health/immigration nexus, with particular attention to social aspects. Material, visual and media issues accompany her research on mental health. Among her publications are: Marianna Scarfone, 'Outpatient facilities, visiting nurses, and propaganda: Spaces, actors and tools of mental hygiene in interwar Italy', *Social History of Medicine* (2023); Marianna Scarfone, 'Psychosis of civilization: A colonial-situated diagnosis', *History of Psychiatry*, 32:1 (2021), 52–68; Marianna Scarfone, 'Lives in storage: Clothes and other personal effects as a way of recovering patients' histories in a psychiatric hospital', in Monika Ankele and Benoît Majerus (eds), *Material Cultures of Psychiatry* (Bielefeld: Transcript, 2020), pp. 314–45.

Florent Serina is a lecturer at the University of Lausanne and researcher at the Institut des Humanités en Médecine (CHUV). His research focuses on the history of the human sciences and social and cultural history of psy-sciences. Among his publications are: Florent Serina, *C. G. Jung en France: Rencontres, passions et controverses* (Paris: Les Belles Lettres, 2021); Florent Serina and Stéphane Gumpper (eds), *Pierre Janet: Les Formes de la croyance* (Paris: Les Belles Lettres, 2021); Florent Serina (ed.), *C. G. Jung: Comptes rendus critiques de la psychologie francophone* (Lausanne: Editions BHMS, 2020).

Marica Setaro is a research fellow at the Gerda Henkel Stiftung in Düsseldorf. Her main research areas are the history of psychiatry and the historical epistemology of scientific concepts. Among her publications are: Beatrice Biagioli, Lucilla Gigli and Marica Setaro (eds), *Uno psichiatra umanista: Tra le carte e gli scritti di Agostino Pirella* (Pisa: Edizioni ETS, 2022); Marica Setaro and Silvia Calamai (eds), *Ci chiamavano matti: Voci dal manicomio (1968–1977), by A. M. Bruzzone* (Milan: il Saggiatore, 2021); Matteo Vagelli and Marica Setaro (eds), 'Introduction: Ian Hacking and the historical reason of the sciences', *Philosophical Inquiries*, 9:1 (2021), 115–20.

Ketil Slagstad (MD) is a postdoctoral researcher at the Institute for the History of Medicine and Ethics in Medicine, Charité – Universitätsmedizin Berlin. His research focuses include the history of clinical research, history of transgender medicine, history of HIV/AIDS and the history of psychiatry. Among his publications are: Ketil Slagstad, 'Bureaucratizing medicine: Creating a gender identity clinic in the welfare state', *Isis*, 113:3 (2022), 469–90; Ketil Slagstad, 'The pasts, presents and futures of Aids, Norway (1983–1996)', *Social History of Medicine*, 34:2 (2020), 417–44; Ketil Slagstad, 'The political nature of sex: Transgender in the history of medicine', *New England Journal of Medicine*, 384:11 (2021), 1070–4.

Henriette Voelker is a research associate at the Institute for the History of Medicine and Ethics in Medicine, Charité – Universitätsmedizin Berlin. Her research focuses on the history of the psy-sciences and patient history. Among her publications are: Henriette Voelker, 'Fürsorge und Psychotherapie an der Charité: Berufspraxis im Wandel in den 1960er und 1970er Jahren', in Ekkehardt Kumbier and Kathleen Hack (eds), *Psychiatrie in der DDR III: Weitere Beiträge zur Geschichte* (Berlin: be.bra, 2023), pp. 301–15; Henriette Voelker, '"Die 'freischaffende' Arbeitsweise des Psychologen zu beseitigen": Politischer Auftrag und Eigenlogik psychologischer Praxis in der Schulpädagogik der DDR', *psychosozial*, 45:169 (2022), 9–21.

Introduction: Just another turn? Practices, doing psychiatry and historiography

Volker Hess and Marianna Scarfone

Sociologists, historians and cultural studies scholars often diagnose another turn in the recent study and historiography of sciences, the 'practice turn' (Schatzki *et al.*, 2001; Soler *et al.*, 2016). Sociologists focus on practices in order to reconstruct routines in organisations and companies; historians analyse practices to grasp the meanings of social activities and their transformations over time; and cultural scholars engage with practices to understand how gender is performed or how (sub)cultures become apparent. Everyday practices, material cultures and the history of small things are currently in vogue, and scholars working on the history of psychiatry are beginning to take these objects and perspectives seriously. This collective volume aims at adding a multifaceted contribution, studying psychiatry in its making and unmaking in the second half of the twentieth century through some of the practices that contributed to its shaping: designing hospital buildings and rethinking more 'human' spaces of care; testing treatments and, ongoingly or exceptionally, employing those treatments; inventing new protocols and new relations to patients and users; opening up new fields of expertise and melding with other professionals. Far from just being a fashionable approach employed to renew historiography, engaging with psychiatric practices allows us to understand what psychiatry and mental health assistance were concretely made up of in a more nuanced and precise manner. They were not merely the result of great men and women's actions and discourses, nor a construct of modern society for the control and isolation of deviant subjects, nor an outgrowth of technical and medical progress in the implementation of neuroscientific laboratory findings.

What we aim to show in the following chapters is the variety of practices covering and expanding the field of psychiatry in Europe after World War II, practices that contributed to shape and misshape the field, to redefine its core questions and to answer new ones. The idea of this volume is not to categorise (e.g. psychiatric, extra-psychiatric, anti-psychiatric) or evaluate (e.g. old-fashioned, avant-garde), but to analyse what psychiatrists and other actors of the field did in their daily work. Using selected case studies from across Europe,[1] we will explore how this 'doing' has changed psychiatry through the invention, routinisation and living of a variety of practices, and how these in turn have produced new methods, tools and even goals. The periodisation and spaces covered are vast, but the contributions for the most part adopt a local scale, allowing for a bigger picture to be drawn which highlights the international, national and local contexts, as well as the exchanges and circulations in terms of ideas and their concrete applications.

Psychiatry has experienced various kinds of disempowerment in the post-war period. Today, it no longer takes the form of a large institution in most European countries. Many of the walled-off, fortified bastions on the periphery of urban agglomerations are closed, empty or have been reused for other purposes. Likewise, the expertise of psychiatrists, which had long been in demand in society, politics and the courts, is being disputed by other professionals: educators, psychologists and neuroscientists, even ethicists and alternative practitioners, are competing for the power to determine the narrative in public discourse and private consultations. The territory of psychiatric diagnosis and therapy also has increasingly blurred borders, as we can see in the case of new terms like 'neurodiversity'. With every new edition of the Diagnostic and Statistical Manual (DSM), it is not only the number of diagnoses that grows, but also the reach of the psychiatric gaze (Frances, 2013). At the same time, some of the new "troubles" do not seem to require a psychiatrist to diagnose, treat or provide an expert opinion (for instance concerning child behaviour). Other professionals take over the job. Now that the institutional fundament, disciplinary contours and professional monopoly have been partly lost, it is becoming increasingly difficult to find an adequate answer to the question: 'What is psychiatry and what does psychiatry do?'

We cannot provide an answer, but we can suggest a way to better understand what actually makes psychiatry what it is today. That is what this book aims to do. We do not seek to uncover the theoretical core of present-day psychiatry, to focus on the prominent and influential players, or to question concepts, institutions or academic representation. Instead, we aim to follow psychiatrists as they navigate the field, as they try to help suffering people, to make diagnoses, to counsel relatives, to provide treatment, to write expert reports, to guide policies and courts, to engage in public health services – in short, as they do psychiatry.

Psychiatry is what psychiatrists do? Psychiatry is the way in which psychiatrists do? This tautology is the argument of our volume? No kidding, what may look trivial at first glance becomes a methodological device as soon as we distinguish between doing and acting (Giddens, 1984). While by 'acting' we mean a directed action, with a clearly definable beginning and end of the executed movement, in the following we want to use 'doing' to refer to those habitual patterns of action or more or less ingrained ways of acting that are characterised by repetition, habituation and habitual customisation, in short: the practices of psychiatric doing as they manifest themselves in admitting or discharging patients, having exchanges with them or creating the conditions for broader relations with other patients or carers (for example, placing chairs in a circle and arranging group meetings), entrusting them to other services or professionals, note-taking, prescribing and so on. Such practices resemble invisible little tools or patterns that are present all the time. Their performance is usually understood by all participants sharing the same social sphere, which cannot be said of deliberate acts. The turn of our historical analysis to such practices should not be misunderstood as a 'reinvention'. Rather, it is an extension of the methodological arsenal necessary to devote adequate reflection to contemporary psychiatry.

If we take up this 'praxeological approach' and follow the psychiatrists, patients, other caregivers and expert figures involved in the psychiatric field, three advantages become apparent. First, the praxeological approach allows us to identify and provide a thick description of many practices that – for a short period of time or settling in as routines – contributed to the profound transformation of psychiatry as an ensemble of institutions and as a discipline. Whether writing an epicrisis, organising the daily life of a therapeutic community or documenting one's experience through the spoken word, some psychiatric practices have apparently proven far more durable and stable than the institutions from which they once emerged. Other 'ways of doing' came from other disciplines or other institutions and were implemented in the psychiatric field as it expanded its skillset or sought new ways to answer old questions (how to cure, how to reduce the symptoms, how to deal with patients). At the same time, we observe that psychiatrists became involved in entirely new fields of activity, such as for example sex therapy (Lišková, 2018), which had little to do with the conception of psychiatry that once made the institution great. Moreover, new practices involved new professionals such as psychologists, psychotherapists, social workers and, more recently, peer support workers. At present, relatives' groups and affected persons' organisations are becoming part of psychiatric work and making their voices heard. If we take a closer look at such practices, we will probably attain a better understanding of what psychiatry has been about since the end of the classical institution and the loss of its power to determine the narrative.

Second, looking at such practices can show how existing structures enabled and mediated certain actions (e.g. forced medication or morning rounds) but, at the same time, how they were simultaneously established and structured by certain activities (e.g. talk therapy, patients' leisure time, use of space). In and through their actions, the actors involved (professionals, patients and relatives) in turn reproduced the conditions that make these actions possible (Giddens, 1984: 2). Power relations presented themselves as more fluid and malleable in such recursive loops. We can more easily trace how they became effective, how they were embedded in the daily lives of psychiatric patients and how they changed or were reshaped.

Third, analysing practices allows us to focus on and explore other fields of activity that have rarely been considered in the context of mental health issues. In this way, aspects reaching beyond institutionalised psychiatry (including facilities that emerged within the multifaceted post-war reform of psychiatry, such as out-patient care, day and night clinics and assisted living) become objects of analysis. Other elements also enter the picture of this renewed historical enquiry, such as public health policy, affected persons' organisations, architecture and sociology. The multiple fields associated with psychiatry form an integrated network that is established and connected through common practices.

If one takes the practices seriously and observes how they are interwoven, how they solidify in routines and liquefy again, and how they occasionally emerge from a patchwork of different activities, it is not only a different history of psychiatry that emerges. Such a reconstruction certainly has implications for our understanding and conception of psychiatry. From a praxeological perspective, psychiatry presents itself less as a science grounded in theory or laboratory research than as an art of doing. Psychiatry can be understood as the outcome of practices and routinised habits. Psychiatry, even in the age of neuroscience, is not so much a science in the strict sense of the word, but a *techne* – a learned craft – characterised by those special skills that make psychiatrists, even today, sought-after professionals: experts who include social aspects, who see their own actions as having a rationale of social responsibility, and, finally, who develop solutions to problems that reach far beyond the threshold of the clinic or laboratory – in short, professionals who make the challenges of modern society manageable. How is that possible?

What all praxeological approaches have in common is that they concede or ascribe an intrinsic value to practices. This means that practices cannot be reduced to the mere 'application' of theoretical concepts, the execution of normative rules or the intentionality of actions. Nor is it sufficient to focus on the fact that theories, rules or norms are subject to some wear and tear or shrinkage in the mangle of practice (Pickering, 1991). Rather, practices are generative or productive, not in the sense of historical epistemology but in the sense of a 'resistance' or material constraint through which cherished habits, entrenched routines and formalised courses of action resist change. They become generative through unacknowledged conditions that produce unforeseen or unintended consequences, which can be articulated in new structures, rules and norms, but also new meanings, habits and routines.

The question remains: What is new about a history of psychiatric practices? Is this not merely a rewriting of the classical history of psychiatry? Are 'psychiatric practices' more than the regularities of action or regulated patterns of intervention whose description and explanation the historiography of psychiatry has pursued from the beginning? Scepticism seems understandable at first glance, but there is a risk of underestimating the innovative value of a well-considered concept of practice. In fact, such a concept entails a changed understanding of what 'acting' is – and thus also of what 'actor' and 'subject' mean. At the same time, and above all, it changes our understanding of psychiatry.

What is the theory of practice?

Science studies and the history of science were the first historical disciplines to adopt praxeological approaches (Lynch, 1993; Buchwald, 1995; Pickering, 1995). By asking what researchers actually do in their laboratories and how scientific facts are produced, the hitherto popular notion of intentional rational experimentation was reduced to absurdity (Knorr Cetina, 1984; Latour and Woolgar, 1986; Fleck, 1993). Many studies in the history of science have been able to show – by reconstructing the practices involved, the constant tinkering with the equipment, the incessant changes in the experimental set-up and the apparent game of trial and error – how a scientific finding emerges, is stabilised and disseminated, and finally accepted. In contrast, the history of medicine understood practice for a long time as the locus where medical treatment was performed, or even the performative dimension of such activities itself. Only under the influence of ethnological considerations has that aspect been problematised which today is at the centre of all praxeological approaches – namely the mediation and production of meaning.

Praxeological approaches feed from quite different disciplines, ranging from anthropology and sociology to philosophy, as well as the already mentioned science studies. For Max Weber, who always understood social sciences as part of cultural studies (*Kulturwissenschaften*), 'no cognition of cultural processes is conceivable other than on the basis of the meaning which the always individual reality of life has for us in specific, individual relationships' (Weber, 2006: 745).[2] Therefore, all cultural expressions are merely a 'finite section of the senseless infinity of the world events, which is considered with meaning and significance'. These considerations have brought the anthropologist Clifford Geertz to the much-quoted formulation that culture is to be understood as a 'self-spun web of meanings' (Geertz, 1973: 5), in which the human being is always entangled.[3]

According to Claude Lévi-Strauss (Lévi-Strauss, 1962), a given practice can be seen as a bricolage, a patchwork created by various elements of action and rules of combination. The early Pierre Bourdieu, drawing on Noam Chomsky, extended this model of a generative grammar of action to the whole field of social practices (Bourdieu, 1977). A finite number of established and routinised elements of action in the psychiatric field (dressing the ill, dispensing medication, patients' work therapy) and an equally finite number of pairings (free choice/uniform (dressing), self-reliant/forced (medication), paid/unpaid (work)) generate and enable, through their recombination, both new possibilities for action and other practices. On this grammar of action, Bourdieu built his theory of practice to establish the concept of habitus and link the microanalysis of individual behaviour with the macroanalysis of society. A praxeological analysis of psychiatric practices can show, for instance, how a traditional element of psychiatric diagnosis (the 'sick person's handwriting sample') combined with a likewise established element of ambulatory psychiatric approaches (the 'talking cure') acquired a dazzling ambiguity through the routine of writing a daily report in a socialist setting, carrying both emancipatory and disempowering meanings. Even the use of hypnosis, formerly considered obsolete, could suddenly appear as a resistant mode of action in a politicised setting.

It is, of course, possible, as many sociologists and philosophers suggest, to specify each individual act in at least one of these respects: purpose, intention and motive. However, this does not yet determine a practice; rather, it conflates the designation of agency with the description of separate purposes (Giddens, 1984). In Giddens's words, any purposive action is not composed of a set of separate intentions, reasons and motives. In practice, each individual action is embedded in a constant flow of conduct. It cannot be separated from its social context of time and space. There are former and subsequent actions. Repetition, practice and habituation not only transform the execution of actions into a practice, they also charge this practice, so to speak, with the context of the original activity, and give the practice a meaning that goes beyond its mere purpose or intention.

This is easier to understand from a historical distance which alienates us from the 'naturalness' of recent patterns of practice. To give an example: the purpose of dressing newly admitted patients in uniforms was to provide each of them with functional, safe and egalitarian clothing. It also served hygiene and was intended to prevent the spread of germs and unwelcome parasites. Over the decades, if patients were redressed upon admission, repetition and habituation inscribed further meanings on this action beyond its original purpose, which were in turn conveyed with each performance of the practice – the undressing, accompanied by the deprivation of personal effects, contributed to the humiliation of the patient, taking away some material expressions of his or her identity, defining him or her as an inmate of a total institution. Defined as purposive acts, practices, including psychiatric practices, reveal themselves to us only incompletely and thus remain underdetermined. They may be theoretically grounded, scientifically justified and rationally legitimated, however, practices are neither adequately described nor even sufficiently understood by theory, science and reason. Rather, they lead – metaphorically speaking – a life of their own, which only opens up to historical analysis if one understands practices as meaning-mediating and meaning-generating, and includes these meanings in the analysis. In this way, the ceremony of dressing newly admitted patients took on a meaning that was presumably not intended, and certainly not adequately reflected or rationalised.

Practices are thus understood as temporally extended events or processes, as both Anthony Giddens (1984) and Joseph Rouse (2018) describe them. However, while for Giddens a practice is characterised by repetition, habituation and routinisation (as opposed to the act as an element of action), Rouse, in a more traditional way, emphasises the rule-governed and normatively set or legitimated constructivity of such practices. In this way, however, rules and norms again become primary. Nevertheless, the normative approach opens up a thought-provoking perspective, since Rouse sees actors themselves (and their actions) as constituted by practices. As a result, practices are the essential mode of interaction with the world through which human action is mediated.[4] Giddens, on the other hand, sees the reflexivity with which actors themselves track, evaluate and correct their actions as the crucial factor for a rationality of action. Some of Geertz's cultural anthropology comes into play when Rouse depicts practices as meaningful configurations of the world – i.e. as the weaving and spinning activity which fabricates that cocoon in which the human being – as a social and cultural being – is trapped.

The conclusion that Bourdieu, Giddens and Rouse draw from their praxeological considerations seems more important for us: practices are a prior or at least more important category than subject and action. The study of practices avoids or defers the inevitable questions of professional historiography, from which the history of psychiatry has emerged over the last decades: Who did this? What is the driving force? Beyond all theoretical differences, we hold that it is more important to consider for which questions a particular praxeological approach can be operationalised, for which sources it is suitable and which pitfalls of previous historiography of medicine and science it helps to avoid.

State of the art

More than a decade ago, it was noted that the history of twentieth-century psychiatry lacked strong narratives comparable to those that have helped us to understand the psychiatry of former times, that is, those produced by historians, cultural scholars, psychiatrists and other professionals (Hess and Majerus, 2011). Instead, the historiography of contemporary psychiatry is still intertwined with the legacies of the nineteenth century, especially in German-speaking countries (Weindling, 1989; Faulstich, 1993; Hohendorff *et al.*, 2010; Fangerau *et al.*, 2017). What is needed, so the programmatic claim, is to take into account new actors and spaces, different methodologies and fresh perspectives. Indeed, the last decade has seen many approaches that transcend the disciplinary narrative while retaining a sense of the dynamics of silencing, the wilfulness (*Eigensinn*) of actors and the rare forms of resistance (Gijswijt-Hofstra *et al.*, 2005; for case studies see Meier, 2007; Lamb, 2014; Göhlsdorf, 2015). Many studies have also overcome the narrative of the single institution while retaining an awareness of the advantages of the micro-level approach (Majerus, 2013) and deconstructed the insane asylum as the only space where psychiatry could develop (Beddies and Dörries, 1999; Henckes, 2011; Beyer, 2016; Klein *et al.*, 2018). Recent research has finally examined the multiple manifestations of psychiatric practice in respect to the places, techniques and activities of doing, particularly for the post-World War II period (Crossley, 2006; Skålevåg, 2006; Eghigian, 2015; Kritsotaki *et al.*, 2019).

Many studies have been carried out on the relation between war and psychiatry. Wars have been seen as an important trigger of mental troubles, which led to innovation in the field of mental health in the military system as well as in civil medicine and society. War brought a rise in new diagnoses like the ancestors of PTSD (post-traumatic stress disorder) and a decline in older ones like neurasthenia and hysteria (Lerner, 1996; Gijswijt-Hoftstra and Porter, 2001; Crouthamel and Leese, 2017; Schöhl and Hess, 2019); the bible of psychiatry in the USA, the DSM (Diagnostic and Statistical Manual of Mental Disorders), was a veritable child of military medicine (Mayers and Horwitz, 2005; Horwitz, 2021). The international mental hygiene movement is being scrutinised in its national and local developments as one of first systematic expressions of the will to deinstitutionalise mental assistance and to make it penetrate the social fabric (Fussinger, 2011; Kritsotaki *et al.*, 2019). Psychiatry's expertise went beyond the asylum walls: homes were visited to detect mental (as well as familial and social) misfunction (Kölch, 2001; Fuchs *et al.*, 2012; Bakker, 2021); dispensaries distributed psychiatric care in urban areas; day clinics extended the former asylum into urban spaces (Hess and Ledebur, 2012); and preventative strategies and counselling developed into new fields of activity with which psychiatry entered the realm of normal everyday life (Henckes *et al.*, 2018; Kritsotaki *et al.*, 2019). While recent psychiatric history now largely agrees on the historiographical evaluation of heroic therapies, the pharmacological revolution remains a challenge (Schmuhl and Roelcke, 2013; Greene *et al.*, 2016). Thus, the apologetic progress stories about the introduction of psychotropic drugs have now given way to a certain thoughtfulness.[5] Although it is indisputable, there has not yet been sufficient research on whether the psychiatric reforms of the post-war decades, especially the dehospitalisation of psychiatric patients and reduction in inpatient length of stay, were greatly aided by the psychopharmacological revolution (Pieters and Majerus, 2011). However, its consequences, especially the economisation of psychiatric treatment and close collaboration between psychiatry and big pharma, are now viewed more critically (Healy, 1997, 2013).[6] This is also due to the fact that the success of psychopharmacotherapy is by no means as convincing in historical analyses as it is in the accounts of the psychiatrists involved (Majerus, 2019).

Deinstitutionalisation has proved to be probably the most enduring buzzword for a new narrative that may do justice to the post-war history of psychiatry. Even if deinstitutionalisation, according to the accounts of its protagonists, often seems to have fallen out of history, given the radical calls in the 1960s and 1970s for an end to the asylum, the beginnings of deinstitutionalisation can be traced back to more or less isolated practices at the end of the nineteenth century (Schmiedebach and Priebe, 2003; Klein *et al.*, 2018; von Bueltzingsloewen, 2020). Thus, it remains topical to ask what deinstitutionalisation meant in concrete terms and how one can analytically grasp and conceptualise those areas of psychiatric action which, beyond the 'boundaries of the institution', resurrected it in a new form – in the form of forensic psychiatric hospitals, institutions for the disabled or homes for the elderly (Brink, 2010; Coché, 2017). Much more intriguing, however, are the attempts to explore the fringes of psychiatric activity since World War II: transcultural psychiatry (Ellenberger *et al.*, 2020; Antic, 2022), sex therapy (Lišková, 2018) and the transformation of psychiatric treatment services into a lifestyle and consumer item (Ehrenberg and Lovell, 2000; Donald, 2001), to name just three examples. Ideological boundaries are also being brought into view. In addition to class and social origin, recent studies have shed light on the role of gender, race and geographical origin in shaping disciplinary assumptions and concrete relations in the field of psychiatry (for instance Studer, 2016; Edwards-Grossi, 2022; Scarfone, 2023).

Greg Eghigian's call for a deinstitutionalisation of the historiography of psychiatry has fallen on receptive ears (Eghigian, 2011; von Bueltzingsloewen, 2015; Guillemain, 2020). However, recent studies have rarely questioned the boundaries of the subject and the academic discipline; instead, they have mostly described the fragmentation and specialisation of knowledge. For one, recent research has 'decentred' a long-held focus on the psychiatric department and identified other spaces and places where psychiatry was also practised or where the actors' actions and activities were guided by the goals and tools of psychiatry. For another, more recent approaches closer to cultural studies are readily adopted to explore the materiality and performativity of institutional practices with an interdisciplinary or even artistic approach (Ankele and Majerus, 2020).

The scene of psychiatry has been enriched by new actors whose invisibility was marked in previous research. Besides psychiatrists, other professionals from the field of care are being considered, from nurses and social workers to psychologists and psychoanalysts (Henckes, 2014; Rzesnitzek, 2015; Tornay, 2016; Marks, 2017; Balz and Malich, 2020; Smith, 2020). Psychotherapy began to play an important role in urban facilities, where social and medical aspects of treatment were dealt with simultaneously, as for instance in drug abuse policy or in the therapeuticisation of 'total institutions' like jail or school. Here, beside the prescription of drugs and other treatments, some of the carers began to devote their time to considering the patients' words, as psychology and psychoanalysis proposed. During the post-war reform of psychiatry, psychoanalytic insights gained a place in some psychiatrists' training and in their approach, not only to patients, but also to institutional issues. The French movement of 'institutional psychotherapy' (Oury, 2016; Robcis, 2021) – at the core of the 'refoundation' of some psychiatric hospitals – is an example of this trend.

Furthermore, psychologists began to perform tests, on which the psychiatrists' diagnostic work in part relied, both in psychiatric hospitals and in other facilities. Through paper technologies and the materiality of the psychologists' tools and tests retrieved from the archives, the professionalisation of psychologists and their integration in public mental health become tangible. Nurses' roles were reshaped as well: to adjust to treating mental patients, they could follow special trainings, as at the *Association de Santé Mentale du 13ème arrondissement* in Paris or at the Heidelberg Psychiatric University Clinic (Henckes, 2007; Prebble and Bryder, 2008; Henckes, 2014; Borsay and Dale, 2015). The social worker, after a shy appearance in the interwar period, became a figure of mediation between the medical sphere and other spheres of the everyday life of mentally affected people, a means of tentative integration in these spheres: self-sufficiency, work, welfare and administrative procedures (Borsay and Dale, 2015; Dickinson, 2015; Nolte and Hähner-Rombach, 2017). Speech and language therapists could also accompany the global care of some psychiatric patients, as could occupational therapists and ergotherapists, who were involved in redesigning the environment within which one evolves and in rehabilitative processes (Mitchell, 2002).

Moreover, the family, relatives and milieu in a broader sense have also found their place in the complex mosaic of the history of psychiatry. They are no longer reduced to their role in the admissions and discharge processes. Rather, they are taken seriously as actors in the patient trajectory, who offer a different perspective on the illness, develop different ways of dealing with it and ultimately have to bear the consequences for the family and the workplace. The patient, too, is given a proper place in this picture. Admittedly, the claim of a history from below cannot be realised in the way some once imagined (Porter, 1985; Condrau, 2007).

The sick person is no longer seen as the more or less passive bearer of a label or conceptualised as the victim of stigma. Instead, there is an attempt to do justice to him or her as the actor of a life of his or her own. More recent histories consider the integration of the patient in treatment as a peer support worker and attempt to grasp their social networks and reconstruct the web of shared experiences in order to gain a more detailed perception of their lives beyond authority: their hardships, but also their joys and freedoms (see Ankele, 2009). This new attention to everyday-life aspects of mental illness beyond the institution sharpens our view of the causes and consequences of social precarity, also as a consequence of migration and discrimination (Nellen, 2007; Guillemain, 2018).

Roy Porter's demand to give importance to the patient's perspective has produced narratives from the bottom up, made possible by a more sensitive way of approaching the archive, which enables the historian to not only see paper technologies as deployed by the psychiatric staff, but also observe the appropriation of these technologies in their dimension as tools of expression. The archive is somehow more stratified, more complex: the now classic clinical files are articulated with interviews, made and registered in the past decades or conducted by the historian nowadays with witnesses or actors (Bruzzone, 2021), with material objects or with spaces and atmospheres (Ankele and Majerus, 2020). A growing importance is given to media, the audiovisual and visual technologies that furnish both new objects of inquiry and precious sources to question how psychiatry represented itself (Berton *et al.*, 2018).

These multiple turns contributing to diversify, decentre and enrich the gaze of the history of psychiatry – the patient's turn, the spatial turn, the visual turn, the material turn – have been taken as an invitation to consider new actors, new perspectives and new sources. The practical turn could be applied likewise to writing the history of mental health. However, this collective volume suggests a slightly different way, because the many turns that the history of psychiatry has endorsed also raise more fundamental questions, especially about the relationship between theory and practice, everyday life and science, the profession at large and experts, and so on. A praxeological approach, this volume argues, contributes to providing insightful answers to these questions through the thick description of experiences.

Of course, practices cannot be observed historically in the field as their actual deployment can be through the immersive ethnological methods of observation and participation. But we can retrieve the traces they have left in the more or less classical material we deal with to write history. In most cases, these traces are not intentionally handed down, but are inscribed in the materiality of the surviving sources, such as arrows, notes and crossed out elements on the cover of a medical record that once steered its way through an institution (Hess and Schlegelmilch, 2016; Hess, 2018). We can also trace the repetition and carrying out of actions that, in their processualism, ground a practice. And we can, finally, reconstruct their meaning and purpose by embedding them in an analysis of the historical context of their development, which once gave them meaning and mediated their purpose.

Outline of the volume

Practices come to life and are performed in very different dimensions: productive, experimental, reflexive or transgressive. In and through practices, new ideas are articulated or visions take shape, but they also open up new options for action, sometimes even new worlds waiting to be realised. Practices are also the acid test in which new concepts prove themselves or become concrete. Reflecting on practices can itself become a self-reflective practice. After all, practices do not adhere to institutional or disciplinary boundaries; on the contrary, they often form the hinge that articulates very different areas of our modern wider world. These dimensions – visions and dreams, experimentation, reflections, crossing boundaries – organise the volume.

The section 'Visions and dreams' focuses on experiences that have been viewed, lived and narrated by the very protagonists as unique and utopian. The four cases presented here cover different spaces and temporalities – from 1980s Greece to 1960s Italy, from 1970s Germany to post-war England. These ways of doing psychiatry are linked to the spaces where they took place as much as to the initiators of these 'groundbreaking' practices. They represent a reformist impetus determined to break with previous entrenched frameworks. The character of novelty assigned by the actors to their creations and experiences is here also seen through the eyes of the patients, as far as the sources allow one to read and interpret how the latter saw these activities and apparatuses primarily addressed at the well-being of each individual, rather than at refreshing discipline and its therapeutic and architectural expressions in se (extraverted sensing). New ethics for mental health professionals – for doctors as well as nurses and new collaborating professions – appeared: democratisation, the exchange of views (of roles in the most extreme cases), reducing distance, allowing empathy to emerge. The newly conceived spaces in the post-war period seemed to reflect these ambitions too.

The first essay of this section is Despo Kritsotaki's, on a facility in Athens that pursued socially and politically oriented mental healthcare in post-dictatorship Greece, combining the models of group analysis and the therapeutic community. Here, the political dimension endorsed by the protagonists contributed to making the project a utopian microcosm. Democratising psychiatry – through emancipation, the absence of hierarchy, equal participation and respect of everyone's personality – was the aim, as well as the ideological and practical framework in which therapeutics and relations were deployed.

Marica Setaro's chapter looks at the general assemblies that took place in the therapeutic community implemented in the 1960s in the psychiatric hospital of Gorizia (Italy). Insofar as it brought together doctors, patients, nurses and volunteers, it presented itself as a democratic tool, a space for non-hierarchical exchange and discussion. However, the chapter shows a cleavage between this stated ambition and its perception by some of the inmates – as a supplementary space for the doctors to scrutinise patients' attitudes and a place where requests remained unanswered. Giving an account of the Gorizia experience – classically described as the departure point of the reform trajectory that led to the closing of mental hospitals in Italy at the end of the 1970s – from a multifocal perspective, this chapter balances visionary intent with more concrete aspects.

Gundula Gahlen's text focuses on the Department of Social Psychiatry and Rehabilitation at the Heidelberg Clinic in the 1960s and 1970s. Here, practices included less systematic use of drugs and shock therapies; an awareness of the importance of patients' expression; daily meetings of medical professionals, staff and patients; new roles, responsibilities and attitudes for the nurses; and continuity in the path of care, from inpatient to outpatient, from bringing people back from acute phases to rehabilitation and reintegration into social life, through work, education and multiple activities in outpatient facilities. Unique and somehow visionary at the beginning of the 1960s, those practices later become routinised here and elsewhere and part of what was expected in a psychiatry ward.

These three chapters focus on visionary ways of doing psychiatry through the development of renewed relations to inmates, the aspiration to democratise and de-hierarchise, and the support of social reintegration paths for the mentally ill. The fourth deals with visionary ways of materially preparing the ground and equipping the space for a renewed psychiatry. Christina Malathouni's chapter is about architectural transformations of psychiatric facilities in 1950s England. It takes the admission unit of a psychiatric hospital situated in what is today Oxfordshire as one of the first examples in which aspirations to reform psychiatric practices and their environment merged with architectural and spatial arrangements through the reflection of a new generation of architects on these topics. The chapter highlights the place that some professionals, who are not psy-specialists, can take in providing the best possible solutions, in a somehow utopistic way, to some aspects of psychiatric doing – namely the spaces, the environment and the atmosphere.

The section 'Experimentation' focuses on some specific cases – one from 1970s Finland, another from 1950s France and the third from post-1956 Hungary – whose protagonists were aware that they were trialling new ways of doing. These have not necessarily become mainstream, but contributed to shaping new frameworks of therapeutic intervention or allowed for feebler protocolar procedures and eclectic appropriations.

Katariina Parhi's chapter captures the functioning of two Helsinki outpatient facilities for the treatment of young drug users. The chapter highlights the experimental character that these non-profit, non-governmental organisations for the prevention of substance abuse embodied. On the one hand, they refused the alcohol abuse model of assistance – namely the imposition of strict rules, as well as the prescription of medication. On the other hand, they tended to abolish rigid ways of understanding sociopsychological mechanisms. In this way, previous psychiatric ways of doing were overturned, making space for non-hierarchical experimentation in the emerging field of the care of young drug users, where psychiatry worked shoulder to shoulder with social work. Experimentation here meant dealing with a new problem – the substance abuse among the youngest – and distancing from the classical hierarchical and prescriptive ways of correcting these styles of life. It also meant giving new value to non-authoritarian expertise, coming more from a place of exchange than imposition, more from listening than redressing.

Florent Serina's chapter is dedicated to the implementation of psychosurgical techniques in the University Psychiatric Clinic of Strasbourg over a decade, from the end of the 1940s. It shows how that innovation was used, routinised and finally excluded from the arsenal of available treatments. The chapter covers experimentation in two ways. Firstly, as a locally situated and locally observed setting up of a technique experimental in se, through an ensemble of actors and what can be retrieved of procedures, mostly from paper technologies, related to the implementation of that technique. Secondly, it focuses on the phases that composed something that remained of the order of the experimental: uncertain beginnings, the peak of uses with a kind of routine, the reduction in the number of operations performed and the growing caution around them.

The last chapter of this section, Gábor Csikós on Hungarian child psychiatry following the 1956 insurrection and repression, focuses on one single treatment case, through which some developments of this young discipline are highlighted. With the backdrop of the political conditions, the chapter considers the question of the

difficult differential diagnosis of mutism, the fitting of electroconvulsive therapy with Pavlovian theories and the therapeutic eclecticism
at the practical level. In the young boy's story, hypnotherapy is
applied when ECT and other biological therapies do not seem to
be successful. This constitutes a shift from active therapies to psy-
chodynamics, although of course hypnosis was considered more in
line with Pavlovian principles than 'bourgeois' Freudianism.

Entitled 'Reflections', the third section aims at showing how the
actors were called to think about the practices in which they directly
or indirectly took part and how they gave them meaning. This
reflective habit questioned the very role of doctors. It was conducive
to a closer empathic and therapeutic exchange with patients, as in
Marietta Maier's chapter, and to the potential role of other professionals, like the sociologists rethinking the asylums' atmosphere and
relations in Monika Ankele's chapter. It also appears in the patients'
perception of a particular way of treating them and of asking them
for a personal written reflection on daily life within the ward, as in
Henriette Voelker's chapter.

Through medical records and treatment protocols filled out in
the Burghölzli clinic in Zurich in the early 1950s, Marietta Maier
gives us access to how a psychotherapeutic trial took place which
intensively involved a team of professionals and a selected number
of patients. A thick description of the new practice is offered: the
time they spent together, the patients' improvement and deterioration
and the critical reflections that doctors and nurses began to have
about themselves, their work and the social role of psychiatry. Here
we can see how the psychiatric self – the self-perception of one's
very role in clinical, professional and human terms – was changed
by experiences. These contributed to place attentive observation,
regular exchanges with the patients, and reflection on day-to-day
actual and mainly relational psychiatric doing at the core of the
professionals' practice. The following chapter by Monika Ankele
shows how sociology became a tool for social criticism and for
sociopolitical change in the years when new ways of doing psychiatry
were sought after. With the aim of observing daily life in the hospital
– living conditions for patients and working conditions for nurses
– the empirical research carried out at the main Vienna psychiatric
hospital in the 1970s resounded with the political will to reform

psychiatry. Although a reflective attitude is palpable here on the sociologists' and decision-makers' side and, further, instilled in psychiatric professional actors, the patients' voices and reflexions remain inaudible in the critical sociological practice. In the last chapter of this section, by Henriette Voelker, we can see how dynamic group psychotherapy practice aimed at empowering patients in socialist East Berlin. Avoiding authoritarian guidance, patients were invited to write reports on their daily experience of this experimental therapeutic milieu. The writing practice, both intimate and relational, resulted in a combination of self-analysis, interpersonal communication and further reflection by therapists on their own role, on the practices implemented and on the efficacity of the therapies for each patient. As a brick in the larger construct of reformed ways of doing psychiatry, this practice tended to make the patients protagonists of their cure and responsible for their attitude – in the spotlight of a medical 'reading gaze'.

The last section, 'Crossing institutional boundaries', shows how disciplines and fields of action other than psychiatry have borrowed practices that were characteristic of psychiatry and how psychiatric expertise has played a central role beyond the treatment of mental diseases, namely in the field of sex reassignment in 1970s Norway and in youth redressing institutions in 1960s Belgium.

Ketil Slagstad's chapter analyses the role of psychiatric expertise in transgender healthcare. In a decade when sexology gained autonomy and public credit, the Oslo Health Council began to offer standardised assistance and accompaniment for trans people. Here, psychiatry crossed the borders of its classic diagnostic and therapeutic terrain to take charge of issues concerning medical transition. In Benoît Majerus and David Niget's chapter, we can see how the use of psychotropics crossed the borders of the psychiatric field, as they were used within the Belgian youth guidance institution of Saint-Servais between 1959 and 1975. 'Difficult' girls were closely observed in the 'Special Section', to which 'troublesome elements' were sent when they disturbed the normal course of life in the pavilions. The quantitative and qualitative analysis shows an entanglement of disciplinary and curative objectives and the ways to achieve them, through the significant – though almost unnoticeable in individual files – use of neuroleptics.

The contributions in this volume emerged from a working group conducted by the Franco-German research project 'Alter Psy' jointly led by the two of us between autumn 2020 and winter 2021. We would like to thank all of the authors, who were willing to present and discuss their contributions again and again in the workshops and to incorporate the suggestions from the joint working meetings into their contributions. We would also like to give special thanks to the commentators who, as external experts, critically reviewed the contributions at the last meeting of the working group, namely Viola Balz, Cornelius Borck, Jean-Christophe Coffin, Susanne Doetz, Alexa Geisthövel, Louise Hide, Bettina Hitzer, Lisa Malich, Sarah Marks, Jörg Niewöhner, Maike Rotzoll and Markus Wahl. For helpful support, we also thank Janik Hollnagel (MA student) and Stefanie Voth, and Brier Field for English proof reading. We also received a great deal of help during the publication process. Many thanks go to the pleasant cooperation with David Cantor as series editor and Meredith Carroll from Manchester University Press, as well as to Jaqueline Sachse from Humboldt University Berlin for her support with the open access publication. Last but not least, we are grateful for the support of this project by the Agence national de la recherche and the Deutsche Forschungsgemeinschaft. For all errors we, the editors, are of course responsible.

Notes

1 In contrast to Doroshow, Gambino and Raz (2019), who studied mostly the USA context.
2 Translation ours.
3 The (retranslated) German translation of Geertz is much more vivid than the original phrase: 'that the man is an animal suspended in webs of significance he himself has spun' (Geertz, 1973: 5). For the German translation see Geertz, 1983: 9.
4 Koo 2017: 95; see also 'practice' in the *Oxford English Dictionary*.
5 For success stories see: Swazey, 1974; McCrae, 2006; in contrast: Speaker, 1997; Greenslit, 2005; Jenkins, 2010; Balz, 2010; Balz, 2011; Tornay, 2016. For patients' perspectives on biological therapies: Majerus, 2019; Guillemain, 2020.
6 For case studies see: Hess, 2015; Meier, König and Tornay, 2019; Wagner, 2019; Hottenrott, 2021.

References

Ankele, Monika, 2009, *Alltag und Aneignung in Psychiatrien um 1900: Selbstzeugnisse von Frauen aus der Sammlung Prinzhorn* (Vienna: Böhlau).

Ankele, Monika and Benoît Majerus (eds), 2020, *Material Cultures of Psychiatry* (Bielefeld: Transcript).

Antic, Ana, 2022, 'Decolonising madness: Transcultural psychiatry, international order, and the birth of a global psyche in the aftermath of WWII', *Journal of Global History*, 17:1, 20–41.

Bakker, Nelleke, 2021, 'From talking cure to play- and group-therapy: Outpatient mental health care for children in the Netherlands *c.*1945–70', *History of Psychiatry*, 32:4, 385–401.

Balz, Viola, 2010, *Zwischen Wirkung und Erfahrung: Eine Geschichte der Psychopharmaka: Neuroleptika in der Bundesrepublik Deutschland, 1950–1980* (Bielefeld: Transcript Verlag).

Balz, Viola, 2011, 'Terra incognita: An historiographic approach to the first chlorpromazine trials using patient records of the Psychiatric University Clinic in Heidelberg', *History of Psychiatry*, 22:2, 182–200.

Balz, Viola and Lisa Malich (eds), 2020, *Psychologie und Kritik: Formen der Psychologisierung nach 1945* (Wiesbaden: Springer).

Beddies, Thomas and Andrea Dörries, 1999, 'Coping with quantity and quality: Computer-based research on case records from the "Wittenauer Heilstätten" in Berlin', *History of Psychiatry*, 10:37, 59–85.

Berton, Mireille, Charlotte Bouchez and Susie Trenka, 2018, *La circulation des images: Cinéma, photographie et nouveaux médias / Die Zirkulation der Bilder: Kino, Fotografie und neue Medien* (Marburg: Schüren).

Beyer, Christof, 2016, '"Islands of reform": Early transformation of the mental health service in Lower Saxony, Germany in the 1960s', in Despo Kritsotaki, Vicky Long and Matthew Smith (eds), *Deinstitutionalisation and After: Post-War Psychiatry in the Western World* (Basingstoke: Palgrave Macmillan), pp. 99–114.

Borsay, Anne and Pamela Dale, 2015, *Mental Health Nursing: The Working Lives of Paid Carers in the Nineteenth and Twentieth Centuries* (Manchester: Manchester University Press).

Bourdieu, Pierre, 1977, *Outline of a Theory of Practice* (Cambridge: Cambridge University Press).

Brink, Cornelia, 2010, *'Grenzen der Anstalt': Psychiatrie und Gesellschaft in Deutschland 1860–1980* (Göttingen: Wallstein).

Bruzzone, Annamaria, 2021, *Ci chiamavano matti: Voci dal manicomio (1968–1977)* (Milan: Il Saggiatore).

Buchwald, Jed Z. (ed.), 1995, *Scientific Practice: Theories and Stories of Doing Physics* (Chicago, IL: University of Chicago Press).

Bueltzingsloewen, Isabelle von, 2015, 'Vers un désenclavement de l'histoire de la psychiatrie', *Mouvement social*, 253:4, 3–11.

Bueltzingsloewen, Isabelle von (ed.), 2020, *La psychiatrie hors de l'asile: Pour une nouvelle histoire de la folie à l'époque contemporaine*, special issue of *Revue d'histoire moderne et contemporaine*, 67/1.

Coché, Stefanie, 2017, *Psychiatrie und Gesellschaft: Psychiatrische Einweisungspraxis im 'Dritten Reich', in der DDR und der Bundesrepublik 1941–1963* (Göttingen: Vandenhoeck & Ruprecht).

Condrau, Flurin, 2007, 'The patient's view meets the clinical gaze', *Social History of Medicine*, 20:3, 525–40.

Crossley, Nick, 2006, *Contesting Psychiatry: Social Movements in Mental Health* (London: Routledge).

Crouthamel, Jason and Peter Leese (eds), 2017, *Psychological Trauma and the Legacies of the First World War* (Cham, Switzerland: Palgrave Macmillan).

Dickinson, Tommy, 2015, *'Curing Queers': Mental Nurses and Their Patients, 1935–74* (Manchester: Manchester University Press).

Donald, Alistair, 2001, 'The Wal-Marting of American psychiatry: An ethnography of psychiatric practice in the late 20th century', *Culture, Medicine and Psychiatry*, 25:4, 427–39.

Doroshow, Deborah, Matthew Gambino and Mical Raz, 2019, 'New directions in the historiography of psychiatry', *Journal of the History of Medicine and Allied Sciences*, 74:1, 15–33.

Edwards-Grossi, Elodie, 2022, *Mad with Freedom: The Political Economy of Blackness, Insanity, and Civil Rights in the US South, 1840–1940* (Baton Rouge, LA: Louisiana State University Press).

Eghigian, Greg, 2011, 'Deinstitutionalizing the history of contemporary psychiatry', *History of Psychiatry*, 22:2, 201–14.

Eghigian, Greg, 2015, *The Corrigible and the Incorrigible: Science, Medicine, and the Convict in Twentieth-Century Germany* (Ann Arbor, MI: University of Michigan Press).

Ehenberg, Alain and Anne Lovell, 2001, *La Maladie mentale en mutation: Psychiatrie et société* (Paris: Odile Jacob).

Ellenberger, Henri F., Emmanuel Delille and Jonathan Kaplansky, 2020, *Ethnopsychiatry* (Montreal: McGill-Queen's University Press).

Fangerau, Heiner, Sascha Topp and Klaus Schepker (eds), 2017, *Kinder- und Jugendpsychiatrie im Nationalsozialismus und in der Nachkriegszeit: Zur Geschichte ihrer Konsolidierung* (Berlin: Springer).

Faulstich, Heinz, 1993, *Von der Irrenfürsorge zur 'Euthanasie': Geschichte der badischen Psychiatrie bis 1945* (Freiburg: Lambertus).

Fleck, Ludwik, 1993, *Entstehung und Entwicklung einer wissenschaftlichen Tatsache: Einführung in die Lehre vom Denkstil und vom Denkkollektiv* (Frankfurt: Suhrkamp).

Frances, Allen, 2013, *Saving Normal: An Insider's Revolt Against Out-of-Control Psychiatric Diagnosis, DSM-5, Big Pharma, and the Medicalization of Ordinary Life* (New York: William Morrow).

Fuchs, Petra, Wolfgang Rose and Thomas Beddies, 2012, 'Heilen und Erziehen: Die Kinderbeobachtungsstation an der Psychiatrischen und Nervenklinik der Charité', in Volker Hess and Heinz-Peter Schmiedebach (eds), *Am Rande des Wahnsinns: Schwellenräume einer urbanen Moderne* (Cologne: Böhlau), pp. 111–48.

Fussinger, Catherine, 2011, '"Therapeutic community", psychiatry's reformers and antipsychiatrists: Reconsidering changes in the field of psychiatry after World War II', *History of Psychiatry*, 22:2, 146–63.

Geertz, Clifford, 1973, *The Interpretation of Cultures: Selected Essays* (New York: Basic Books).

Geertz, Clifford, 1983, *Dichte Beschreibung: Beiträge zum Verstehen kultureller Systeme* (Frankfurt: Suhrkamp).

Giddens, Anthony, 1984, *The Constitution of Society: Outline of the Theory of Structuration* (Cambridge: Polity Press).

Gijswijt-Hofstra, Marijke, Harry Oosterhuis, Joost Vijselaar and Hugh Freeman (eds), 2005, *Cultures of Psychiatry and Mental Health Care in the Twentieth Century: Comparisons and Approaches* (Amsterdam: Amsterdam University Press).

Gijswijt-Hoftstra, Marijke and Roy Porter (eds), 2001, *Cultures of Neurasthenia: From Beard to the First World War* (Amsterdam: Rodopi).

Göhlsdorf, Novina, 2015, 'Wie man aufschreibt, was sich nicht zeigt: Autismus als Widerstand und Anreiz früher kinderpsychiatrischer Aufzeichnungen', in Cornelius Borck and Armin Schäfer (eds), *Das psychiatrische Aufschreibesystem* (Paderborn: Wilhelm Fink), pp. 225–44.

Greene, Jeremy A., Flurin Condrau and Elizabeth Siegel Watkins (eds), 2016, *Therapeutic Revolutions: Pharmaceuticals and Social Change in the Twentieth Century* (Chicago, IL: University of Chicago Press).

Greenslit, Nathan, 2005, 'Depression and consumption: Psychopharmaceuticals, branding, and new identity practices', *Culture, Medicine and Psychiatry*, 29:4, 477–502.

Guillemain, Hervé, 2018, *Schizophrènes au XXe siècle. Des effets secondaires de l'histoire*, Paris, Alma éditeur.

Guillemain, Hervé, 2020, 'Les effets secondaires de la technique. Patients et institutions psychiatriques au temps de l'électrochoc, de la psychochirurgie et des neuroleptiques retard (années 1940–1970)', *Revue d'histoire moderne & contemporaine*, 67:1, 72–98.

Healy, David, 1997, *The Antidepressant Era* (Cambridge, MA: Harvard University Press).

Healy, David, 2013, *Pharmageddon* (Berkeley, CA: University of California Press).

Henckes, Nicolas, 2007, 'Le nouveau monde de la psychiatrie française: Les psychiatres, l'Etat et la réforme des hôpitaux psychiatriques de l'après-guerre aux années 1970'. PhD thesis, Ecole des hautes études en sciences sociales, Paris.

Henckes, Nicolas, 2011, 'Reforming psychiatric institutions in the mid-twentieth century: A framework for analysis', *History of Psychiatry*, 22:2, 164–81.

Henckes, Nicolas, 2014, 'Learning constraint: Exploring nurses' narratives of psychiatric work in the early years of French community psychiatry', *Culture, Medicine and Psychiatry*, 38:4, 597–617.

Henckes, Nicolas, Volker Hess and Marie Reinholdt, 2018, 'Exploring the fringes of psychopathology: Boundary entities, category work and other borderline phenomena in the history of 20th century psychopathology', *History of the Human Sciences*, 31:2, 3–21.

Hess, Volker, 2015, 'Beyond the therapeutic revolution: Psychopharmaceuticals crossing the Berlin Wall', in Matt Savelli and Sarah Marks (eds), *Psychiatry in Communist Europe* (London: Palgrave), pp. 153–79.

Hess, Volker, 2018, 'A paper machine of clinical research in the early 20th century', *Isis*, 109:3, 473–93.

Hess, Volker and Sophie Ledebur, 2012, 'Psychiatrie in der Stadt: Die Poliklinik als urbaner Schwellenraum', in Volker Hess and Heinz-Peter Schmiedebach (eds), *Am Rande des Wahnsinns: Schwellenräume einer urbanen Moderne* (Cologne: Böhlau), pp. 19–56.

Hess, Volker and Benoît Majerus, 2011, 'Writing the history of psychiatry in the 20th century', *History of Psychiatry*, 22:2, 144–54.

Hess, Volker and Sabine Schlegelmilch, 2016, 'Cornucopia officinae medicae: Medical practice records and their origin', in Martin Dinges, Kay Peter Jankrift, Sabine Schlegelmilch and Michael Stolberg (eds), *Medical Practice, 1600–1900: Physicians and Their Patients* (Leiden: Brill), pp. 11–38.

Hohendorff, Gerit, Petra Fuchs, Paul Richter, Christoph Mundt and Wolfgang U. Eckardt (eds), 2010, *Die nationalsozialistische 'Euthanasie'-Aktion 'T4' und ihre Opfer: Geschichte und ethische Konsequenzen für die Gegenwart* (Paderborn: Schöningh).

Horwitz, Allan V., 2021, *DSM: A History of Psychiatry's Bible* (Baltimore, MD: Johns Hopkins University Press).

Hottenrott, Laura, 2021, 'Arzneimittel und klinische Studien', in Heiner Fangerau, Anke Dreier-Horning, Volker Hess, Karsten Laudien and Maike Rotzoll (eds), *Leid und Unrecht: Kinder und Jugendliche in Behindertenhilfe und Psychiatrie der BRD und DDR 1949 bis 1990* (Cologne: Psychiatrie Verlag), pp. 216–68.

Jenkins, Janis H., 2010, 'Psychopharmaceutical self and imaginary in the social field of psychiatric treatment', in Janis H. Jenkins, *Pharmaceutical*

Self: The Global Shaping of Experience in an Age of Psychopharmacology (Santa Fe, NM: School for Advanced Research Press), pp. 17–40.

Klein, Alexandre, Hervé Guillemain and Marie-Claude Thifault, 2018, *La fin de l'asile? Histoire de la déshospitalisation psychiatrique dans l'espace francophone au XXe siècle* (Rennes: Presses universitaires de Rennes).

Knorr Cetina, Karin, 1984, *Die Fabrikation von Erkenntnis: Zur Anthropologie der Naturwissenschaft* (Frankfurt: Suhrkamp).

Kölch, Michael Gregor, 2001, 'Theorie und Praxis der Kinder- und Jugendpsychiatrie in Berlin 1920–1935: Die Diagnose 'Psychopathie' im Spannungsfeld von Psychiatrie, Individualpsychologie und Politik'. Doctoral thesis, Freie Universität Berlin.

Koo, Jo-Jo, 2017, 'Rouse's conception of practice theory and existential phenomenology', *Phänomenologische Forschungen*, 93:2, 93–111.

Kritsotaki, Despo, Vicky Long and Matthew Smith (eds), 2019, *Preventing Mental Illness: Past, Present and Future* (Cham: Springer International Publishing).

Lamb, S. D., 2014, *Pathologist of the Mind: Adolf Meyer and the Origins of American Psychiatry* (Baltimore, MD: Johns Hopkins University Press).

Latour, Bruno and Steve Woolgar, 1986, *Laboratory Life: The Construction of Scientific Facts* (Princeton, NJ: Princeton University Press).

Lerner, Paul Frederick, 1996, 'Hysterical Men: War, Neurosis and German Mental Medicine, 1914–1921'. PhD thesis, Columbia University, New York.

Lévi-Strauss, Claude, 1962, *La pensée sauvage* (Paris: Plon).

Lišková, Kateřina, 2018, *Sexual Liberation, Socialist Style: Communist Czechoslovakia and the Science of Desire, 1945–1989* (Cambridge: Cambridge University Press).

Lynch, Michael, 1993, *Scientific Practice and Ordinary Action: Ethnomethodology and Social Studies of Science* (Cambridge: Cambridge University Press).

Majerus, Benoît, 2013, *Parmi les fous: Une histoire sociale de la psychiatrie au XXe siècle* (Rennes: Presses universitaires de Rennes).

Majerus, Benoît, 2019, 'A chemical revolution as seen from below: The "discovery" of neuroleptics in 1950s Paris', *Social History of Medicine*, 32:2, 395–413.

Marks, Sarah, 2017, 'Psychotherapy in historical perspective', *History of the Human Sciences*, 30:2, 3–16.

Mayers, Rick and Allan V. Horwitz, 2005, 'DSM-III and the revolution in the classification of mental illness', *Journal of the History of the Behavioral Sciences*, 41:3, 249–67.

McCrae, Niall, 2006, '"A violent thunderstorm": Cardiazol treatment in British mental hospitals', *History of Psychiatry*, 17:1, 67–90.

Meier, Marietta, 2007, *Zwang zur Ordnung: Psychiatrie im Kanton Zürich, 1870–1970* (Zurich: Chronos).

Meier, Marietta, Mario König and Magaly Tornay, 2019, *Testfall Münsterlingen: Klinische Versuche in der Psychiatrie, 1940–1980* (Zurich: Chronos).

Mitchell, Duncan, 2002, 'A contribution to the history of learning disability nursing', *Journal of Research in Nursing*, 7:3, 201–10.

Nellen, Stefan (ed.), 2007, *Paranoia City: Der Fall Ernst B.: Selbstzeugnis und Akten aus der Psychiatrie um 1900* (Basel: Schwabl).

Nolte, Karen and Sylvelyn Hähner-Rombach (eds), 2017, *Patients and Social Practice of Psychiatric Nursing in the 19th and 20th Centuries* (Stuttgart: Steiner Verlag).

Oury, Jean, 2016, *La psychothérapie institutionnelle de Saint-Alban à La Borde* (Paris: Editions d'une).

Pickering, Andrew, 1991, 'Objectivity and the mangle of practice', *Annals of Scholarship*, 8, 409–25.

Pickering, Andrew, 1995, *The Mangle of Practice: Time, Agency and Science* (Chicago, IL: University of Chicago Press).

Pieters, Toine and Benoît Majerus, 2011, 'The introduction of chlorpromazine in Belgium and the Netherlands (1951–1968): Tango between old and new treatment features', *Studies in History and Philosophy of Biological and Biomedical Sciences*, 42:4, 443–52.

Porter, Roy, 1985, 'The patient's view. Doing medical history from below', *Theory and Society*, 14:2, 175–98.

Prebble, Kate and Linda Bryder, 2008, 'Gender and class tensions between psychiatric nurses and the general nursing profession in mid-twentieth century New Zealand', *Contemporary Nurse*, 30:2, 181–95.

Robcis, Camille, 2021, *Disalienation: Politics, Philosophy, and Radical Psychiatry in Postwar France* (Chicago, IL: University of Chicago Press).

Rouse, Joseph, 2018, *Engaging Science: How to Understand its Practices Philosophically* (Ithaca, NY: Cornell University Press).

Rzesnitzek, Lara, 2015, '"Psychologische Mitarbeit" in der Psychiatrie: Die Etablierung der "Klinischen Psychologie" am Beispiel von Lilo Süllwolds diagnostischen Bemühungen um die beginnende Schizophrenie', *Medizinhistorisches Journal*, 50:4, 357–92.

Scarfone, Marianna, 2023, 'La psychiatrie française face aux migrants au milieu du XXe siècle', *L'Autre*, 24:1, 49–58.

Schatzki, Theodore, Karin Knorr Cetina and Eike von Savigny, 2001, *The Practice Turn in Contemporary Theory* (London: Routledge).

Schmiedebach, Heinz-Peter and Stefan Priebe, 2003, 'Open psychiatric care and social psychiatry in 19th and early 20th century Germany', in Eric J. Engstrom and Volker Roelcke (eds), *Psychiatrie im 19. Jahrhundert:*

Forschungen zur Geschichte von psychiatrischen Institutionen, Debatten und Praktiken im deutschen Sprachraum (Basel: Schwabe), pp. 263–81.

Schmuhl, Hans-Walter and Volker Roelcke (eds), 2013, '*Heroische Therapien*': *Die deutsche Psychiatrie im internationalen Vergleich, 1918–1945* (Göttingen: Wallstein).

Schöhl, Stephanie and Volker Hess, 2019, 'War imprisonment and clinical narratives of psychiatric illness, Psychiatric Hospital Charité, Berlin, 1948–1956', *Journal of the History of Medicine and Allied Sciences*, 74:2, 145–66.

Skålevåg, Svein Atle, 2006, 'The matter of forensic psychiatry: A historical inquiry', *Medical History*, 50:1, 49–68.

Smith, Kylie, 2020, *Talking Therapy: Knowledge and Power in American Psychiatric Nursing* (New Brunswick, NJ: Rutgers University Press).

Soler, Léna, Sjoerd Zwart, Michael Lynch and Vincent Israel-Jost (eds), 2016, *Science After the Practice Turn in the Philosophy, History, and Social Studies of Science* (New York: Routledge).

Speaker, Susan L., 1997, 'From "happiness pills" to "national nightmare": Changing cultural assessments of the minor tranquilizers in America, 1955–1980', *Journal of the History of Medicine*, 52:3, 338–76.

Studer, Nina Salouâ, 2016, *The Hidden Patients: North African Women in French Colonial Psychiatry* (Cologne: Böhlau Verlag).

Swazey, Judith P., 1974, *Chlorpromazine in Psychiatry: A Study of Therapeutic Innovation* (Cambridge, MA: MIT Press).

Tornay, Magaly, 2016, *Zugriffe auf das Ich: Psychoaktive Stoffe und Personenkonzepte in der Schweiz, 1945 bis 1980* (Tübingen: Mohr Siebeck).

Wagner, Sylvia, 2019, *Arzneimittelversuche an Heimkindern zwischen 1949 und 1975* (Frankfurt am main: Mabuse Verlag).

Weber, Max, 2006, 'Die "Objektivität" sozialwissenschaftlicher und sozialpolitischer Erkenntnis [1904]', in Daniel Lehmann (ed.), *Politik und Gesellschaft* (Frankfurt: Zweitausendeins), pp. 719–772.

Weindling, Paul, 1989, *Health, Race and German Politics Between National Unification and Nazism, 1870–1945* (Cambridge: Cambridge University Press).

I

Visions and dreams

1

New practices, new institutions: group psychotherapy in Greece and the Open Psychotherapy Centre of Athens, 1960s–1980s

Despo Kritsotaki

In the early 1950s, Samuel Slavson, one of the pioneers of group psychotherapy in the USA, detected its origins in 'classes' of patients with tuberculosis at the turn of the nineteenth century (Slavson, 1975). Others went further back, to the groups of mental patients created in mental hospitals since the late eighteenth century (Schiffer, 1983). However, the first systematic attempts at group psychotherapy as a psychodynamic method can be traced to the interwar period – Slavson himself started his first groups in the 1930s – and to World War II, with the work of Maxwell Jones and John Rickman, Wilfred Bion, and S. H. Foulkes at the Mill Hill and Northfield military hospitals in Britain. Following these experimental approaches, group psychotherapy spread after the war, in North America and in Europe (Shorter, 1997; Blok, 2005; Fussinger, 2010; Marquet, 2013), on both sides of the Iron Curtain, as group techniques were practised also in communist Europe (Leuenberger, 2001; Savelli, 2018).[1]

In Greece, the history of group psychotherapy remains untold. This chapter intends to remedy this omission by exploring Greek group practices, starting with the first experiments of the late 1950s and moving to more extensive and standardised practices of the 1980s. I approach practices as 'dreaming' ways of doing psychiatry in a twofold sense. First, the group therapy practices I examine took into consideration and commented upon the socio-economic condition of the patients and, to a degree, Greek post-war society, and proposed a reform of therapeutic and social relationships, thus having political implications. Second, while I use a variety of written sources and oral history interviews from mental health professionals, as well as the testimonies of former patients, most of the information originates from the practices' initiators.[2] These self-narratives, especially the retrospective accounts of professionals, tend to focus on the pioneering, even visionary, aspects of the practices, and to emphasise successes rather than shortcomings.

This is manifest in the case of the Open Psychotherapy Centre (OPC), on which the chapter concentrates. A private mental health institution founded in 1980 in Athens, the OPC made group therapy its main treatment method. As we will see, its self-narratives praise its ground-breaking and unique nature, while narratives stemming from other sources provide a different view. In order to make sense of these contrasting accounts, the chapter places the history of the OPC within the context of previous group experiences – in particular, the Centre for Mental Health and Research, which is also examined here – contemporary Greek mental healthcare reforms, and the broader social and political changes in Greece after the fall of the seven-year military dictatorship in 1974. Through this analysis, the chapter argues that the OPC was a distinct, or even peculiar, institution, which, at the same time, constituted an example and vehicle of both the expansion of psychotherapies and the politicisation taking place in Greece in the late 1970s and early 1980s.

Group psychotherapy in Greece

In Greece, psychotherapy of any form was only practised sporadically for most of the twentieth century, and training on psychotherapeutic methods was practically non-existent. Psychiatry was a unified specialty with neurology until 1981, and biological understandings and treatments of mental illness prevailed in both public hospitals and private clinics. Nevertheless, psychoanalysis had been known since the 1910s (Atzina, 2004; Karydaki, 2018), and Adler's individual psychology since the 1930s (Papagianni, 2013). From the 1960s, different psychotherapeutic methods were being tried and developed, including psychoanalytical psychodrama, systemic therapy and psychoanalytical psychotherapy (Ierodiakonou, 1967; Sakellaropoulos *et al.*, 1971). In the last decades of the century, although biological psychiatry remained dominant, psychotherapy was starting to be partially covered by some insurance funds, thus becoming slightly more available to the non-wealthy (*Η Ελευθερία Είναι Θεραπευτική*, 1993).

Group psychotherapy methods were probably first tried at Dromokaitio Hospital in Athens in the late 1950s, as part of the hospital's reform through the therapeutic community model (Lyketsos, 1998: 261–8; Kritsotaki and Ploumpidis, 2019). Group methods were also applied at a couple of private institutions: the Athenian Institute of Anthropos, established in 1963, which introduced group image therapy, a technique based on the use of free artistic creation (Vassiliou, 1968); and the Centre for Mental Health and Research, which was founded in 1956 in Athens, and moved to state funding and supervision in 1969. The centre was a hub of psychotherapies in Greece; there are indications that group therapy had been practised in the Athens branch at least since 1960.[3] It also ran outpatient mental healthcare services for children and adults, and four welfare centres, the social aid stations, in four cities: Athens, Thessaloniki, Piraeus and Patra (Kritsotaki, 2018).

One of the centre's innovations was the establishment of a therapeutic club in the annex of Thessaloniki in 1965. The psychiatrist in charge of the annex, Efstathios Liberakis, practised psychotherapy and was influenced by social psychiatry, an approach that highlighted the social causes and consequences of mental illness, focused on the social relationships and (re)integration of patients and often incorporated group psychotherapy (Shorter, 1997; Smith, 2016).[4] Liberakis explicitly referred to US social psychiatry and to the psychotherapy services for lower-class patients of the 1960s (Bernard, 1965; Yamamoto and Kraft Goin, 1965; Zwerling, 1965, in Liberakis, 1966). He also underlined that Freud himself had argued that welfare assistance could and should be combined with psychotherapy (Liberakis, 1966). This view had led to the establishment of clinics with low-cost or free psychotherapy in different European countries during the 1920s and 1930s by analysts who made a case for psychoanalysis as a socially active discipline (Danto, 2005; Gaztambide, 2012).

These inter- and post-war developments resonated with the work of the centre in Thessaloniki, which had started out in the late 1950s as a social aid station, offering welfare and mental health services to disadvantaged social strata, and was turned into a social psychiatry service by the end of the 1960s (Kritsotaki, 2018). The therapeutic club aimed at the socialisation, rehabilitation and therapy of patients of low socio-economic status through occupational therapy, recreational activities and group psychotherapy. In group psychotherapy, the members, usually women, talked about their everyday life, their financial and practical difficulties, their problems with their husbands and children and their health issues. Liberakis, as the therapist, was meant to have a minimal, non-directive role, reflecting on statements, encouraging participation and interpreting attitudes. While group psychotherapy was more economical than individual psychotherapy, Liberakis noted that, similarly to individual psychotherapy, it was not always effective for lower-class patients. Many had not heard of psychotherapy before and did not see the need for it, insisting on somatic approaches – mainly medication. According to Liberakis, they had trouble verbalising their problems, often kept silent and avoided active participation, or used defence mechanisms, such as 'conversion' (of mental to somatic symptoms). Another reason for the inefficacy of group psychotherapy was that only one group was formed because few patients were willing to participate and because the centre did not have the financial means to establish more groups. Thus, the group was heterogenous, including neurotic and psychotic patients of different ages, and most patients soon left with no benefit (Liberakis, 1966).

In any case, Liberakis suggested that psychotherapy was not suitable for all members of the group, some of whom would have benefited from a more 'authoritative' approach and 'placebo treatments' instead of the non-directive approach of group psychotherapy. He underlined that similar issues and the need for the flexible application of psychotherapy had been raised in the USA, but also in the USSR (Yamamoto and Kraft Goin, 1965; Liberakis, 1966; Ziferstein, 1966). By stressing that psychotherapy had to fit the special characteristics of the poor, 1960s social psychiatry often ended up stereotyping them. Some psychiatrists, like Viola Bernard (1965), warned against the oversimplification of the poor as lacking the necessary personality traits to be fit for intensive psychotherapy, such as psychological-mindedness and the capacity for introspection and abstract thinking. Despite these pitfalls, social psychiatry was vested with sociopolitical meaning, as it strove to make psychotherapy – often through group psychotherapy – available to those whose sole treatment options were until then biological methods and the asylum. In Greece, the configuration of group psychotherapy as a social and political endeavour continued in the next years, when a mental health reform movement emerged in a more systematic way and psychotherapy became more widespread, as new services (Hatzidaki, 1983; Stefanis, 1989) and scientific societies were founded, including the Greek Society of Group Analysis and Family Therapy, established in 1988. The Open Psychotherapy Centre was a chief promoter of socially and politically orientated mental healthcare through group psychotherapy.

The Open Psychotherapy Centre

Foundation and orientation

The OPC was founded in February 1980 on the initiative of the psychiatrist Ioannis Tsegos, who had been trained at the Institute of Group Analysis of London (founded in 1971 by Foulkes and colleagues), and was an active member of the Group Analytic Society International, a learned society founded among others by Foulkes in 1952 (Morarou, 2007; Kakouri-Bassea and Moschonas, 2007b). In 1978, Tsegos returned from England and became director of the Social Psychiatry Service of the Centre of Mental Health and Research in Athens, where he started his first analytic group. After disagreeing with the administration of the centre regarding his methods for the formation of psychotherapeutic groups, he resigned and founded the OPC with some of his former co-workers: his future wife, social worker Eleni Morarou, and the psychiatrist Athanasia Kakouri-Bassea, who had recently returned from her studies in Rome, where she had gained experience in social psychiatry and psychiatric reform (Kakouri-Bassea, 2019). Another co-founder of the OPC was psychologist Zoe Voyatzaki, who had studied at the Valparaiso University of Indiana (USA) and the US International University of California, where she obtained a master's in family and clinical psychology (Voyatzaki, 2019). The remaining founders were another psychologist, two more psychiatrists, one occupational therapist, and four non-professionals: a former patient, a relative of a patient, and two interested friends, who were put in charge of the administration and finances of the OPC.

The OPC aimed at providing mental illness prevention, treatment and rehabilitation, according to its protagonists, in a 'humanitarian and modern way', without confinement, limitation of freedom, and insult to human dignity (Karapostoli and Skandaliari, 2007: 146; Kakouri-Bassea and Moschonas, 2007b). Targeting mostly patients of low socio-economic status with serious mental disorders (psychoses, personality disorders and affective disorders), it predominantly used psychotherapy and avoided drugs, although these were prescribed 'sensibly'.[5] The main form of treatment was group therapy: there were analytic groups, sociotherapy groups (enhanced with the principles of group analysis), and group analytic psychodrama groups, along with group activities for families, couples, children and adolescents. Group therapy was favoured not for economic reasons, but because it was deemed necessary for the reconstruction of the personality: the treatment of psychiatric disorders had to involve many people, mainly non-experts, as the members of the groups were (Kakouri-Bassea and Moschonas, 2007a: 39 and *passim*).

Group therapy at the OPC was based on the combined use of two models: group analysis and the therapeutic community. Historically, the two models had been distinct or even conflicting, mainly in cases of therapeutic communities that opposed psychoanalysis, but in some cases they had been combined (Blok, 2005; Geyer, 2011a; Chapter 10 in this volume). Tsegos, who shaped the approach of the OPC, being initially the only one who had the training and experience to work with groups and train his co-workers, regarded the two models as related and complementary, and stressed that they were both created by psychoanalysts. On the one hand, group analysis was understood as Foulkes had defined it in 1975 – namely as a form of psychotherapy of the whole group, including the coordinator, by the group. The coordinator was not to guide but to trust the group, and was allowed to express his own experiences (Tsegos, 2007a). On the other hand, the therapeutic community, which endorsed the democratisation of the relationships between patients and professionals (Fussinger, 2011), was understood as an international movement that emerged in the 1950s but shrank in the 1970s without evolving into a systematic therapeutic method due to its unclear, sometimes hostile, stance towards psychotherapy and the lack of organised training. The OPC claimed to have combined the therapeutic community with group analysis for the first time in Greece (Karapostoli and Skandaliari, 2007), introducing the Group Analytical Community Model of Psychotherapeutic Community (Karapostoli, 2007).[6]

The OPC approached the two models critically and developed them freely, aiming to adjust theory to the benefit of the patients, not the other way around (Kakouri-Bassea and Moschonas, 2007b). Tsegos presented as the main OPC theory the principles of tolerance and permissiveness and the use of common sense (Tsegos, 2007a). This was a manifestation of his experience from Britain, where an empirical type of group psychotherapy dominated, with the focus shifting from analytical training to humanistic values, such as sincerity and respect for the personality of the patient. This meant that group psychotherapy could be undertaken not only by trained physicians but also by other professionals, such as nurses and patients (Fussinger, 2011), which was the case in the OPC, as we will see. Furthermore, while group psychotherapy was inspired chiefly by psychoanalysis, it adopted models beyond classical psychoanalysis. The OPC claimed to have revised the classical psychoanalytical model, adopting an approach of empowerment of the ego through the elevation of the person (Tsegos, 2007a), while stressing the therapeutic importance of informal activities among group members outside of the therapeutic process, such as parties, cooking breaks and coffee meetings (Tsegos, 2007d).

'An action of political content'

These methodological innovations corresponded to a broader restructuring of the handling of mental illness, which was seen as a political issue. As Tsegos already stated in 1981, the OPC was 'founded in order to constitute an action of political content for the Greek psychiatric field' (Tsegos, 2007c: 19). In line with radical psychiatric thinking, which had been circulating since the mid-1970s in Greece, challenging psychiatry not only as a medical action but also as a social institution, the OPC was alert to the ideological and political core of psychiatry: its role in repressing those who were different, its entanglement with political parties and pharmaceutical companies in pursuit of profit and power, and the way it discriminated along class lines, treating the upper social classes with psychotherapy and the lower social classes with drugs (Tsegos, 2007c). Such issues were discussed in the OPC's group on 'ideo-political problematisation' (Karapostoli and Skandaliari, 2007), but more importantly motivated its attempt to change mental healthcare organisation and therapeutic practice. The attempted changes were based on the principles of autonomy, non-hierarchical relationships, equal participation, provision of low-cost psychotherapy, and the respect of the professionals' and patients' personalities and rights. In this context, the chapter employs the analytical concept of democratisation, even if it did not appear in the OPC's self-representation, because it grasps the meaning of the transformations ventured by the institution.[7]

More specifically, the OPC stressed that it objected to the 'regulatory' and 'normative' character and 'hierarchical and authoritative' structure of 'most therapeutic spaces', where the mentally ill were considered incurable, incompetent, inferior or dangerous, and in need of lifelong treatment and supervision, and where the staff were classified by specialisation and tasks (Tsegos, 2007d). In the OPC, patients and staff (both scientific and administrative) were meant to be equal, have friendly relationships, and enjoy themselves. Patients – who were called 'therapees'– were deemed very sensitive and often very smart individuals, who could and should be responsible for and actively involved in their treatment, and help themselves (Mitroutsikou, 2007; Karapostoli, 2019).[8] They could participate in the OPC's seminars and coordinate groups, such as the self-esteem group and the magazine group (Skandaliari and Tzotziou, 2007), or even create their own therapeutic, artistic, or socially engaged groups without the participation of professionals. The active and equal role of patients in groups was meant to destigmatise and mobilise them, facilitate their trust in the group and community, and enable them to develop their creativity, take up responsibilities, and gain freedom (Karapostoli, 2007; Papadakis and Kouneli, 2007).

The epithet 'open' did not only mean that the OPC provided extra-mural treatment to patients who freely decided to receive it, but also that its financial and administrative organisation was based on the principles of 'open systems' and the 'community approach'. Every staff member was supposed to be aware of and participate in decision-making (Kostopoulos *et al.*, 2003), salaries were equal, and working conditions enabled communication (Papadakis and Kouneli, 2007; Kakouri-Bassea and Moschonas, 2007b; Tsegos, 2007c). To achieve this type of organisation, the OPC's founders opted for the form of a non-profit and self-funded company. This was unusual for mental health services at the time, but the founders considered it the only alternative to the rigid atmosphere of state mental hospitals and the profit-making of private clinics, but also to what they claimed to be the stigma-inducing character of charitable institutions. The OPC emphasised that by not receiving any funding, either from public or private/charitable actors, no 'superstructure', such as the state, could intervene in the work, limiting the group's dynamism and affecting the therapeutic relationships (Kakouri-Bassea, 2007: 19). The insistence on independence was grounded in Tsegos's previous experience at the Centre for Mental Health and Research, where he had felt that the administrative board was intervening in his therapeutic work. The initial capital for the OPC was provided by each of the founders equally, and subsequently the expenses were covered by the patients' fees, which, however, were kept low to prevent the exclusion of patients for economic reasons. To the same end, the OPC offered reduced prices to those who needed it, as long as they contributed to the work – for example, helping out in the secretariat, doing chores, or coordinating a group. If the patients created their own group, they received treatment for free during the time they acted as coordinators (Karapostoli and Skandaliari, 2007; Kakouri-Bassea and Moschonas, 2007b; Karapostoli, 2019).

Along with these organisational elements, the therapeutic principles and methods of group analysis and the therapeutic community served well what I describe as the democratisation of psychiatric practice in the OPC. Instead of the hierarchical model of other psycho-analytically orientated psychotherapies, group analysis was seen as favouring the equal relationships of group members (Voyatzaki, 2007) and the weakening of the power tendencies of the therapist, to allow the therapeutic dynamic of the group to emerge and to help activate the mental state of the patients and restructure their personalities (Kakouri-Bassea and Moschonas, 2007b). The therapeutic community model was based on democratic principles, respect and participation, and enabled authentic communication. In the therapeutic communities, group roles were not rigidly defined (Mitroutsikou, 2007; Voyatzaki, 2019) and there was not a specific discussion agenda: members were supposed to discuss their feelings, concerns and opinions freely (Papadakis and Kouneli, 2007). In combination with group analysis, the therapeutic community created a community atmosphere that, according to the OPC, contrasted permissiveness, playfulness and the joy of relationships and entertainment with the pretence of seriousness and cultivated common sense (Markezinis, 2007, citing Kakouri-Bassea).

An integral part of what I designate the democratisation of psychiatric organisation and therapeutic practice was the inclusion of non-professionals. As already noted, patients had an active role in the groups and could even be group coordinators. In addition, non-professionals were not only among the OPC founders, but were included as members of the non-profit company and contributed to OPC seminars, in particular the seminar of social psychiatry (Karapostoli and Skandaliari, 2007; Karapostoli, 2019). The involvement of non-professionals did not just serve the OPC theory that non-experts facilitated psychiatric treatment; it also aimed at offering another view on mental illness, one not strictly professional, but social and political (Karapostoli, 2019). This approach was further manifested in the OPC's links to the first formal association in which mental patients participated, the Motion for the Rights of the 'Mentally Ill'. The association aimed at securing the rights of mental patients and making their voices heard. Although the OPC and the Motion were distinct, they had common activities and members, and the OPC encouraged its patients to join the motion (Kritsotaki, 2021).

'Peculiarities' and 'deviations'

The OPC saw itself as a 'deviation' from contemporary handlings of mental illness, with deviations understood as 'integral and very useful features of nature' (Tsegos, 2007e: 13). It proudly stressed its 'peculiarities' as related to its uniqueness, longevity and autonomy (Kakouri-Bassea, 2019). In the volume *Open Psychotherapy Centre: Activities and Peculiarities*, the founders described themselves as a group of romantics, who without thinking about it too much placed their cheerfulness and creativity (Mitroutsikou, 2007; Kakouri-Bassea and Moschonas, 2007b) against the 'modern obsession with objectivity', 'the persecution of the irrational', 'the devaluation of emotions', the intolerance of difference and the lack of consideration of the personality of the patient and therapist, which led to incomplete diagnoses and treatments (Tsegos, 2007b: 49). In particular, Tsegos emerges as an unconventional individual, with no concern for forms and types, stressing the key role of humour as a natural and healthy part of one's mental state, and using provocative discourse (Tsegos, 2007d) – for example, the phrase 'media of mass influence' instead of 'media of mass information', as the media are called in Greek (Tsegos, 2007c).

However, it was not just the personality of the OPC key figure and other members that gave rise to its 'peculiarities'. The OPC staff noted that the post-dictatorship period – mainly the years from 1974 to the early 1980s – was a time of progressiveness (Tsegos, 2019), when novel and anti-conformist activities were encouraged (Kakouri-Bassea and Moschonas, 2007b; Kakouri-Bassea, 2019; Voyatzaki, 2019). Some OPC members explained the participation of non-professionals using the same frame – the zeitgeist of the 1980s, when people were more socially and politically engaged and active (Karapostoli, 2019). Certainly, the fall of the seven-year military dictatorship in 1974 signalled a period of politicisation and rising demands for the protection of human rights and social emancipation, when social movements, such as the feminist, homosexual, ecological and disability movements, developed. The left, after being persecuted for most of the twentieth century, gained an officially recognised and increasingly prominent political and social place.[9]

The politicisation and liberalisation of the time had an impact on and was reflected in the work of mental health professionals, especially young and leftist ones, who had studied abroad and were influenced by radical psychiatry, the French experience of the 13th arrondissement (Henckes, 2005), and Italian democratic psychiatry (Foot, 2015).[10] They saw mental healthcare as a locus of political intervention and a break with the past, represented by the infamous public asylums, and chiefly Leros.[11] The mental health reform movement that emerged in late 1970s Greece had a political and ideological edge; it was critical of what it saw as the repressive functions of psychiatry and promoted the rights of the patients (Tzanakis, 2008). A few pilot projects were initiated, such as the Centre of Community Mental Hygiene of Vyronas-Kaisariani, an open service of the Psychiatric Clinic of the University of Athens

(1978); the Society for Social Psychiatry and Mental Health (1981), which promoted the adaptation of psychoanalysis to public mental healthcare; and the first mobile psychiatric unit in Fokida, in central Greece (1981). In 1981, with the establishment of the National Health Service (one of the seminal post-dictatorship reforms), new public mental health services, most notably mental health centres, were envisioned, and a few years later, in 1984, the first official psychiatric reform policy started with funding and advice from the European Economic Community, which Greece had joined three years earlier. The aim was to downsize and reform, not shut down, the asylums, to establish community services and to promote social rehabilitation. All these initiatives were inspired by social psychiatry and many had a strong psychotherapeutic, and even psychoanalytical, orientation.[12]

Hence, the OPC was not exactly unique. On the one hand, there had been antecedents of group psychotherapy, most notably in the therapeutic club of the Centre for Mental Health and Research in Thessaloniki, which advanced socially engaged psychiatric practice. On the other hand, and more significantly, since the late 1970s a number of professionals and organisations introduced a social psychiatry and/or open services approach and launched therapeutic communities and group psychotherapy. Even so, it can be argued that the OPC did stand out among both previous and contemporaneous innovative services, if anything because it insisted on remaining self-funded in a period when almost any mental health reform in Greece was at least partially backed by the European Economic Community and/or the Greek state.

This distinctiveness, though, had another side. Although there were instances of dissemination of the OPC's practices by members of the staff who moved to different services,[13] the OPC emerges as relatively secluded within the Greek mental health landscape. Professionals who were working in other mental health services during the 1980s did not have much to comment on its work, claiming that they were not familiar with it. The psychiatrist Dimitris Ploumpidis, who had worked from 1988 to 2015 in the Psychiatric Clinic of the University of Athens, and in its Centre of Community Mental Hygiene of Vyronas-Kaisariani, stressed that the OPC's staff did not have outside collaborations, although they presented their work at the conferences of the Hellenic Psychiatric Association (Ploumpidis, 2020). Grigoris Ampatzoglou, a psychiatrist who worked at the Society for Social Psychiatry and Mental Health in the 1980s and later became professor of child psychiatry at the University of Thessaloniki, was aware of positive assessments of the OPC from people who were near it, but he did not think that it had a role in the scientific community and was critical of its ideological orientation, at least as it had evolved since the 1990s (Ampatzoglou, 2021). Indeed, in the 1990s and 2000s there was controversy over some aspects of the OPC's views. For example, in the 2000s a piece of OPC research claimed that learning ancient Greek was of preventive and therapeutic value for learning difficulties. In the ensuing debate, linguists and psychiatrists outside the OPC argued that the research was methodologically flawed, and its claims were ideological rather than scientific (Harris, 2006).

The patient perspective

While those outside the OPC were ambivalent towards its distinctiveness, two former patients, to whom I was introduced by members of the OPC staff, described it in unquestionably positive ways. Dionysis Perros, who in the early 1990s joined the everyday therapeutic community – the music therapy, writing and magazine groups – was very emotional about it. 'For the first time in my life, I met so many people important to me, who played a big part in my life, in such as small place', he said, and described the years he spent in the therapeutic community from 1992 to 1995 as among the best of his life. Psychotherapy there did not just help him get back to his everyday activities, it was a life-changing experience – his 'personal rebirth'. He highlighted that psychotherapy does not change people, but teaches them to control their stress and change their behaviour. 'Psychotherapy is a feeling', it cannot be easily described, he added. Another major factor in his recovery was that he was not treated as disabled but as an equal. He was never diagnosed, and he was given the chance to attend the seminar on group analysis and psychodrama. Finally, he stressed that although in his working-class neighbourhood people were surprised that he was having psychotherapy, considering it an upper-class treatment, the OPC was not very expensive, and he even got a discount for the six months when he was the editor of the magazine (Perros, 2020).

Georgia Nassiakou was an OPC patient in the early 1980s for about six years. After a short period of individual therapy, she joined the analytic group and the 'games' (play therapy), magazine, 'painting' (art therapy) and mythology groups, and later the fortnightly psychotherapeutic community. She also participated in the social psychiatry seminar, which she described as a pleasant and intense group that discussed various issues – for example, ancient philosophy and the role of religion. Nassiakou attended various conferences organised by the OPC and other actors, and she underlined that it was important that the OPC invited patients to these conferences. Like Perros, she was passionate about the OPC. She described it as a 'hug' of safety and relaxation, a place to talk to somebody, learn to talk about oneself, and feel that everyone had problems to different degrees. She too, like Perros, stressed that patients were not pitied, but helped to fight. They were informed about everything happening in the OPC, and trusted it, as it had stable structures. The professionals knew what they were doing, and, despite their differences, they all functioned within a common framework. Finally, she stressed that the OPC was not aiming at profit: it did not treat people just to get their money, but took patients who really needed treatment, patients with more or less serious disorders (Nassiakou, 2020).

Forming a view of the exact practices of group therapy during the 1980s and early 1990s is not easy. Neither Perros nor Nassiakou talked in detail about their sessions. They both noted though that in group therapy one talked about whatever one wanted – personal, professional or other issues. According to Nassiakou, everyone said what they thought, joking, arguing or disagreeing. It was important for the group to let off steam, not to be afraid to have a quarrel, and therapists encouraged patients to react and express their thoughts. Different groups had different activities. For example, in the magazine group, therapy was undertaken through the members' work to publish a 'proper magazine' (Nassiakou, 2020); in the music group, they listened to music and relaxed (Perros, 2020). In all groups, however, anyone could be leader, which Nassiakou deemed significant, although she only occasionally took this role because she thought it was stressful to deal with whatever came up in the group, even an intense dispute. Another instance of patients taking the initiative was the organisation of parties in cooperation with the therapists. Parties, as well as the lunch break, were mentioned as opportunities for patients to participate, joke, laugh and talk (Nassiakou, 2020).

Conclusion

In exploring the history of group psychotherapy practices in post-war Greece, 'visions and dreams' surfaced in two ways. First, the self-narratives of the OPC depict an image of uniqueness, innovation and achievements. This possibly idealised portrayal is also put forward by former patients – whom I met through the OPC – and is contradicted by more ambivalent or even negative depictions of the OPC by professionals outside it. Probably, the awareness of being part of an extraordinary reform project, shared equally by the protagonists and the patients interviewed, and reinforced by the factor that (group) psychotherapies were only used to a very limited extent in Greece, played a decisive role here. This made everyday difficulties and wrong decisions fade into the background in the memories. Nevertheless, this does not apply to the other case study of the present chapter, the Centre for Mental Health and Research. The self-narrative of Liberakis, the founder of the therapeutic club, not a retrospective account, but one given shortly after the club's foundation in 1965, was rather modest, and underlined the shortcomings of the experiment, perhaps because it was too soon for him to be overconfident about the method.

The second dimension of visionary and dreaming ways of doing psychiatry emerged in both case studies of the chapter: the intent to address social issues or even have an impact on society through psychiatric practices. In the therapeutic club of the Centre for Mental Health and Research, group therapy was applied to underprivileged patients with no other access to psychotherapy and aspired to promote their autonomy and less authoritative relationships with the middle-class staff. However, the psychiatrist in charge soon became uncertain about the possibility of attaining this goal. The interconnection of psychiatric practices with the social and the political was more pronounced in the case of the OPC, where group therapy was proposed not only as therapeutically innovative and effective, but also as politically and ideologically appropriate, in line with the endeavour to highlight the political aspects of psychiatry and generate changes in the approach to mental illness. Through the discourse on autonomy, freedom, rights, equality, and the erosion and diffusion of the therapist's authority, group therapy was elevated from a treatment method to a political endeavour, which, as this chapter argued, aimed at the democratisation of therapeutic and, by extension, social relationships. Significantly, this new way of handling mental illness was accessible to the less well-off. The former patients, while mostly stressing the effects of therapy in the OPC on their personal lives and behaviour, also hinted at its political, democratic aspects: they reminisced about the equality and cooperation among patients and staff, the sharing of knowledge, the participation of patients in therapy, education and entertainment, and the cultivation of free expression, initiative and responsibility.

In order to better understand this visionary aspect of psychiatric practices, more apparent in the case of the OPC, the chapter situated them within the psychiatric, social and political conditions of their time. The therapeutic club of the Centre for Mental Health and Research was influenced by inter- and post-war trends that used (group) psychotherapy for the treatment of the underprivileged. The OPC continued this tradition but was mostly an example and vehicle of the politicisation and democratisation, of the mental healthcare reforms, and of the expansion of psychotherapies in Greece after the fall of the dictatorship in 1974. Albeit distinct, even peculiar, the OPC was not really 'deviant', as its self-narratives contended. During this time of social and political change and demands for social liberation and rights, a politicised and ideological mental health reform movement emerged in Greece. The OPC, with its conception of mental illness and healthcare as political issues, was one of the reform agents that envisioned a social and political mission for (group) psychotherapy.

Funding

This project has received funding from the European Union's Horizon 2020 research and innovation programme under the Marie Skłodowska-Curie grant agreement No 793875.

Acknowledgments

I am grateful to the organisers of the book workshop 'Contemporary History of Psychiatric Practices in Europe' for accepting my proposal and granting me access to its fascinating papers and discussions. I would like to thank all participants and contributors, as well as the editors and the anonymous reviewers of this volume for their insightful suggestions and comments on the various versions of this chapter. Finally, I am thankful to all the professionals and 'therapees' who gave oral history interviews, sharing their stories, memories and thoughts with me. This chapter is dedicated to them.

Notes

1 Group therapy practices are also explored in this volume by Gundula Gahlen (in West Germany) and Henriette Voelker (in East Germany). See Chapters 3 and 10. It needs to be stressed that the interest in the history of group psychotherapies is part of a broader expansion of the historiography of psychotherapies, not just psychoanalysis, in recent years. See, indicatively, Geyer, 2011b; Marks, 2017, 2018. The last two are introductions to two special issues of the *Journal of the Human Sciences* on the history of psychotherapies.

2 Informed consent was obtained for all interviewees who participated in the research.

3 Archive of Panayiotis Sakellaropoulos, Athens, A01_S04_F06, Minutes of Staff Meeting, Centre for Mental Health and Research, 1960.

4 On social psychiatry in the Federal Republic of Germany in the 1960s and 1970s, see Chapter 3.

5 It must be noted that for this research I did not have access to the OPC's records and thus did not obtain any precise information on the patients' social and medical condition.

6 On the therapeutic community in other national contexts, see the contributions by Gundula Gahlen, Katariina Parhi (for the treatment of drug use) and Henriette Voelker in Chapters 3, 5 and 10 in this volume. The therapeutic community in the OPC was inspired by the British model.

7 The relationship of psychotherapy to democracy and the construction of a 'democratic self' in the post-war world is a fascinating subject recently explored by Alexander (2016) and Shapira (2013). While this

literature refers to psychoanalysis in the West, Voelker's chapter in this volume touches upon the ways in which the democratic connotations of group psychotherapy and the therapeutic community were understood and reworked in a socialist country (the German Democratic Republic). See Chapter 10.

8   The Greek word for therapy is 'θεραπεία' and for therapist 'θεραπευτής'. 'To be under therapy' is the verb 'θεραπεύομαι' and the participle of this verb is 'θεραπευόμενος', a person being under therapy, a 'therapee'.

9   A landmark of this process was the 1974 legalisation of the Communist Party of Greece, which had been outlawed since 1947. For a compelling trajectory of the Greek left in the twentieth century, see Karamanolakis, 2019. The importance of the fall of the dictatorship (1967–74) can only be appreciated in the broader frame of post-war Greek history. After the civil war (1946–49) between the state's army, supported by the UK and the USA, and the Democratic Army of Greece, supported by the Soviet Union and other countries of the Eastern bloc, an autarchic regime – the 'sickly democracy' (Nikolakopoulos, 2001) – was established: under the official anti-communist and nationalist agenda and in the context of the Cold War, the state curtailed personal freedoms, imprisoning, exiling and socially, politically and economically excluding a great segment of the population on the basis of their political beliefs and activities (Kornetis, 2013). A short period of democratisation in the 1960s was halted by the military dictatorship in 1967, which heightened the oppression and exclusion of the previous years. Thus, the establishment of democracy in 1974 signalled a break with the past and the beginning of a transformation process, in political, social and cultural terms. Moreover, as historian Danae Karydaki aptly argues, the period that followed the fall of the dictatorship can be interpreted as 'the satisfaction of a popular demand for healing the accumulated and unspoken traumas caused by ... the "interminable wars": World War II, the Nazi occupation, the Civil War, the ideological conflict of the 1950s and 1960s, and the seven-year military junta' (Karydaki, 2018: 21).

10   See also Chapter 2.

11   The Leros Psychiatric Hospital was founded in 1957 as a 'colony for psychopaths' on a remote island of Greece and received many of the chronic patients of the public asylums of Athens and Thessaloniki. In the 1960s and 1970s patient numbers increased constantly, surpassing 2,700 in 1974. Even though the initial revelations of the inhumane conditions in which the patients were kept were made in the late 1970s, the hospital was first reformed in the early 1990s and closed in 1997 (Mitrosyli, 2015).

12 After the fall of the dictatorship, and especially since the late 1970s, psychoanalysis and psychoanalytic psychotherapy were becoming more accepted and grounded in Greece: the first professional societies were founded in 1977 and 1982, and in the 1980s psychoanalysts who had trained abroad were employed in the National Health Service, contributing to the reform of public mental healthcare. Here again we can discern a strong political element, as psychoanalysis and psychoanalytic psychotherapy were conceptualised as a 'social good' and were meant to reach the 'non-privileged' (Karydaki, 2018).

13 An example of the dissemination of the OPC's practices was the transfer of the therapeutic community to the psychiatric clinic of the Naval Hospital of Salamis (Markezinis, 2007).

References

Alexander, Sally, 2016, 'D. W. Winnicott and the social democratic vision', in Matt Ffytche and Daniel Pick (eds), *Psychoanalysis in the Age of Totalitarianism* (Abingdon: Routledge), pp. 114–30.

Ampatzoglou, Grigoris, 2021, Interview by Despo Kritsotaki Athens, 25 January.

Atzina, Lena, 2004, *Η μακρά εισαγωγή της ψυχανάλυσης στην Ελλάδα: Ψυχαναλυτές, ιατρικοί θεσμοί και κοινωνικές προσλήψεις (1910–1990)* [The long introduction of psychoanalysis in Greece: Psychoanalysts, medical institutions and social perceptions (1910–1990)] (Athens: Exantas).

Bernard, Viola, 1965, 'Some principles of dynamic psychiatry in relation to poverty', *American Journal of Psychiatry*, 122:3, 254–67.

Blok, Gemma, 2005, 'Madness and autonomy: The moral agenda of anti-psychiatry in the Netherlands', in Marijke Gijswijt-Hofstra, Harry Oosterhuis and Joost Vijselaar (eds), *Psychiatric Cultures Compared: Psychiatry and Mental Health Care in the Twentieth Century: Comparisons and Approaches* (Amsterdam: Amsterdam University Press), pp. 103–15.

Danto, Elizabeth Ann, 2005, *Freud's Free Clinics: Psychoanalysis and Social Justice, 1918–1938* (New York: Columbia University Press).

Foot, John, 2015, *The Man Who Closed the Asylums: Franco Basaglia and the Revolution in Mental Health Care* (London: Verso).

Fussinger, Catherine, 2010, 'Eléments pour une histoire de la communauté thérapeutique dans la psychiatrie occidentale de la seconde moitié du 20e siècle', *Gesnerus*, 67:2, 217–40.

Fussinger, Catherine, 2011, '"Therapeutic community", psychiatry's reformers and antipsychiatrists: Reconsidering changes in the field of psychiatry after World War II', *History of Psychiatry*, 22:2, 146–63.

Gaztambide, Daniel J., 2012, '"A psychotherapy for the people": Freud, Ferenczi, and psychoanalytic work with the underprivileged', *Contemporary Psychoanalysis*, 48:2, 141–65.

Geyer, Michael, 2011a, 'Ostdeutsche Psychotherapiechronik 1970–1979', in Michael Geyer (ed.), *Psychotherapie in Ostdeutschland: Geschichte und Geschichten 1945–1995* (Göttingen: Vandenhoeck & Ruprecht), pp. 245–56.

Geyer, Michael (ed.), 2011b, *Psychotherapie in Ostdeutschland: Geschichte und Geschichten 1945–1995* (Göttingen: Vandenhoeck & Ruprecht).

Η Ελευθερία Είναι Θεραπευτική, 1993, 'Εναλλακτικές θεραπείες στην Ελλάδα' [Alternative treatments in Greece], *Η Ελευθερία Είναι Θεραπευτική* [Freedom is therapeutic], 10, 39–40.

Harris, Giannis, 2006, 'Το καρκινογόνο αντιγριππικό' [The carcinogenic flu vaccine], *Τα Νέα* [The news] (8 July 2006).

Hatzidaki, Rena, 1983, 'Ψυχιατρική "περίθαλψη" και ψυχιατρική "μεταρρύθμιση" στην Ελλάδα: το έγκλημα με τη φορεσιά της αθωότητας' [Psychiatric 'care' and psychiatric 'reform' in Greece: The crime with the cloak of innocence], *Σύγχρονα Θέματα* [Contemporary issues], 6:19, 61–70.

Henckes, Nicolas, 2005, 'Réformer la psychiatrie, organiser les pratiques de secteur: La construction de la psychiatrie de secteur dans "l'expérience du treizième arrondissement"', Centre de Recherche Médecine, Sciences, Société, Santé, https://hal.archives-ouvertes.fr/hal-01163556/document (accessed 7 August 2023).

Ierodiakonou, C. S., 1967, 'Greece', *American Journal of Psychotherapy*, 21:3, 712–15.

Kakouri-Bassea, Athanasia, 2007, 'Η διαμορφωτική περίοδος' [The defining period], in Ioannis Tsegos, Natasa Karapostoli, Maroula Mitroutsikou and Youla Pantou (eds), *Ανοικτό Ψυχοθεραπευτικό Κέντρο (1980–2007): Δραστηριότητες και Ιδιοτροπίες* [Open Psychotherapy Centre (1980–2007): Activities and peculiarities] (Athens: Enallaktikes Ekdoseis), pp. 15–19.

Kakouri-Bassea, Athanasia, 2019, Interview by Despo Kritsotaki, Athens, 4 December.

Kakouri-Bassea, Athanasia and Dimitris Moschonas, 2007a, 'Αδρομερής περιγραφή του θεραπευτικού τομέως' [Sketch of the therapeutic sector], in Ioannis Tsegos, Natasa Karapostoli, Maroula Mitroutsikou and Youla Pantou (eds), *Ανοικτό Ψυχοθεραπευτικό Κέντρο (1980–2007): Δραστηριότητες και Ιδιοτροπίες* [Open Psychotherapy Centre (1980–2007): Activities and peculiarities] (Athens: Enallaktikes Ekdoseis), pp. 86–100.

Kakouri-Bassea, Athanasia and Dimitris Moschonas, 2007b, 'Γενική θεώρηση' [General view], in Ioannis Tsegos, Natasa Karapostoli, Maroula Mitroutsikou and Youla Pantou (eds), *Ανοικτό Ψυχοθεραπευτικό Κέντρο*

(1980–2007): Δραστηριότητες και Ιδιοτροπίες [Open Psychotherapy Centre (1980–2007): Activities and peculiarities] (Athens: Enallaktikes Ekdoseis), pp. 35–41.

Karamanolakis, Vangelis, 2019, *Ανεπιθύμητο παρελθόν: Οι φάκελοι κοινωνικών φρονημάτων στον 20ό αιώνα και η καταστροφή τους* [Undesirable past: The files of social beliefs in the 20th century and their destruction] (Athens: Themelio).

Karapostoli, Natasa, 2007, 'Κοινωνικοθεραπεία: Η χρήση της δραστηριότητας στην ψυχοθεραπεία' [Social therapy: The use of activity in psychotherapy], in Ioannis Tsegos, Natasa Karapostoli, Maroula Mitroutsikou and Youla Pantou (eds), *Ανοικτό Ψυχοθεραπευτικό Κέντρο (1980–2007): Δραστηριότητες και Ιδιοτροπίες* [Open Psychotherapy Centre (1980–2007): Activities and peculiarities] (Athens: Enallaktikes Ekdoseis), pp. 75–82.

Karapostoli, Natasa, 2019, Interview by Despo Kritsotaki Athens, 7 November.

Karapostoli, Natasa and Themelina Skandaliari, 2007, 'Οι ψυχοθεραπευτικές κοινότητες' [The psychotherapeutic communities], in Ioannis Tsegos, Natasa Karapostoli, Maroula Mitroutsikou and Youla Pantou (eds), *Ανοικτό Ψυχοθεραπευτικό Κέντρο (1980–2007): Δραστηριότητες και Ιδιοτροπίες* [Open Psychotherapy Centre (1980–2007): Activities and peculiarities] (Athens: Enallaktikes Ekdoseis), pp. 135–50.

Karydaki, Danae, 2018, 'Freud under the Acropolis: The challenging journey of psychoanalysis in 20th-century Greece (1915–1995)', *History of the Human Sciences*, 31:4, 13–37.

Kornetis, Kostis, 2013, *Children of the Dictatorship: Student Resistance, Cultural Politics and the 'Long 1960s' in Greece* (New York: Berghahn Books, 2013).

Kostopoulos, C., Natasa Karapostoli, N. Polyzos, V. Bardis, D. Bartsokas, G. Pierrakos and Ioannis Tsegos, 2003, 'Το κόστος των υπηρεσιών μιας ημερήσιας ψυχοθεραπευτικής μονάδας' [The cost of services of a day psychotherapy unit], *Psychiatriki*, 14:2, 121–35.

Kritsotaki, Despo, 2018, 'From "social aid" to "social psychiatry": Mental health and social welfare in post-war Greece (1950s–1960s)', *Palgrave Communications*, 5:1, 1–9.

Kritsotaki, Despo, 2021, 'Changing psychiatry or changing society? The Motion for the Rights of the "Mentally Ill" in Greece, 1980–1990', *Journal for the History of Medicine and Allied Sciences*, 76:4, 440–61.

Kritsotaki, Despo and Dimitris Ploumpidis, 2019, 'Progressive science meets indifferent state? Revisiting mental health care reform in post-war Greece (1950–1980)', *Dynamis: Acta Hispanica Ad Medicinae Scientiarumque Historiam Illustrandam*, 39:1, 99–121.

Leuenberger, Christine, 2001, 'Socialist psychotherapy and its dissidents', *Journal of the History of the Behavioural Sciences*, 37:3, 267–373.

Liberakis, Efstathios, 1966, *Group Techniques in a Therapeutic Club* (Athens: Centre for Mental Health and Research).

Lyketsos, Georgios, 1998, *Το μυθιστόρημα της ζωής μου* [The novel of my life] (Athens: Gavriilidis).

Markezinis, Efthimios, 2007, 'Ινστιτούτο Ομαδικής Ανάλυσης Αθηνών: Η εκπαίδευση ψυχαναλυτών ομάδας' [Institute of Group Analysis of Athens: The training of group analysts], in Ioannis Tsegos, Natasa Karapostoli, Maroula Mitroutsikou and Youla Pantou (eds), *Ανοικτό Ψυχοθεραπευτικό Κέντρο (1980–2007): Δραστηριότητες και Ιδιοτροπίες* [Open Psychotherapy Centre (1980–2007): Activities and peculiarities] (Athens: Enallaktikes Ekdoseis), pp. 223–44.

Marks, Sarah, 2017, 'Psychotherapy in historical perspective', *History of the Human Sciences*, 30:2, 3–16.

Marks, Sarah, 2018, 'Psychotherapy in Europe', *History of the Human Sciences*, 31:4, 3–12.

Marquet, Jérémie, 2013, 'Contribution à un certain mouvement vers une psychothérapie institutionnelle: Entre pérennité fragile et pérenne fragilité'. Doctoral thesis, Université du droit et de la santé, Lille.

Mitrosyli, Maria, 2015, *Ψυχιατρείο Λέρου και μεταρρύθμιση: Δημόσιες πολιτικές, ίδρυμα, ασθενείς, κοινότητα* [The mental hospital of Leros and reform: Public policies, institution, patients, community] (Athens: Papazisis).

Mitroutsikou, Maroula, 2007, 'Η γραμματεία του Ανοικτού Ψυχοθεραπευτικού Κέντρου' [The administration of the Open Psychotherapy Centre], in Ioannis Tsegos, Natasa Karapostoli, Maroula Mitroutsikou and Youla Pantou (eds), *Ανοικτό Ψυχοθεραπευτικό Κέντρο (1980–2007): Δραστηριότητες και Ιδιοτροπίες* [Open Psychotherapy Centre (1980–2007): Activities and peculiarities] (Athens: Enallaktikes Ekdoseis), pp. 309–20.

Morarou, Eleni, 2007, 'Το Τμήμα Σεμιναρίων και Συνεδρίων' [The Department of Seminars and Conferences], in Ioannis Tsegos, Natasa Karapostoli, Maroula Mitroutsikou and Youla Pantou (eds), *Ανοικτό Ψυχοθεραπευτικό Κέντρο (1980–2007): Δραστηριότητες και Ιδιοτροπίες* [Open Psychotherapy Centre (1980–2007): Activities and peculiarities] (Athens: Enallaktikes Ekdoseis), pp. 185–201.

Nassiakou, Georgia, 2020, Interview by Despo Kritsotaki Athens, 12 July.

Nikolakopoulos, Ilias, 2001, *Η καχεκτική δημοκρατία: Πολιτικά κόμματα και εκλογές, 1946–1967* [The sickly democracy: Political parties and elections, 1946–1967] (Athens: Patakis).

Papadakis, Thalis and Ersi Kouneli, 2007, 'Το Τμήμα Θεραπείας Οικογένειας και Παιδιών' [The Department of Family and Children Therapy], in Ioannis Tsegos, Natasa Karapostoli, Maroula Mitroutsikou and Youla Pantou (eds), *Ανοικτό Ψυχοθεραπευτικό Κέντρο (1980–2007): Δραστηριότητες και Ιδιοτροπίες* [Open Psychotherapy Centre (1980–2007): Activities and peculiarities] (Athens: Enallaktikes Ekdoseis), pp. 105–19.

Papagianni, Ioanna, 2013, *Μα τους τράβηξε ο Άντλερ ... Η πορεία της ατομικής ψυχολογίας στην Ελλάδα* [But they were drawn by Adler ... The course of individual psychology in Greece] (Athens: Plethron).

Perros, Dionysis, 2020, Interview by Despo Kritsotaki, Athens, 13 June.

Ploumpidis, Dimitris, 2020, Interview by Despo Kritsotaki, Athens, 21 December.

Sakellaropoulos, Panayiotis, Lilian Svarna, M. Nassiakos, A. Nassiakou, G. Mpotonakis and Froso Karapanou, 1971, 'Η συναισθηματική μεταβίβαση στο ψυχαναλυτικό ψυχόδραμα' [Emotional transference in psychoanalytical psychodrama], *Εγκέφαλος: Αρχεία Νευρολογίας και Ψυχιατρικής* [Encephalos: Archives of neurology and psychiatry], 8, 185–94.

Savelli, Mat, 2018, '"Peace and happiness await us": Psychotherapy in Yugoslavia, 1945–85', *History of the Human Sciences*, 31:4, 38–57.

Schiffer, Mortimer, 1983, 'S. R. Slavson (1890–1981)', *International Journal of Group Psychotherapy*, 33:2, 131–50.

Shapira, Michal, 2013, *The War Inside: Psychoanalysis, Total War and the Making of the Democratic Self in Postwar Britain* (Cambridge: Cambridge University Press).

Shorter, Edward, 1997, *A History of Psychiatry: From the Era of the Asylum to the Age of Prozac* (New York: J. Wiley & Sons).

Skandaliari, Themelina and Anna Tzotziou, 2007, 'Η καθημερινή ψυχοθεραπευτική κοινότητα' [The daily psychotherapeutic community], in Ioannis Tsegos, Natasa Karapostoli, Maroula Mitroutsikou and Youla Pantou (eds), *Ανοικτό Ψυχοθεραπευτικό Κέντρο (1980–2007): Δραστηριότητες και Ιδιοτροπίες* [Open Psychotherapy Centre (1980–2007): Activities and peculiarities] (Athens: Enallaktikes Ekdoseis), pp. 151–7.

Slavson, S. R., 1975, 'Current trends in group psychotherapy', *International Journal of Group Psychotherapy*, 25:2, 131–40.

Smith, Matthew, 2016, 'A fine balance: Individualism, society and the prevention of mental illness in the United States, 1945–1968', *Palgrave Communications*, 2:1, 1–11.

Stefanis, Kostas, 1989, 'Ψυχιατρική περίθαλψη και κοινωνική ψυχιατρική' [Psychiatric care and social psychiatry], in Serge Lebovici and Panayiotis Sakallaropoulos (eds), *Ελληνογαλλικό Συμπόσιο Κοινωνικής Ψυχιατρικής* [Greek–French Symposium of Social Psychiatry] (Athens: Kastaniotis), pp. 82–95.

Tsegos, Ioannis, 2007a, 'Το Περί-εγώ και τα εμπρόσωπα ψυχοθεραπευτικά σχήματα' [The around-ego and the face-to-face psychotherapeutic schemata], in Ioannis Tsegos, Natasa Karapostoli, Maroula Mitroutsikou and Youla Pantou (eds), *Ανοικτό Ψυχοθεραπευτικό Κέντρο (1980–2007): Δραστηριότητες και Ιδιοτροπίες* [Open Psychotherapy Centre (1980–2007): Activities and peculiarities] (Athens: Enallaktikes Ekdoseis), pp. 43–8.

Tsegos, Ioannis, 2007b, 'Ανάδειξη της ετερότητας και αξιοποίηση της προσωπικότητας' [Emphasising the distinctness and utilising the personality], in Ioannis Tsegos, Natasa Karapostoli, Maroula Mitroutsikou and Youla Pantou (eds), *Ανοικτό Ψυχοθεραπευτικό Κέντρο (1980–2007): Δραστηριότητες και Ιδιοτροπίες* [Open Psychotherapy Centre (1980–2007): Activities and peculiarities] (Athens: Enallaktikes Ekdoseis), pp. 49–52.

Tsegos, Ioannis, 2007c, 'Ιδεολογικοπολιτικοί προβληματισμοί περί την ψυχιατρική και την ψυχοθεραπεία κατά τη Μεταπολίτευση' [Ideological and political concerns about psychiatry and psychotherapy during the post-dictatorship period], in Ioannis Tsegos, Natasa Karapostoli, Maroula Mitroutsikou and Youla Pantou (eds), *Ανοικτό Ψυχοθεραπευτικό Κέντρο (1980–2007): Δραστηριότητες και Ιδιοτροπίες* [Open Psychotherapy Centre (1980–2007): Activities and peculiarities] (Athens: Enallaktikes Ekdoseis), pp. 19–28.

Tsegos, Ioannis, 2007d, 'Οι αδόμητες δραστηριότητες' [Unstructured activities], in Ioannis Tsegos, Natasa Karapostoli, Maroula Mitroutsikou and Youla Pantou (eds), *Ανοικτό Ψυχοθεραπευτικό Κέντρο (1980–2007): Δραστηριότητες και Ιδιοτροπίες* [Open Psychotherapy Centre (1980–2007): Activities and peculiarities] (Athens: Enallaktikes Ekdoseis), pp. 53–8.

Tsegos, Ioannis, 2007e, 'Πρόλογος' [Preface], in Ioannis Tsegos, Natasa Karapostoli, Maroula Mitroutsikou and Youla Pantou (eds), *Ανοικτό Ψυχοθεραπευτικό Κέντρο (1980–2007): Δραστηριότητες και Ιδιοτροπίες* [Open Psychotherapy Centre (1980–2007): Activities and peculiarities] (Athens: Enallaktikes Ekdoseis), pp. 13–14.

Tsegos, Ioannis, 2019, Interview by Despo Kritsotaki Athens, 7 November.

Tzanakis, Manolis, 2008, *Πέραν του ασύλου: Η κοινοτική ψυχιατρική και το ζήτημα του υποκειμένου* [Beyond the asylum: Community psychiatry and the issue of the subject] (Thessaloniki: Koinos Topos Psychiatrikis, Nevroepistimon ke Epistimon tou Anthropou).

Vassiliou, George, 1968, 'Certain basic aspects of transactional group image therapy', *Group Analysis*, 1:2, 65–8.

Voyatzaki, Zoe, 2007, 'Ευρωπαϊκό Δίκτυο Ομαδικο-Αναλυτικών Εκπαιδευτικων Οργανισμών (EGATIN)' [European Group Analytic Training Institutions Network (EGATIN)], in Ioannis Tsegos, Natasa

Karapostoli, Maroula Mitroutsikou and Youla Pantou (eds), *Ανοικτό Ψυχοθεραπευτικό Κέντρο (1980–2007): Δραστηριότητες και Ιδιοτροπίες* [Open Psychotherapy Centre (1980–2007): Activities and peculiarities] (Athens: Enallaktikes Ekdoseis), pp. 295–305.

Voyatzaki, Zoe, 2019, Interview by Despo Kritsotaki, Athens, 16 December.

Yamamoto, Joe and Marcia Kraft Goin, 1965, 'On the treatment of the poor', *American Journal of Psychiatry*, 122:3, 265–71.

Ziferstein, Isidore, 1966, 'The Soviet psychiatrist: His relationship to his patients and to his society', *American Journal of Psychiatry*, 123:4, 440–6.

Zwerling, Israel and Institute of Pennsylvania Hospital, 1965, *Some Implications of Social Psychiatry for Psychiatric Treatment and Patient Care* (Nutley, NJ: Roche Laboratories).

2

The Gorizia experiment: the genesis of therapeutic practices in Basaglia's psychiatric community (1962–68)

Marica Setaro

Breaking the boundaries in a frontier asylum

The 'general assembly' of the therapeutic community at the Gorizia Psychiatric Hospital, Italy, near the border with what was then Yugoslavia (today Slovenia) organised during the directorship of Franco Basaglia from 1961 to 1968, became the most important daily practice of this community. We cannot be certain when the first general assembly was held; in fact, we do not even know for certain that 'general assembly' was its official name.[1] Primary and secondary sources seem to concur in indicating November 1965 as the inception of a collective practice which, every morning from ten to eleven o'clock, brought together patients, doctors, nurses, auxiliary staff and visitors. The content of the meetings was not planned in advance, but the subjects for discussion, decided by the assembly that was presided over each time by a different patient, always regarded the communal life of the hospital. The discussion of problems related to the practical management of the wards reflects the social relations within the therapeutic community in Gorizia and gives an insight into the decision-making aspects that were essential to the experiment of gradually opening up the psychiatric hospital until 1968. Basaglia's reforms in Gorizia gave rise to a national psychiatric reform movement in Italy, which resulted in the passing of law no. 180 in 1978. Commonly known as the 'legge Basaglia', this was the first legal framework mandating the definitive closure of civil psychiatric hospitals and regulating compulsory treatment in Italy by establishing a regional public mental health service.

In order to reconstruct in detail the motivation for the establishment of the general assembly as well as the practices that characterised the meetings, we will first look at its 'prehistory', starting from late 1961 when Basaglia took over the management of the psychiatric hospital in Gorizia. The following is an analysis of how these community assemblies functioned: the setting and events, who spoke, what the subject for discussion was, who took the minutes and how and why people participated. Exploring the mechanisms of this practice, through whatever remains in documentary terms over a limited period, 1962 to 1968, allows us to reconstruct Gorizia's fundamental therapeutic experience as well as to understand the difficulties and potential conflicts associated with this practice. This contribution analyses not only the therapeutic significance of Gorizia's general assembly, but also if and to what extent it established the epistemological bases for a 'new' psychiatric practice.[2]

There is a thread that the present analysis intends to weave, focusing on the scientific, political and practical significance of the 'experiment' within the Gorizia case. The transformative aspect of this experimentation, especially the development of a 'transformation of relations',[3] defines the identity of the collective body founded on the premises of the Gorizia Psychiatric Hospital. This transformation did not develop without risk, and in particular the risk of failure of the experiment itself, as one of its protagonists wrote: 'There was a great risk for us as well as for the patient ... There was tension about the innovation: we were involved in a unique and unrepeatable experience' (Venturini, 2020: 143).

To reconstruct how and why the therapeutic community, of anglophone inspiration,[4] at Gorizia became an example to follow, I propose here to use several sources, some unpublished, which offer a viewpoint beyond theoretical and practical psychiatric perspectives. I will therefore analyse material from *Il Picchio: Organo dei degenti dell'Ospedale Psichiatrico Provinciale* (The woodpecker: Journal of the patients of the Provincial Psychiatric Hospital), a magazine written by a group of patients, beginning publication just a few months after the arrival of Franco Basaglia and Antonio Slavich and continuing until 1966.[5]

Looking closer to the assembly practice in Gorizia hospital, this chapter aims at contributing to a comprehensive account of the Italian struggle against institutionalisation, which was sparked, historically, by Basaglia's experience in this hospital. Works on it are numerous: books such as *L'istituzione negata* (The institution denied) and other contemporary texts, together with historical research and more recent testimonies,[6] underline the essential features of the social dissent that, in accordance with the political culture of the period, had a tangible result in the approval of law no. 180 of 1978. A widespread shift in public opinion supported this victory. There is no doubt that the charisma of the movement's leader Franco Basaglia (1924–80), together with the influence of mass media, namely television, radio and newspapers, ensured that the experiment, initiated in an asylum built on the wall that divided Italy and Yugoslavia like a fresh scar, found an echo of global concern. Many have written of their memories of the Gorizia asylum as a mecca to be reached in order to see for themselves the profound effect of change (Babini, 2009: 178; Foot, 2014: 237). Many of those who did so were students, volunteers, writers, photographers, journalists, intellectuals and artists.[7]

The disruptive force of the events which gradually changed the reality of asylums in Italy should be read in the political and ideological context of the Italian Republic of the 1960s and 1970s. It would, however, be wrong to circumscribe the anti-institutionalisation movement within an exclusively medical or ideological frame of reference. From the outset, the daily practices, as well as the essays and articles produced for conferences, books, magazines, international congresses and public meetings by the protagonists, a handful of psychiatrists, had raised the stakes. It was not merely a question of denouncing the inhumane and degrading conditions in which the anonymous inmates of asylums were held, nor simply of opening a path towards the reform of psychiatric institutions.[8] That Italian psychiatry was a sort of 'desolate cathedral' in a still immature republic was an assumption made even in those academic circles less inclined to radical change. However, in Basaglia's view, 'backwardness and laziness' (Basaglia, 2018: 41) were seen as barely keeping alive a culture that intertwined musty organicism, of positivist imprint, with a sort of ineluctability of the closed hospital. These were the aspects that had led to a delay in, if not to actual rejection of, the introduction of anthropo-phenomenological and psychoanalytic orientations, already active in other countries in Western Europe.[9]

In many cases, including at the hospital of Gorizia, this 'backwardness' was the result of a continuous deterioration in psychiatric facilities, especially after World War II, and 'laziness' indicated the acceptance of this situation, the absence of any willingness to change. The asylum in Gorizia, inaugurated in the 1930s during the height of the fascist regime, was more closed off and peripheral than others in the country, not only for geopolitical reasons. The wards were overcrowded, the human and economic resources completely insufficient.[10] Gorizia was a place of 'second choice', even for those psychiatrists and doctors who had not found a place in academia.

When, in 1947, the Allies redefined Italy's eastern border, the hospital suffered the effects of the partition of the Isonzo territory with Yugoslavia. Many patients of Slovenian origin, who could not be discharged, found themselves stateless, facing a long internment aggravated by linguistic barriers and forced 'Italianisation'. Of the six hundred internees, more than a third were Slovenian, and for these the Italian government was obliged to pay a daily fee in reparation for war damages to the Yugoslav People's Republic.[11]

We might imagine that for Franco Basaglia the directorship of this hospital, gained by passing a public examination in November 1961, seemed like exile. Basaglia had not chosen Gorizia as a career move; his friend and first collaborator, the psychiatrist Antonio Slavich, remembers that Gorizia was an unexpected and unrequested destination (Slavich, 2018: 21). After years spent as assistant at the neurological clinic of the University of Padua, where he obtained a professorship and was given the title of 'philosopher' by his teacher Giovanni Battista Belloni, Basaglia hoped to continue his research, albeit from a different theoretical perspective. His first scientific papers, published in the 1950s, focus on the analysis of psychopathological subjectivity. The influence of Jaspers and Binswanger is evident (Basaglia, 2017: 45–91; Colucci and Di Vittorio, 2020: 27–79). The diagnostic repertoire observed in the Paduan clinic became an opportunity to explore, in anti-reductionist form, the relationship between biological therapeutic approaches and those which Basaglia describes as anthropo-phenomenological.

This signalled a new critical approach to the organicist model of psychiatry. Belloni, professor of neurology at the University of Padua, found himself in the uncomfortable position of having to 'settle' this brilliant but unconventional student.[12] Basaglia was at this point fully aware that he was in the humiliating predicament of academic limbo.

The opening for an asylum director in Gorizia came about by chance in March 1961. Director Antonio Canor had died in a road accident and the provincial administration of Gorizia began to seriously consider the possibility of a management change for the hospital, the maintenance of which had become barely sustainable, especially in financial terms. At the time of his appointment in November 1961 the asylum had about 630 inmates, distributed among eight wards.

'When Franco arrived in Gorizia, the impact with the asylum was violent', to the point of Basaglia not excluding his imminent resignation (Terzian, 1980: 2). On his first tour, zigzagging between courtyards, working colonies and wards, Basaglia described the asylum as 'the dunghill' where human beings lost all dignity (Basaglia, 2017: 663). Men and women in uniform, with shaven heads, slumped on the benches of the courtyards; others, the most 'agitated', were in fenced yards tied to trees during their daily hour of outdoor access. The interior of each ward held from fifty to one hundred beds. In wards B and C many inmates were restrained in their beds within divided cells. Others wandered, in perpetual motion and with blank eyes, around enormous, unadorned rooms. The most docile, under the supervision of workers and nurses, filled the workshop, the carpentry shop and the colonies, working according to the dictates of ergotherapy.

The abrupt encounter with this grim reality evoked in Basaglia an urgent need to break with previous standards and invent new practices: an uncertain and arduous endeavour. An almost legendary anecdote recounts that his first great gesture, made from his position of command at the end of that November morning, was his refusal to sign the register of restraints. '*E mi no firmo!*' (And I will not sign!) he declared in Venetian dialect. A symbolic gesture, quite unexpected, that affronted his staff and marked a first caesura, foreshadowing, if somewhat obliquely, a change of pace for the hospital.

Knock like a woodpecker's beak: a newsletter as documentary evidence

In one of his most important academic contributions, *Le istituzioni della violenza* (Institutions of violence), Franco Basaglia gives a brief history of the early years of the Gorizia experiment. These are not primarily theoretical elaborations supported by practical experience, but rather Basaglia's recounting of his observations in the preceding years:

> The situation we faced ... was highly institutionalised in all sectors: patients, nurses, doctors ... An attempt was made to provoke a situation of rupture that could help the three poles of hospital life emerge from their crystallised roles, placing them in a game of tension and counter-tension in which everyone would find themselves involved and responsible. It meant entering the 'risk', which alone could put doctors and patients, patients and staff on the same level, united in the same cause, tending towards a common purpose (Basaglia, 1968: 131).

What did it mean, materially, to 'provoke a situation of rupture'? Where and how should it begin? How could risk and tension be made productive? Plunging into the alienating experience of asylum life was the only way to appreciate what the outdated exercise of scientific knowledge had produced. These results were not the occasional distortion of a malfunctioning institution but a sign that the entire Italian psychiatric system was collapsing. The small hospital of Gorizia triggered that first essential earthquake: the raw reality that presented itself required careful consideration of the theoretical basis on which it had been formed. It had now become necessary to place theory at the service of practice. And that was no simple matter. 'Bracketing mental illness' (Basaglia, 2017: 315) was more than just an anti-psychiatric slogan. It meant abrading the surface of the dominant psychiatric model and ascertaining the human, social, medical and cultural outcomes of its application. 'Dirty' and risky work, which could change nothing if carried out in complete solitude. The medical staff needed to be rebuilt from scratch, the work of the paramedical staff needed to be reorganised and reim-agined, and this was undoubtedly one of the most delicate and complex aspects: in fact, the only continuous relationships that patients had previously established in that environment were with the nurses, nuns, labourers and caretakers; certainly not with the doctors.

August 1962 saw the publication of the first issue of the monthly magazine *Il Picchio*. Produced on an old in-house printing press and strongly endorsed by the new director, the first issue was composed of four sheets. There was no comment within on the choice of the name, although it referred, metaphorically, to the characteristic activity of its namesake bird – that of beating with insistence on hard, apparently unbreakable bark, every day.

The idea of printing a patients' magazine was not in itself original. By the end of the nineteenth century such initiatives had already been introduced in several European psychiatric institutions.[13] Often their function was to provide a diversion, an activity that could be an expression of asylum ergotherapy as well as a vehicle of self-expression. Not infrequently, however, articles favoured a paternalistic tone and emphasised the positive aspects of asylum life on which doctors and staff agreed. Such journals resembled a bulletin that documented and praised the successful operation of a well-functioning village asylum. *Il Picchio* was not completely immune to this style, but it nonetheless became the first instrument to publicise the radical change inside the hospital of Gorizia. Soon, issues were sent not only to other psychiatric hospitals, but also to discharged patients, doctors, volunteers and others who requested it. One patient above all, 'Furio', became the driving force of this initiative and would a few years later become one of the key figures of the general assembly. The first issue of the journal opens with an invitation from the editorial staff, initially composed only of male patients, mainly from ward A:

> This is our newspaper and all of us, patients, men and women, must collaborate in its drafting. We especially invite women, whom we have not, for obvious reasons, been able to contact directly, to send us their contributions (*Il Picchio*, 1 (1962): 1).

The 'obvious reasons' referred to the clear separation of the sexes within the wards, aggravated by internal architectural boundaries which were difficult to overcome. The courtyards between the pavilions were surrounded by high wire mesh. Along the border with Yugoslavia, the hospital grounds were closed off by a high boundary wall. Reducing internal distance, especially that of gender,

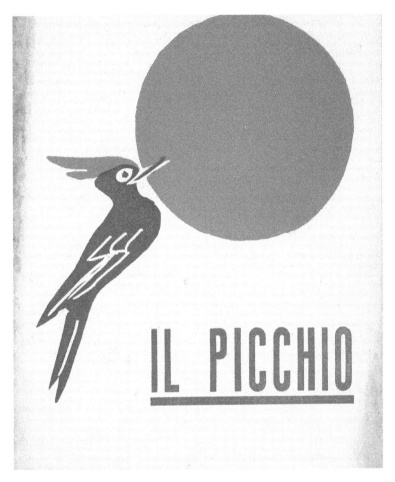

Figure 2.1 One of the illustrations used for the cover of *Il Picchio*. Courtesy of Archivio Agostino Pirella della Biblioteca di Area Umanistica di Arezzo – Università degli Studi di Siena.

was one of the first decisions shared with patients by the new director between November and December 1962. This is how the news was reported and commented on:

> One of these days we will witness an epoch-making event. The barriers surrounding the courtyard-walks will be dismantled. [...] We applaud the dynamic directorship that with this action initiates a series of

measures that will render our hospital similar to other civilian hospitals. In our humble opinion, this event should be celebrated (*Il Picchio*, 4 (1962): 1).

The following month, after the removal of the fences, an article, signed by the editorial staff, was headlined 'The Barriers Fall':

The 'overturning' of the fences is important not only in itself, but also in re-establishing serenity in the surrounding environment, in restoring the dignity and trust of the patients, for contact with the outside world, … for the new psychiatric conception to which it gives rise. … Its usefulness will be even more significant if the general principle is extended to each and every person, and includes civil and legal rights (*Il Picchio*, 5 (1962): 4–5).

The dismantling of the fences in December 1962 was publicised through a film that, fortunately, is still preserved.[14] Both Basaglia (2017: 261–9) and Slavich (2018: 150) emphasised the importance of removing the internal and external constraints in the departments, even though the opening of those for chronic inmates, such as in C ward, came about gradually. And yet the dismantling of the fences was not merely symbolic. Several words used in the *Il Picchio* article highlight two fundamental aspects. On the one hand, to materially topple the fences meant to initiate the practical exercise of small freedoms regained by the patients in their daily lives. On the other, torn down fences did not mean immediate freedom of movement for the bodies of men and women long confined to bed or in a contained environment. This required further measures aimed at redefining the relationship between body, time and space within that environment.

One of the most important steps in the redefinition of this relationship was the introduction of psychotropic medication, as Basaglia himself remembered during his first communication on the experience of Gorizia at the International Congress of Social Psychiatry (London, 1964): 'If the sick man has lost his freedom because of illness, this freedom to repossess himself has been given to him by his medication' (Basaglia, 2017: 264).

The introduction of psychotropic drugs therefore supported a greater but still limited freedom of patients' bodies and an innovative and often successful treatment of the most serious forms of regression.

Nevertheless, Basaglia emphasised that medication could not be raised to thaumaturgical power: 'If, in conjunction with the action of a drug, the hospital does not implement measures to defend freedom, whose loss the patient already suffers, the drug, activating a wider range of consciousness, will increase in him the conviction of being now definitively lost' (Basaglia, 2017: 264). Here, in the first experimental stage, an attitude emerges that would become a motto and part of everyday practice in Trieste a few years later: 'Freedom is therapeutic'.[15]

The second important aspect in the article 'The Barriers Fall' is the term 'overturning'. The use made of it by *Il Picchio* is not casual. It is a clear reference to a new dictum that the radical reformers in Gorizia adopted. 'The practical overthrow of the institution of the psychiatric asylum'[16] became a central slogan of the anti-institutional dialectic, along with its radical implications. In the patient-writer's view, the overturning of the fences only made sense if the civil and legal system of the psychiatric institutions was also overturned and thus, in the process, the necessity of the institution would also disappear. In addition, it reflects a political position of a Hegelian-Marxist character, which was already expressed in Gorizia's first collective writings (see Basaglia, 1967: 433).

For forty-two issues, from 1962 to 1966, *Il Picchio* kept track of the daily upheavals in Gorizia, often registering setbacks and failures. It remains the most detailed documentary testimony of the first contacts of patients with the outside world through day trips, the exploration of deeply felt problems such as alcoholism, the need to discuss the possible social reintegration of patients through work, the difficulties of re-establishing family relationships, the entry of a new generation of nurses, doctors and social workers into the hospital, and the renovation and opening up of the wards to create a more comfortable and less degrading environment. The journal also contained reports on the film forum, the choir, the library, music therapy, the bar, festivals and celebrations as well as personal stories of patients, poems and interviews with visitors from 'outside'. Thus, the magazine presented a hospital trying to create and increase spaces of encounter, and addressed the daily contradictions and clashes those relationships, involving different and asymmetrical roles, created.

Although it is impossible to render here the rich variety of all the newspaper's monthly columns, for the present examination it is worth focusing on three elements which present the prototype of the general assembly: group psychotherapy, the birth of the 'Let's help each other to heal' committee, and the institution of meetings of the wards and the newspaper's editorial staff, spanning 1962 to 1965.

From asylum to hospital community: helping each other heal

The new year of 1963 began under new auspices for *Il Picchio*. For starters, the cover changed.

In the 1963 issue, under the ever-present image of the hammering bird, appear two silhouettes of people shaking hands. The caption contains a strong message: 'Let's help each other to heal.' And the article within elaborates: 'Each must be the friend, the adviser of the other. In this way we can find what the disease has made us lose. ... It is not only our disease that is our damage' (*Il Picchio*, 6 (1963): 2).

The call to help each other was made to those in the hospital who did not yet participate in the activities of the newspaper or in other common occupations and was addressed to the decision-makers: the doctors, the administrators, the bursar and the nurses. This binary relationship between staff and patients would remain ineluctable. The daily exercise of patients' self-determination and the reconstitution of one's own subjectivity was closely related to a redefinition of distinct roles and tasks both inside and outside the hospital.

This aspect did not escape any of the actors, especially doctors, patients and nurses, and became an integral part of therapeutic relationships in the community:

> However, our position of privilege with respect to a sick person who has been rendered inferior in our eyes will not be easily overcome, but we can try to live the needs that are part of the patients' reality by establishing a relationship based on a process of mutual risk and contestation (Basaglia, 2017: 331).

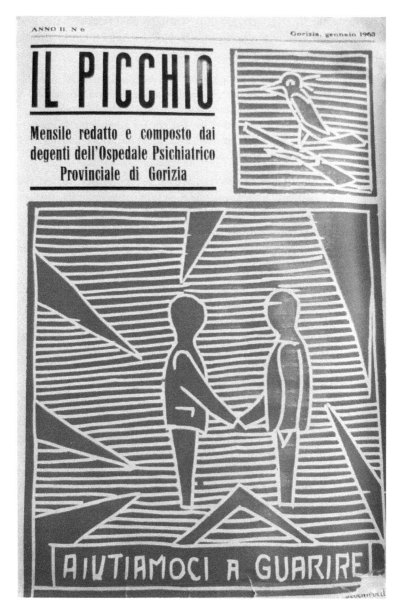

Figure 2.2 *Il Picchio*. Magazine written and composed by the patients of the Provincial Psychiatric Hospital of Gorizia. Slogan: 'Let's help each other to heal'. Courtesy of Archivio Agostino Pirella della Biblioteca di Area Umanistica di Arezzo – Università degli Studi di Siena.

The dialectic of that relationship strongly characterised the first reflections on group psychotherapy in Gorizia, which could also be found in the pages of *Il Picchio* in 1962:

> A mentally ill person will certainly not recover from treatment alone, but psychotherapy, as our doctors understand it, will have a beneficial effect on his personality. ... In this group, which should be nothing other than a miniature society, the patient encounters his fellows, freeing himself, speaking, at first with great difficulty and then, overcoming emotional resistance, fluently (*Il Picchio*, 5 (1962): 1).

Furio, the soul of the newsletter, was also spokesperson for the patients in this phase, which suggests their participation in discussions with doctors concerning psychotherapy. How was psychotherapy understood, and how would it be practised starting from 1963? It is again a short article from the newsletter that commented on the introduction of group psychotherapy:

> Group psychotherapy has begun. This therapy consists in bringing together groups of patients, who are selected a priori, and in giving them ample opportunity to converse among themselves on problems which they choose spontaneously, that is, which most affect all those present, while the function of the doctor is to listen and to guide, in order to stimulate the conversation and, if necessary, lead it back to the right track (*Il Picchio*, 6 (1963): 4).

The article is signed 'L.V.'; we do not know if it was a male or a female patient, but it is certain that all monthly issues of both 1963 and 1964 are rich in articles about group psychotherapy, a sign that members of the 'Let's help each other to heal' committee were increasingly writing about their experiences for the magazine. From issue nine of 1963, the editorial staff began to methodically publish the internal patient movements of the hospital, highlighting the relationship between discharged and hospitalised patients, and noting the progressive increase of patients participating in different work activities. In March 1963, of 563 patients (273 men and 290 women), 319 were employed either inside or outside the hospital. Here the usual statistics for male and female employment were reversed, seeing 200 women employed compared to only 119 men.[17] But what was the meaning of work in this context? In Gorizia, the reformers criticised traditional ergotherapy, regarding it as degrading labour, unremunerated or bartered for cigarettes and sweets, with the work done there only serving the asylum-related needs of nurses and doctors. In 1964, work in the hospital changed fundamentally when, through an internal cash system, a weekly wage was paid to meet certain basic needs of patients. So it was that workshops were created: sewing, knitting, chair upholstering, printing and even a hairdressing salon. No less important was the creation of a library and the opening of a school that was recognised by the state. From 1965 there was another step forward: it was made possible for inmates to work at simple artisanal tasks for external companies and factories through conventions stipulated by the psychiatric hospital. Thus, day by day, it became feasible to realise at Gorizia what Basaglia's team had seen and known mainly through the English experiment of Maxwell Jones at Dingleton.[18] Yet, none of these changes were obsequious emulations of facile sociotherapy prescriptions or tried-and-tested forms of occupational therapy. Many problems remained, such as the doubts and contradictions that Antonio Slavich expressed as follows:

> Perhaps ergotherapy was a necessary beginning, but it risked increasing internal institutionalisation. It was necessary to go beyond ... to organise occupational therapy or play therapy. All were aspects of the asylum technique, of course, but at the beginning we did not disdain organising them in Gorizia, on the condition that the tendency was to gradually involve the whole hospital. ... In short, one could do anything, but not call any of these activities 'therapy' (Slavich, 2018: 97).

The process was one of trial and error, guided according to Slavich by 'a healthy empiricism' (Slavich, 2018: 98). Nor can we consider the changes in the years 1963 to 1965 as the most radical. These resulted from the constitution of the 'Let's help each other to heal' committee and the initiation of psychotherapy, a complete transition from the reality of the asylum to that of the hospital. Several elements co-existed in the same space, given the objective limits imposed by both the lack of staff and of specific skills and resources. Basaglia was aware of this in 1964, when he wrote in the editorial for *Il Picchio*:

> Asylum, Hospital and Therapeutic Community are the stages of our journey in these years. This does not mean that these three stages do not exist at one and the same time in our institution. We have tried to destroy the asylum as a place of exclusively forced admission, but

there are still many elements that remind us of it (*Il Picchio*, 28–9 (1964): 1).

The differences in the equipment of the wards were often substantial. As a group of patients wrote to *Il Picchio* in July 1963, in reference to the renovation of ward A compared to the inferior conditions in ward B: 'Passing from the ground floor to the first floor is like passing from darkness to light' (*Il Picchio*, 12 (1963): 4). Two years later, the women of the female ward D wrote:

> Dearest Woodpecker, we, although once sick, today, thanks to care and goodwill, feel healed, and we show it in the attention with which we carry out our work, for which they pay us but little. ... Secondly, we do not enjoy freedom: in perpetually closed wards, accompanied everywhere, we think we should have the same rights as our friends in ward B (*Il Picchio*, 38–9 (1965): 19).

Finally, there was the last frontier of the pathogenic germ of institutionalisation, ward C, housing chronic patients whose mental and physical condition had deteriorated over the years. For them, it was difficult to imagine a future outside the hospital as well as to integrate into the therapeutic community. In ward C, the railings would remain up and the doors would remain closed for several more years, while therapeutic microcommunities, both male and female, emerged between 1965 and 1966, bringing together patients from the other wards.

The first steps of a therapeutic community: the general assembly as a practical experiment of the excluded

What, then, was the therapeutic community of Gorizia and what was its therapy? From what has been written so far, and as testified in *Il Picchio*, it is clear that every change until 1964 both inside and outside the hospital was oriented towards community principles and methods, applied equally to the 'Let's help each other to heal' committee, to editorial meetings of *Il Picchio* and to group psychotherapy. Yet, something different characterises the first appearance of the therapeutic community officially formed on 6 October 1964, in men's ward B.

The chosen patients from different wards made up 53 out of about 600 inmates, while the selection criteria considered both

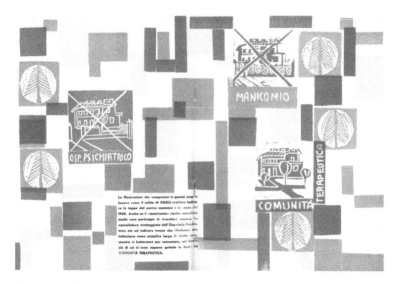

Figure 2.3 *Il Picchio*, 28–9 (1964): 18–19. The illustration for this issue was created by a patient named Velio T. Courtesy of Archivio Agostino Pirella della Biblioteca di Area Umanistica di Arezzo – Università degli Studi di Siena.

diagnostic differentiation and individual patient backgrounds. In ward B, the so-called 'agitated ward' in the old nomenclature, room was made for the community welcoming male patients from other departments. Slavich, director of ward B, recalls that it was far from easy to transfer the patients who were not destined to take part in the experiment to other wards: 'It was necessary to communicate to everyone the reasons for our choice, and to explain to some of the ward B inmates, even to those who probably would not have comprehended or approved, the reasons for their necessary transfer to other wards' (Slavich, 2018: 147).

The selection of nursing staff was another object of careful consideration. The beginning of this community life was not left to chance. Rather, there was a small-scale trial run in September 1964 when twenty-two patients (ten women and twelve men), with the consent of the provincial administration, stayed for a week in a house in Bagni di Lusnizza, a mountain resort not far from Gorizia. There were enthusiastic reports on this from patients in *Il Picchio*: 'The experiment – the first of its kind in Italy – was, we can affirm, a positive success. Immediately on arrival the daily schedule was established in a general meeting and then everyone was at work' (*Il Picchio*, 25–6 (1964): 2). This is how Velio T. remembered 'the holiday': 'The moral atmosphere was something I cannot even begin to express; it was so different from what I have been used to for the last ten years' (*Il Picchio*, 25–6 (1964): 2). And Francesca S. wrote: 'Everything was so beautiful, the scenery, the walks, the meetings, the meals, being together ... everything was discussed freely' (*Il Picchio*, 25–6 (1964): 2).

In his memoirs, Slavich emphasised the intramural changes that were necessary for the establishment of the first therapeutic community in Gorizia. Beyond the need to improve the material conditions of ward B through renovations that would facilitate meetings and collaboration, it was also necessary to provide special care for the inmates who would participate: 'The choice of the group of collaborators was a difficult task, because we well knew the disruptive effect on the cared-for of any tensions and disharmonies within the team of caretakers' (Slavich, 2018: 147).

The programme of daily activities was rigorous and structured around both the individual and the group. In addition to self-government of the common areas, care was also taken to verify the individual therapeutic approach within the community through a substantial review of patients' medications, as well as with the implementation of twice-weekly ward and staff meetings. *Il Picchio* also became an important factor in informing and educating inmates about the innovations introduced by the therapeutic community. Beginning with issue twenty-seven of 1964, in fact, the journal introduced a new section with an unequivocal title and matching content: 'Therapeutic Community'. The initial considerations of the editorial leave no room for doubt as regards the distinction between the experiences of a traditional hospital and those of the community of Gorizia. Thus, the editorial wrote that the traditional hospital was based on:

> the principle of authority: an authority that is distributed in different degrees among the staff and asserted in different ways. The patients, however, are completely without authority: they have nothing to say, to predict, to organise, the environment is made for them but not by them. Deprived of any possibility of decision, they are simply objects of those norms (*Il Picchio*, 27 (1964): 3).

The existence of therapeutic communities, on the other hand, reverses the principle of authority, according to the editorial:

> A therapeutic community is a psychiatric ward organised by the patients together with the staff, so that, through this collaboration, they establish ... bonds of mutual knowledge and trust; ties that also have a therapeutic value. ... These communities are small societies: if it is true that mental suffering results from disharmony ... it is legitimate to expect that a spontaneous and orderly reconstruction of a social life within the community can mitigate and resolve this suffering by becoming a therapeutic instrument (*Il Picchio*, 27 (1964): 4).

In the early months of 1965, in women's ward B, in a similar manner and under the coordination of the only female psychiatrist present in the team, Maria Pia Bombonato, a second nucleus of the therapeutic community, was established. The opening of all wards and the inclusion of all patients in subgroups of the therapeutic community was completed three years later, in 1968, with women's ward C.

The community organisation increasingly required continual discussions and decisions, together with a participation of staff and patients that could not always be taken for granted. The proliferation of meetings led to a systematic choice as early as 1965 – that of establishing a general assembly which aimed to resolve four problems in particular. Firstly, it was necessary to avoid unwanted dispersion of the topics addressed, as sometimes happened in ward meetings; secondly, the possibility of participation in the assembly should be extended not only to the individual wards of the community but to the whole hospital; thirdly, the structure of the agendas of the assembly should be improved by empowering patients, who took turns in presiding and taking minutes; and fourthly, it was necessary to increase and facilitate the participation and intervention of the patients on constantly recurring issues, such as the improvement of living conditions in the hospital community, as a condition necessary to better prepare patients for discharge from the hospital.

The proposal to establish a general assembly came from the psychiatrist Agostino Pirella in 1965 (Pirella, 1989: 13–17). Pirella had recently joined the Gorizia staff, taking over the management of ward D and later men's ward C. The daily rhythm of the general assembly had made it one of the most often represented and narrated symbols of Gorizia's spirit of reform in the outside world. Visitors who attended the first general assemblies were often disconcerted by the proceedings; the topics for discussion were all-encompassing, the private life of the medical team effectively disappeared, while the demarcation of the medical team and patients was effectively removed, becoming one collective unit. Franco Pierini, an Italian journalist, wrote in 1967: '[Patients] are better than us in the technique of discussion, in the dialectics of opposing opinions, in the conclusions reached without scapegoats, without losers.'[19]

But how did the general meetings work? What do we know about the topics, the techniques of discussion and the proceedings that took place every day for several years? We know for certain that the historical archive of Gorizia Psychiatric Hospital contains no recorded accounts of the assemblies; these have probably been lost.[20] However, traces remain in several sources. Some accounts are known through the books *What is Psychiatry?* and *The Institution Denied* because assembly discussions appear in the texts, written by different authors between 1967 and 1968. For previous assemblies, in 1965 and 1966, *Il Picchio* is always a valuable source. The last two issues, forty and forty-one,[21] included summaries of the minutes of assemblies held from 1 April to 30 July 1966.

Analysing the reports published in *Il Picchio*, it is possible to understand the course and the outcome of the discussions in this year. Participation, in numerical terms, fluctuated, especially in the spring of 1966: '[We go] from 60 to 130 participants and we do not always get to reach conclusions on the topics discussed' (*Il Picchio*, 40 (1966): 8). On 5 April 1966, an item on the agenda directly concerned the decrease in number and disaffection of those attending the assembly: 'From many of the opinions expressed: it seems that many patients do not intervene because they think that the doctors are present to "scrutinise" their behaviour, that many people do not intervene out of shyness or fear of being judged in public' (*Il Picchio*, 40 (1966): 10).

In many cases, the criticism voiced by patients in the general assembly addressed the forced conditions in the hospital in general, while personal problems brought up by individual patients received much less attention. From the beginning, the most pressing and objectively unresolved issue, at least until the approval of the Mariotti Law of 1968 on voluntary hospitalisation,[22] was that of discharge, which required the signed guarantee of a family member, and which was all too often denied. In the light of the families' refusal to care for their hospitalised relatives and in the absence of external psychiatric services that might have offered an alternative to hospitalisation, most patients saw no prospect of discharge and developed anxiety, disillusionment and discontent, which they directed at doctors during the assemblies. As a result, defiant silences or angry outbursts of emotion occurred from time to time, which the team did not try to limit. It was the task of the patient chairing the respective session of the general assembly to deal with this kind of disorder without overt intervention by hospital staff members or doctors.

It is perhaps surprising that, in the minutes of the general assembly that have been preserved, the same topics were discussed repeatedly. The main topics were always the organisation of parties, management of the bar and life in the wards. At first reading these minutes might therefore appear boring or insubstantial. And yet, this theme clearly reveals the great value that the participants attributed to community life.

As noted by John Foot, in those years more than fifty weekly meetings were held, including those of the wards, of staff, with volunteers and of the newspaper (Foot, 2017: 119). 'Assemblarism', that is, the concrete possibility that the discussion would end without finding effective solutions, was the other side of the coin. In the summer of 1966, this ineffectiveness led to tension and fatigue, which one patient clearly highlighted in an *Il Picchio* article, although he stressed the fundamental value of the meetings:

> During all this time, in which we held assemblies, we have obtained very little, not to say almost nothing, basically here we do nothing but study each other: doctors study us and we can study them. ... The press should be invited [to] change the opinion of those outside who must think of us as their fellow men, only tried by misfortune. If our assemblies have not yielded results in this sense, they are still important to us because they serve to help each other and in this I also include the nursing staff. We must unite to fight. To make ourselves heard (*Il Picchio*, 41 (1966): 21–2).

Overall, both the patients' testimonies and the psychiatric team's own texts highlight the therapeutic value of this reciprocal 'study' (Basaglia, 2017: 395). It can therefore be stated that the assemblies took over the task of group psychotherapy from 1965 onwards and that individual psychotherapeutic approaches played less and less of a role in Gorizia. As one patient, Maria, makes clear:

> Some say that doctors tend to the sick more generally and do not dwell long on each individual case. That is true, but the reason must be analysed. During the meetings group psychotherapy is practised which allows the doctor to observe the patients' attitude regarding problems that concern the life of the hospital, organised as a small town. The protagonists of these meetings are precisely the patients [who] can express and demonstrate their true personality in front of the doctor, who, through a long dialogue, aims to guide, direct, encourage and make them responsible for their own existence. A climate so conceived, along with the psychotherapeutic advantage, also offers a pedagogical one. It seems to me that this dual character can well be considered as helping achieve the freedom that is the goal to which everyone aspires (*Il Picchio*, 40 (1966): 25).

The exercise of taking charge of themselves and others and actively shaping institutional change led to a new process of subjectification for many patients. They became more used to talking and making decisions again, although this was far from an obvious achievement. Granting patients these rights was related to the fact that mental illness was largely seen as the result of internalisation and institutionalisation. In Gorizia, however, this also led to patients increasingly denouncing the exclusion and restrictions imposed by life in hospital. The daily minutes of the general assembly make it clear that those involved in the Gorizia experiment did not attempt to hide therapeutic contradictions and ideological limits but rather that they were very aware of this basic problem in Gorizia and allowed discussion about it: the absence of an alternative to the psychiatric hospital risked perpetuating what already existed, creating a sort of 'good' institutionalisation: well conducted, less traumatic. An internal community could thus become 'a golden cage' (Basaglia, 2017: 267) that risked transforming political mobilisation into technical management.

Conclusion

The last issue of *Il Picchio* was published in 1966. There were many reasons for the end of this experience, not all in line with the official position expressed in *The Institution Denied*. In Nino Vascon's interview of the patient Furio, included in *The Institution Denied*, it is reported that publication 'has not been renewed because the liberalisation of the hospital has made communication media pointless' (Basaglia, 1968: 88). More importantly, the magazine's editorial collective was dwindling and eventually consisted only of Furio himself. The general assemblies, on the contrary, continued through ups and downs in the following years, but there are no records of the minutes during this period, apart from a few extracts.

We can, however, say that the world outside the Gorizia Psychiatric Hospital recognised the central and unprecedented role of community life within the hospital. Public interest in the Gorizia experiment exploded between 1967 and 1968. The collected editions *Che cos'è la psichiatria?* (What is psychiatry?) and *L'istituzione negata* (The institution denied) edited by Basaglia received a large readership. Added to this came a widespread national and international press campaign. The issue of asylums was no longer just a matter for experts to be entrusted with, providing technical and health solutions. Through the volition of the movement that promoted it, it had instead become a high-profile democratic and political issue, and wide sectors of the public responded well to the radical and fundamental idea that closing asylums was as possible and necessary for overcoming the exclusion of the mentally ill.

It is, perhaps, no surprise that the media and cultural representation of this experiment favoured an oversimplistic view, imagining the entire Gorizia Psychiatric Hospital as a therapeutic community. Paradoxically, at the very moment when Gorizia found national and international recognition, Basaglia's team itself encountered signs of crisis and points of no return. Gorizia's path to fame was, therefore, a troubled process with a not entirely favourable outcome. In fact, during the experiment's greatest period of public prominence (1967–68), the relationship between the provincial administration and the medical team became increasingly complicated.[23] The psychiatrists of Gorizia demanded decisive steps regarding the establishment of mental health services external to and different from the hospital, without which they believed the experiment would fall short of its goals. Their demands encountered apparently insurmountable political and normative obstacles. This conflict eventually put an end to the therapeutic community, which was established by Basaglia but continued without interruption under the direction first of Pirella and then of Casagrande until 1971.

The microcosm of the liberalised hospital community clashed with harsh reality. The libertarian potential expressed in the construction of free speech and community action collided with the demands that logically resulted from this. 'When do I get home? When will I be discharged?' became repetitive questions in the last years of Gorizia, but they could not find a definitive answer in the assembly. There was, in fact, an increase in the number of patients discharged, but, in the total absence of external assistance, the management's goal of continual admissions and discharges met with limited success.

The forced choice, first of Basaglia, then of the whole team, to leave Gorizia had a double effect: on the one hand, it meant that this experiment could take root elsewhere, extending the possibility of effecting the transformation of psychiatric practices and the closure of asylums. On the other hand, it was a heavy blow to Gorizia's patients, interrupting certain community life practices.[24] This was particularly true of those with a history of long-term care in the C wards, who resigned themselves to indefinite internment when faced with uncertainty, abandonment and denial.[25]

Ultimately, the experimental nature of these practices remained the most innovative aspect of Gorizia. It was a founding act, necessary but not sufficient for a radical epistemological change in psychiatry. As his friend and colleague Hrayr Terzian wrote, Basaglia

> realised a conceptual operation that was his true scientific work, coherently Galilean. He thought that in the impossibility of examining an object one examines what contains it. ... And this intuition led him to bracket disease, and to examine its many encrustations in the hope of eventually finding the disease itself (Terzian, 1980: 3).[26]

Basaglia's experience at Gorizia has, on several occasions, been criticised as unscientific, and in some quarters the question of the scientific nature of his psychiatry is still a thorny question for debate. Terzian, however, while explaining the experimental matrix of Basaglia's practices, makes clear his belief in their indubitably scientific character.

During Basaglia's tenure, the general assembly was one of the instruments best able to reveal the apodeictic evidence of psychiatry's contradictory nature. Its practical response to the violence of the asylums, by humanising them at an early stage, was an attempt to prevent the effects of institutionalisation on mental illness.[27] Thus, the Gorizia experiment can only be understood if one assumes as a precondition the radically different meaning that therapeutic action assumed within that community. The practices of the therapeutic community during this first Italian implementation were characterised by its highly utopian and ideological orientation. To compare these with subsequent developments in other mental hospitals, whether run along Basaglia's lines or not, is the challenge that awaits us.[28]

Notes

1 Antonio Slavich, the first psychiatrist in Basaglia's team at Gorizia who joined the hospital in 1962, notes that they initially used the English expression 'community meeting' taken from the English model of Maxwell Jones's therapeutic community: 'which everyone later called more modestly *assemblea generale* [general assembly]' (Slavich, 2018: 168). John Foot (2014: 237, 241) talks of both 'general meetings' and 'general assemblies'. I propose keeping the literal translation 'general assembly' to highlight the centrality of this moment.

2 A much-debated aspect of the relationship between practice and theoretical models in Basaglia's approach was the definition of the actual methodology of psychiatric rehabilitation. After Basaglia's death in 1980, by which point the experience gained at Gorizia was being disseminated by members of his team in other psychiatric hospitals (for instance by Arezzo, Parma and Trieste), a more urgent theme emerged; not merely the importance of ending hospitalisation in favour of a less 'concealing' psychiatry, but also 'the possibility of making it a science' (see Castelfranchi, *et al.*, 1995: 39). For the epistemological bases of 'new psychiatry', see Pirella, 1999: 63–71.

3 In an interview with Pirella, conducted by M. S. Goulart on 2 February 2001, published in Venturini (2020: 140), Pirella said: 'Without the Gorizia experience, in Italy we would still have a situation like that of Germany. We would have smaller and more humanised psychiatric hospitals, but with a great difference in terms of power between the psychiatrists, the psychiatric operators and the patients; we would still have … a concept favouring control over care' (Venturini, 2020: 139).

4 This refers to the experience of Maxwell Jones's therapeutic community, which represented a model for Gorizia to explore. On the comparison between different therapeutic community models and that of Gorizia,

see Colucci and Di Vittorio, 2020: 153–60 and Foot, 2017: 84–94. For a more exhaustive historical reconstruction of therapeutic community models in Europe, see also Fussinger, 2010: 217–40.

5 Issues 3–7, 13–14, 17–19 and 22–4 of *Il Picchio* are accessible at the Archivio dell'Ospedale Psichiatrico Provinciale di Gorizia (Historical archive of the Provincial Psychiatric Hospital of Gorizia), Gorizia (hereafter referred to as ASOPPGo); issues 1, 8–12, 15–16, 20–1, 35 and 34–41 can be consulted at the Biblioteca Statale Isontina (Isontine State Library), Gorizia; issues 25–34 are held in the Archivio 'Agostino Pirella' (Agostino Pirella archive) of Arezzo University in Siena. I have been unable to consult issue 2, which today is extremely difficult to locate.

6 See Basaglia, 1967, 1968 and 2017; Jervis, 1977; Corbellini and Jervis, 2008; Slavich, 2018. For principal historical reconstructions see Babini, 2009; Sforza Tarabochia, 2013; Trivelli, 2013; Foot, 2014; Burns and Foot, 2020; Colucci and Di Vittorio, 2020; Bruzzone, 2021.

7 On the role of Gorizia volunteers see Setaro and Calamai, 2019: 43–60; Setaro, 2021: 391–9; of artists and architects see Scavuzzo, 2020; of the media and photographers see Guglielmi, 2018, Sforza Tarabochia, 2021: 209–27.

8 On the immobility and conservatism of Italian psychiatry see Babini, 2009: 130–42; Galli, 2014: 79–90.

9 From the 1960s, Basaglia and his team had already begun to learn about therapeutic experiences in the UK (Dingleton Hospital, Melrose, 1961), Germany (Würzburg and Gütersloh, 1964), France (Sector Psychiatry by Duchêne and Daumezon, XIII Arr.) and Switzerland (L'hôpital psychiatrique de Cery, Lausanne, 1965). Important intermediaries in this process were the psychiatrists Edoardo Balduzzi, Giampaolo Lai, Michele Risso, Gian Franco Minguzzi and Pier Francesco Galli. See Babini, 2009; Foot, 2014; Slavich, 2018.

10 The inventory and documentary introduction of the ASOPPGo is currently being prepared for publication by Sara Fantin, the archivist of the Cooperativa La Collina who has supervised the reorganisation. I consulted the inventory and some of the documentary sources for this article with her invaluable support.

11 On the economic contributions that Yugoslavia granted to Italy to support Slovenian internees see Foot, 2009: 16; Slavich, 2018: 75.

12 See Basaglia *et al.*, 2008: 103. See also Visintini, 1983: 168–9; Giannichedda, 2005: xviii; Colucci and Di Vittorio, 2020: 19–20.

13 The ASOPPGo contains, though still unsorted, many similar magazines from other European institutions. *Il Picchio* provides a detailed overview in the section entitled 'Leggendo la nostra stampa' (see, for example, *Il*

Picchio, 20–1 (1964): 19–21). Among them are *L'information* (Vinatier, France), *Coney Clarion* (Gloucester, England), *Là Haut* (Marsens, Switzerland) and *O Arauto* (Telhal, Portugal).

14 The films, without sound, of the first demolition of fences in the asylum, are now kept at the Mediateca 'Ugo Casiraghi' in Gorizia as part of the Giorgio Osbat Collection.

15 This slogan was written on the walls of the San Giovanni Psychiatric Hospital in Trieste, of which Basaglia was the director from 1971. The inventor of the slogan was Ugo Guarino, an artist who had set up the Rainbow Art Collective in the hospital: see Gallio *et al.*, 1983 and Giannichedda, 2016.

16 This expression occurs frequently in both assembly minutes and the writings of Basaglia's team: see Pirella, 1999; Basaglia, 2017.

17 *Il Picchio*, 9 (1963): 19. Patient movement tables were published in all subsequent issues, up to issues 36–7 of 1965.

18 Regarding this, Foot writes: 'Gorizia had a model for their revolution, and it came from the United Kingdom' (Foot, 2017: 85). On the importance of the English model of therapeutic community, see also Pirella, 1999; Millar, 2000.

19 Pierini was a journalist at L'Europeo, a weekly magazine read widely in Italy. The investigation under his byline was published in *Il Picchio*, 34 (1967): 14, entitled *Se il malato è un uomo* (If the patient is a man).

20 The ASOPPGo inventory gives no indication of any minutes of assemblies or ward and staff meetings among the documents in its possession.

21 The newspaper ended publication in 1966 with issue 41, to which should be added a special edition in December 1962.

22 Law no. 431 of 1968 took its name from the then minister of health, Luigi Mariotti, who had compared asylums to 'German concentration camps'. The law eliminated forced hospitalisation, introducing voluntary hospitalisation for the first time. It was the first concrete act of reform of psychiatric hospitals in Italy and created the preparatory groundwork for law no. 180 of 1978.

23 For an analysis of the last years of the Basaglian experience at Gorizia, when the hospital was under the direction of the psychiatrist Nico Casagrande, see Venturini, 2020.

24 The resignation of Nico Casagrande and his team was welcomed by the Isonzo provincial authority, which offered no possibility of realising the reforms requested over the years by Basaglia's movement (including the formation of a regional mental health service, for example). Subsequently, a psychiatrist from Padua, Giuseppe Carucci, was appointed director, but his experience was very brief. At this point, the general assembly was interrupted. See Foot, 2017: 243; Venturini, 2020: 183.

25 Letizia Comba, the psychologist in charge of the female ward C at Gorizia, defined it as 'a frozen island with no history' (Comba, 1968: 233). Certainly, the cages around the beds had been removed and the spaces reordered, but it remained a confined ward until 1968.

26 Regarding the difficulties of the Gorizia experiment, Edoardo Balduzzi, Basaglia's friend as well as the leading exponent of sector psychiatry in Italy, says: 'The community that "heals by healing itself" has become the only therapeutic background ... in an institutional context. We are in the presence of genuine experimentation' (Balduzzi, 1968: 127).

27 On this aspect see Colucci and Di Vittorio, 2020: 117–34.

28 On therapeutic communities in other European locations see also Chapters 1, 3, 5 and 10.

References

Babini, Valeria, 2009, *Liberi tutti* (Bologna: il Mulino).

Balduzzi, Edoardo, Giorgio Alberti and Paolo Saccani, 1968, 'Psichiatria nella comunità e politica di settore', *Note e riviste di psichiatria*, 61:1, 118–55.

Basaglia, Franco (ed.), 1967, *Che cos'è la psichiatria?* (Turin: Einaudi).

Basaglia, Franco (ed.), 1968, *L'istituzione negata* (Turin: Einaudi).

Basaglia, Franco, 2017, *Scritti: 1953–1980* (Milan: il Saggiatore).

Basaglia, Franco, 2018, *Conferenze brasiliane* (Milan: Raffaello Cortina editore).

Basaglia, Franco, Franca Ongaro Basaglia, Agostino Pirella and Salvatore Taverna, 2008, *La nave che affonda* (Milan: Cortina).

Bruzzone, Annamaria, Marica Setaro and Silvia Calamai, 2021, *Ci chiamavano matti* (Milan: il Saggiatore).

Burns, Tom and John Foot (eds), 2020, *Basaglia's International Legacy: From Asylum to Community* (Oxford: Oxford University Press).

Castelfranchi, Cristiano, Paolo Henry and Agostino Pirella, 1995, *L'invenzione collettiva* (Turin: Gruppo Abele).

Colucci, Mario and Pierangelo Di Vittorio, 2020, *Franco Basaglia* (Merano: Alpha Beta Verlag).

Comba, Letizia, 1968, 'C donne: l'ultimo reparto chiuso', in Franco Basaglia (ed.), *L'istituzione negata* (Turin: Einaudi), pp. 231–3.

Corbellini, Gilberto and Giovanni Jervis, 2008, *La razionalità negata* (Turin: Bollati Boringhieri).

Foot, John, 2009, *Fratture d'Italia* (Milan: Rizzoli).

Foot, John, 2014, 'Franco Basaglia and the radical psychiatry movement in Italy, 1961–78', *Critical and Radical Social Work*, 2:2, 235–49.

Foot, John, 2017, *La 'repubblica dei matti'* (Milan: Feltrinelli).

Fussinger, Catherine, 2010, 'Eléments pour une histoire de la communauté thérapeutique dans la psychiatrie occidentale de la seconde moitié du 20e siècle', *Gesnerus*, 67:2, 217–40.

Galli, Pier Francesco, 2014, 'Psychotherapy, psychoanalysis, and psychiatry in the early 1960s: Annotations for a history', *Trauma and Memory*, 2:3, 79–90.

Gallio, Giovanna, Maria Grazia Giannichedda, Ota De Leonardis and Diana Mauri, 1983, *La libertà è terapeutica?* (Milan: Feltrinelli).

Giannichedda, Maria Grazia, 2005, *L'utopia della realtà* (Turin: Einaudi), pp. vii–lii.

Giannichedda, Maria Grazia, 2016, 'Testimonianze dall'abisso', *il manifesto*, 6 May, https://ilmanifesto.it/testimonianze-dallabisso (accessed 22 September 2023).

Guglielmi, Marina, 2018, *Raccontare il manicomio* (Florence: Franco Cesati).

Jervis, Giovanni, 1977, *Il buon rieducatore* (Milan: Feltrinelli).

Millar, Kate (ed.), 2000, *The Story of a Community: Dingleton Hospital, Melrose* (Melrose: Chiefswood Publications).

Pirella, Agostino, 1989, 'Chi ha paura dell'assemblea generale?', in L. Attenasio and G. Filippi (eds), *Parola di matti* (Verona: Bertani), pp. 13–28.

Pirella, Agostino, 1999, *Il problema psichiatrico* (Pistoia: Centro di documentazione).

Scavuzzo, Giuseppina, 2020, *Il parco della guarigione infinita* (Syracuse, NY: Lettera Ventidue).

Setaro, Marica, 2021, 'Le vite di dentro: Anna Maria Bruzzone e i testimoni della follia', in Annamaria Bruzzone, *Ci chiamavano matti*, ed. Marica Setaro and Silvia Calamai (Milan: il Saggiatore), pp. 391–9.

Setaro, Marica and Silvia Calamai, 2019, 'Pazzi sonori: L'archivio di Anna Maria Bruzzone come orecchio della memoria', *Mefisto*, 3:2, 43–60.

Sforza Tarabochia, Alvise, 2013, *Psychiatry, Subjectivity, Community* (Bern: Peter Lang).

Sforza Tarabochia, Alvise, 2021, 'Claustrophobic visions of the asylum', *Between*, 11:22, 209–27.

Slavich, Antonio, 2018, *All'ombra dei ciliegi giapponesi* (Merano: Alpha Beta Verlag).

Terzian, Hrayr, 1980, 'Ricordo di Franco Basaglia', *Uomo, città, territorio*, 59:60, 1–7.

Trivelli, Elena, 2013, 'Assembling Memories and Affective Practices around the Psychiatric Hospital of Gorizia'. PhD thesis, University of London.

Venturini, Ernesto, 2020, *Mi raccomando non sia troppo basagliano* (Rome: Armando).

Visintini, Fabio, *Memorie di un cittadino psichiatra* (Naples: ESI, 1983).

3

Social psychiatry in the making: practices at Heidelberg's Psychiatric University Clinic in the 1960s and 1970s

Gundula Gahlen

In the Federal Republic of Germany, psychiatric reform began rather late compared to other Western countries. It took until the 1960s for a broad theoretical and practical critique of psychiatry to begin here. And it was not until the Psychiatry Enquete of 1975[1] that outpatient care structures were strengthened and a reform process initiated, which remains incomplete to this day. In contrast, in Canada, the USA, the Netherlands, Great Britain and Scandinavia, social psychiatric reforms in this regard had already been adopted fifteen years earlier (Kersting, 1998; Kersting, 2003).

The Heidelberg psychiatrists Walter Ritter von Baeyer (1904–87), Heinz Häfner (1926–2022) and Karl Peter Kisker (1926–97) were among the key figures in the reform of psychiatry in the Federal Republic of Germany. As early as 1965, they wrote a memorandum entitled 'Urgent Reforms in Psychiatric Health Care in the Federal Republic of Germany', in which they made criticisms that psychiatric hospitals in the Federal Republic were underfunded, that there was a shortage of personnel and rigid clinical hierarchies, and that there were no rehabilitation pathways. As a way out, they proposed the establishment of 250 'psychiatric community centres' with inpatient wards, night and day clinics, outpatient clinics and rehabilitation services. Most of these demands were taken up by the Psychiatry Enquete. This recommended nationwide reforms, which were largely implemented step by step in the years that followed (Häfner, 2003).

Baeyer, Häfner and Kisker worked at the Psychiatric University Clinic in Heidelberg.[2] Baeyer was clinic director from 1955 to 1972, Häfner and Kisker were his senior physicians. Since its foundation in 1878, this clinic, located in the oldest German university town, has been considered one of the most renowned psychiatric institutions in Germany. From the early 1960s, it developed into a pioneering location for psychiatric reform and, along with Frankfurt, into the leading centre of social psychiatric research and practice in the Federal Republic (Rotzoll, 2012: 135). At that time, Heidelberg formed a model institution in which a 'reform before the reform'[3] took place (Häfner, 1979: 154; Schmuhl, 2003: 15).

The literature on social psychiatry in Heidelberg in the era of the clinic director Walter von Baeyer, written mainly by those involved themselves, focuses on reform programmes and the high importance of senior psychiatrists and political developments.[4] It emphasises the early establishment of social psychiatry in Heidelberg in the early 1960s as well as the broad impact of the Heidelberg experiment in the Federal Republic. This occurred, on the one hand, through the staff members who moved to other places of activity and built up social psychiatry there, and on the other hand, through Baeyer, Kisker and Häfner, who were very committed to psychiatric reform and had developed national and international scientific and political networks. Finally, it is claimed that various personnel and structural changes and political events put an end to this heyday of social psychiatry in Heidelberg at the beginning of the 1970s. The decisive factors considered here are the exit of two key figures of the reforms, Kisker and Häfner, the departure of the Department of Social Psychiatry from Heidelberg for the neighbouring city of Mannheim twenty kilometres away, the anti-psychiatric agitation of the Socialist Patient Collective (SPK) in the Heidelberg Clinic in 1970–71 and the change in the directorship from Baeyer to the more conservative Werner Janzarik in 1973 (Häfner, 1979: 154; Pross, 2017: 50).[5]

In contrast, this chapter focuses on practices in the clinic and how these evolved. It analyses the social psychiatric practices in the Heidelberg Clinic in the 1960s and 1970s using medical records, the annual reports of the Department of Social Psychiatry from 1968 to 1974, administrative files, and written records of the medical and nursing staff. By doing so, social psychiatric practice is not reduced to the question of the extent to which the social psychiatric ideas of the leading figures were implemented in the clinic. Rather, the focus is also on those social psychiatric practices in Heidelberg which cannot be explained by the leading physicians' guidelines. In a psychiatric clinic, as in other institutions, everyday practice in some areas is only loosely linked to normative instructions, or completely independent of them, and has its own rules and routines which influence clinic staff and patients in their actions (Weick, 1995: 10).[6] Besides, the clinic staff, below the management level, also made use of their scope for action in everyday treatment and were in turn guided here by their own ideas and interests.

In addition to analysing the senior doctors' social psychiatric ideas and goals, this chapter also examines the organisation of work in the Department of Social Psychiatry and in the psychiatric clinic as a whole. In this way, insights into effective structures and the scope of action can be gained, to which one would not become attentive by the sole investigation of the implementation of social psychiatric goals. Through this, the functioning of the Department of Social Psychiatry, but also the embedding of the influential Heidelberg figures in this setting, becomes visible. And finally, patient records are used in this chapter to analyse when and to what extent psychiatric treatment changed for patients.

The chapter will first investigate what patient treatment looked like in the Department of Social Psychiatry in the 1960s and 1970s. It will then explore to what extent social psychiatric approaches were implemented in other wards of the Heidelberg Clinic during this period. In closing, the significance of personnel changes in the clinic, political events and the parting of ways with the Department of Social Psychiatry in the 1970s, will be examined.

The development of the Department of Social Psychiatry in Heidelberg

Karl Peter Kisker and Heinz Häfner, supported by the clinic director Walter Ritter von Baeyer, pushed for the expansion of social psychiatric facilities and treatment methods at the university clinic from 1960 onward, inspired by the international reform debates and based on Anglo-Saxon models. The most important institutional innovation was the establishment of the first two rehabilitation

Table 3.1 Diagnoses in the rehabilitation wards 1968–73

	1968	1970	1971	1972	1973
Schizophrenic disorders	70	62	58	59	33
Manic-depressive disorders	39	17	13		
Neuroses	29	28	51	38	32
Other diagnoses	24	35	22	46	28
Total recorded	162	142	144	143	93

Jahresbericht, 1968: 21; Jahresbericht, 1970: 19; Jahresbericht, 1971: 33; Zweijahresbericht, 1973: 59–60.

wards in the Federal Republic in 1960, which were housed in pavilion-style buildings that had been completed shortly before. Each pavilion had twelve beds for women and twelve beds for men, divided into rooms with two to four beds.

Statistical information is available on the patients admitted there from 1968 to 1973.[7] Most patients were quite young, the average age being under 30 years. The duration of treatment averaged four to six weeks for patients who came to the ward for the first time; for multiple admissions, which were primarily crisis interventions, the treatment time was much shorter. The medical records show, however, that significantly longer stays of half a year were not uncommon.[8]

The number of patients admitted hovered around 150 before dropping to 93 in 1973 due to the impending move of the ward to Mannheim in 1974 accompanied by Häfner's appointment to the chair of psychiatry there. Barely half of the patients had schizophrenic disorders; other frequently represented diagnoses were manic-depressive disorders and neuroses. The men's pavilion was managed by Kisker, the women's pavilion by Häfner. Here, for the first time in the Heidelberg Psychiatric University Clinic, there were no isolation rooms and closed areas and the dormitories were only used at night. The group rooms were shared by male and female patients and therapies and activities were also mixed.[9]

The rehabilitation wards were joined by a small night clinic with an initial total of twelve beds, which opened as the first transitional facility between inpatient and outpatient treatment in 1962 in the basement rooms of the pavilions and was expanded to seventeen beds by 1968. In 1965, the newly established institutions were merged into the Department of Social Psychiatry and Rehabilitation, headed by Häfner. The first goal of this new department was research and teaching, and the second was psychosocial treatment of patients and aftercare for outpatients (Rotzoll, 2012: 138). The great importance of research is particularly evident in the interdisciplinary special research division Social Psychiatry, which had been located in Heidelberg since 1968, as well as in the high number of scientific guests who came to Heidelberg for study visits from Germany and abroad.[10]

In the second half of the 1960s, the department expanded by establishing transitional facilities outside the hospital grounds, following the US concept of community mental health centres.[11] The integration of patients into the urban space was seen as an important component in dealing with psychosocial problems, and the solution to such problems was not sought solely by optimising and disciplining the individual, but also in designing the social environment. Thus, in 1966, a day clinic for twenty people was established in Heidelberg's city centre, and in 1968, in cooperation with services provided by the Church, the first transitional home, with eight living areas, was built in the Heidelberg neighbourhood of Rohrbach.[12] In addition to the institutional innovations, outpatient aftercare was established on the ward for a gradual, psychiatrically accompanied and stable return to life outside the clinic. After discharge, outpatient consultation hours were offered and the newly created 'patients' club' of the ward with cultural community activities was open not only for inpatients but also for discharged patients. Furthermore, cooperation was established with the social services of the city of Heidelberg and non-profit organisations, and a lay helpers' association for discharged patients was set up (Häfner, 1979: 155).

Sociotherapy

The sociotherapy practised in Heidelberg emphasised the importance of social influences on the development and chronification of mental illness, especially in the areas of socialisation, work and living. The first pillar of the social psychiatric therapy process was the treatment of mental illness during hospitalisation in the framework of a 'therapeutic community', a concept developed in the early 1950s by the British psychiatrist Maxwell Jones (Jones, 1953).[13] The 'therapeutic community' included the entire therapeutic staff and all patients who were supposed to support each other in their therapeutic process. The environment thus created was intended to be therapeutic and was considered more important than individual therapeutic measures. The focus of treatment was that psychiatrists, psychologists, nurses and social workers consciously talked to patients about underlying difficulties and conflicts rather than individual symptoms. In this way, the affected person should learn to understand their symptoms as the product of these difficulties and inner conflicts, and to communicate and discuss them in one-to-one conversations or in groups. The administration of psychotropic drugs and the use of electroconvulsive therapy was done cautiously. They were primarily seen as a prerequisite for acutely psychotic or depressed patients to become capable of communication and thus receptive to the decisive therapy, the community and the activation programmes of the department (Häfner, 1966: 90–1).

In the medical records, the treatment methods on the pavilion ward in the 1960s clearly stand out, since here the focus was not on medication and electroconvulsive therapies as in most of the other wards, but on the psychotherapeutic forms of treatment and social learning processes described above. For each patient, the doctor decided whether medication was necessary, showing a particular reluctance to use electroconvulsive therapies, which was even more pronounced than that for medication.[14] In the epicrisis of most medical records, group therapy as well as the activation programme and the therapeutic community were highlighted as primarily promoting healing (see also Häfner, 1969: 90).

The therapeutic discussion rounds were supplemented by an activation programme with occupational therapy, joint leisure activities, the patients' club and daily ward meetings of doctors, nursing staff and patients, in which mainly organisational issues were dealt with. Behind this was the therapeutic conviction that all these measures would reduce the pathological symptoms and promote social skills (Häfner and von Zerssen, 1964).

However, the patient files reveal the darker side of this therapeutic community, especially in the early years. There are entries that some patients found it too noisy and restless, others suffered from not being taken seriously by more highly educated patients or being ridiculed for their problems. In 1962, a doctor noted in the case of a male patient: 'The patient's marked lack of talent gives his fellow patients, who virtually conspire among themselves for this purpose, repeated opportunities to amuse themselves at his expense. Apart from that, the patient is exposed to the no less unpleasant influence of some of his fellow patients.'[15]

The second pillar of the social psychiatric therapy process was the rehabilitation of the patients – i.e. the psychiatrically accompanied, gradual return of the patients to self-determined living outside the clinic – for which the transitional facilities described above were seen as crucial aids, and to employment. Transitions between rehabilitation facilities were fluid in this regard. For example, on 27 September 1963 clinic director Baeyer and the senior physician Walter Bräutigam reported on the transition from an inpatient stay to the night clinic as the first transitional facility:

> Overall, the combination of relative freedom and the possibility of being attached has proved very successful. After returning from the night clinic, the patients seek out the familiar community of the ward at evening meals and home discussions, they also remain in contact with the doctors they know, and in most cases they also continue to receive medication support.[16]

Professional rehabilitation was provided on the one hand by work therapy, and on the other hand by supervision of the job search in the open labour market. Work therapy was thus clearly distinguished from occupational therapy (*Beschäftigungstherapie*), which was also offered. Whereas in occupational therapy patients were free to choose their activity, work therapy aimed to enable patients to test themselves at experimental workplaces inside and outside the clinic, which were oriented towards their former profession (Böker, 1966; Dörner and Plog, 1999: 83–4). For this purpose, they were mainly employed in the technical and administrative departments of the university hospital and, depending on the activity, were instructed by nurses, technical and administrative staff (Häfner, 1966: 90).

The high significance of the British model of 'industrial units' in the work therapy efforts of the Department of Social Psychiatry is particularly evident in the fact that in 1964 a printing shop was set up for the patients of the pavilion to produce forms for the needs of the clinic. From 1968, an 'industrial rehabilitation unit' also existed in the corrugated cardboard factory in nearby Wiesloch, where six to eight patients did paid part-time work. A minibus took the patients to their place of work, accompanied by nursing staff (Dörner and Plog, 1999: 83; Rotzoll, 2012: 140–1). The reference 'corrugated cardboard in the morning, occupational therapy in the afternoon' was since then often recorded in the medical files. Housewives, office workers and students were also employed in the corrugated cardboard factory, often as an intermediate step before they started work according to their training.[17] When patients complained about this, it was emphasised that the work was primarily intended to get them used to a workload under real conditions and that they should consider the time in the corrugated cardboard factory as part of the therapy.[18]

Heinz Häfner emphasised in 1966 that after the initial medical consultations with the patient, the therapeutic staff discussed all observations and findings together and used this to develop an individual treatment plan, which was then negotiated with the patient by the head physician of the department (Häfner, 1966: 90). However, neither the corresponding plans nor a discussion of treatment were documented in the medical records until the end of the 1960s. For the most part, the sociotherapeutic programme was merely mentioned in general terms without describing individual psychotherapeutic treatment strategies. A typical doctor's letter reads: 'The patient participated in our comprehensive sociotherapeutic programme throughout his inpatient stay, which included group psychotherapy, individual therapy, occupational and work therapy, and meetings.'[19]

It is only in the medical records of the 1970s that individual therapy plans and the formulation of a therapy goal increasingly appear.[20] Often, the documentation reveals that the therapy plan was justified to the patient and that details were negotiated with him or her. For example, a patient who was hospitalised in 1972 and 1974 for 'paranoid ideation and suspected psychosis' received a three-month treatment plan in 1974, divided into the three sections 'planned diagnostic measures', 'medication', and 'sociotherapeutic goals'. The last is elaborated as:

> Connecting with groups, promoting hobbies (linoleum cutting, photography), reducing feelings of unworthiness, reducing paranoid fears, professional reintegration. Restriction of pedantry. Prepare detachment from mother. Training of contact skills, possibly reestablish relationship with youth friend. Participation in games in the ward. Training of work ability; especially speed.[21]

One patient diagnosed with 'neurotic development with obsessive depressive features' in 1975 had among the treatment goals to be achieved: 'Promoting sociability in the context of group therapy, training assertive behaviour, and encouraging greater independence and personal responsibility.'[22]

Another innovation was that the progress reports in the 1970s increasingly described routines that governed interaction on the social psychiatric ward. For example, it was now reported that the actual condition of the patients was made visible for all on the ward by equipping each patient with a red, yellow or green cardboard sign. The assignment of these signs was made at the ward meetings and could be discussed. The granting of freedoms and the rules for living together were regulated via these signs. Only patients with a green sign were given free exit. Patients with red signs were considered unstable and in need of special care. The other patients were asked to pay special attention to them.[23]

New roles for psychiatrists, nurses and social workers

The Heidelberg reformers saw a new understanding of roles and an expansion of the training of psychiatrists and nurses as central to the social psychiatric tasks and establishment of a 'therapeutic community'. The idea was to build a therapeutic team in which different opinions counted, in which nursing staff were trained in social psychiatry, and social workers also played an important role. The psychiatrist's role was to tie these threads together (Häfner et al., 2011: 197).

From the beginning, the leading figures of Heidelberg social psychiatry emphasised the high therapeutic relevance of the nursing staff, who spent most of the time with the patients and shaped the treatment environment. Here, they referred to concepts from the USA, where the nursing staff were given a key position in sociopsychiatric treatment (Häfner *et al.*, 1965: 108–9). In the reformers' view, psychiatric nursing in Germany had until then been limited to a purely custodial function and care for the physical well-being of the patients. This applied to the asylums as well as to the university clinics, including the Heidelberg Clinic. The reformers' distrust of the older nursing staff in Heidelberg is particularly evident from the fact that, in the mid-1960s, senior physician Karl Peter Kisker appointed a medical student to work as an assistant nurse on the closed ward he headed (Männer Gartenhaus), to covertly observe the role of the nurses. Together they published his report under the accusatory title 'The Masters of the Clinic'. The report emphasised the nurses' custodial attitude, their superficial subservience to the physicians, their therapeutic inaction and their undermining of modern therapeutic measures, as well as the violence they exerted (Hemprich and Kisker, 1968). It was an impetus for the nationwide reform movement, but led to heated debates in the Heidelberg Clinic as to whether such actions and the resulting publication were disloyal or justified by the abuses (Pross, 2017: 42–3).

In the sociotherapeutic wards, too, the psychiatrists complained in the early days that the nuns and lay nurses working there initially had a custodial attitude and only insufficiently fulfilled the required new understanding of their roles and the new and diverse tasks. They observed with concern that the nursing staff had difficulties with the younger and more intelligent schizophrenic patients who expressed criticism and questioned their authority in group discussions. And they criticised that nurses reacted to the new system with anxiety, aggression and jealousy about the close therapeutic contact between patients and doctors (Rave-Schwank and Kallinke, 1973; Rotzoll, 2017: 108–9).

In the women's pavilion in Heidelberg, Häfner therefore established a pilot project in April 1963. For the first time in Germany, a social-psychiatric oriented two-year specialised training for fully qualified female nurses with eight places was introduced. In the following years male nurses and social workers could also participate (Rave-Schwank and Kallinke, 1973; Rave-Schwank and Lersner, 1974). Because of the initial difficulties, Häfner made an effort to recruit new nurses for the specialised training instead of the experienced nursing staff who had been working there until then. Young, freshly trained nurses, especially those with high school diplomas, were to be moulded for the new tasks (Häfner *et al.*, 1965: 108–9).

The medical records of the department contain reports by student nurses about individual patients and their dealings with them, which they had to write as part of their training. These reports reveal their intention to respond to the patient, to take on not a maternal but a comradely role, to help and to stimulate.[24] The medical records also show how nurses were given a more and more important voice in ward responsibilities as well as within communication and in writing the medical history. Already, at the end of the 1960s, nurses occasionally wrote parts of the medical history.[25] From 1972, the medical records contained sheets in which the nursing staff entered their observations about the patient as well as treatment measures as a standard feature. In the 1972/73 annual report, this innovation was justified. A new chart scheme had been introduced in which each professional group was to enter its observations about patients as well as intended and achieved measures, thus making these measures easily available and verifiable for the other staff members and ensuring the closest possible information flow between team members.[26] In the 1970s, it came to pass that nurses sometimes even wrote the 'doctor's letters'. For example, the medical file of a patient contains a letter dated 1972 from a nurse in the pavilion ward in which he took over communication with out-of-town physicians and reported to a resident from Mannheim about the patient on behalf of the director. The file contains the assistant physician's reply letter, in which he addressed the nurse directly – a procedure that would have been unthinkable in the past due to deeply rooted professional thinking.[27]

The third pillar in the sociotherapeutic treatment and rehabilitation of mentally ill patients was formed by social workers, who were accorded an important role, especially in the reintegration of patients into their social and professional environment. Here, too, the USA, England, but also Scandinavia and France, served as models, where care sectors, communal treatment centres and psychiatric social work had existed since the 1950s. The Heidelberg Department of Social Psychiatry had two female social workers from 1966, whereas in the Federal Republic of Germany social work only increasingly found its way into clinical psychiatry after the Psychiatry Enquete of 1975 (Brückner and Kersting, 2021). Their main task was to arrange work for the patient awaiting discharge that was appropriate for their capacity and social behaviours. The social worker first consulted with the doctor, who gave their own opinion on the case and provided her with psychiatric and sociopsychological data. Then she contacted the patient and their family to find out what the patient wanted, but also to make them aware of their integration problems and to motivate and support them in finding a job. If this did not lead to clear results, the social worker organised psychological assessments for the patient at the Psychological Service of the Heidelberg Labour Office.[28] In addition, the social worker assisted the patient during the initial period of integration into their new workplace (Dörner and Plog, 1999: 58–60). Finally, she made regular home visits to support the family and broaden their understanding of the family member with a mental illness.[29]

The medical records of the 1960s and 1970s show the important role played by social workers. For example, the medical record of a 17-year-old schoolgirl who had excelled in competitive sports before her admission to the social psychiatric ward in 1968 reports:

> Since the patient seemed to have little interest and was not able to go to grammar school or to obtain the Abitur, efforts were made to initiate a change of profession. The social worker looked for a job where the patient would be involved in sports. After this job seemed to be secured to some extent and because of pressure from the parents, the patient was discharged.[30]

The medical records reveal that the nursing staff were heavily involved in social work alongside the social workers – for example by organising patients' clubs, working in day and night clinics and providing telephone services and home visits. Even the psychiatrists invested a great deal of time here and took an active part in providing organisational support for the rehabilitation of their patients. They discussed the patients' future career plans with them in detail and took care of night clinic or day clinic placements, 'sheltered' jobs and places in residential homes. They also encouraged patients to come regularly to outpatient aftercare and to the patients' club and wrote them letters or made phone calls if they did not show up.[31]

The importance of social psychiatry throughout the clinic in the 1960s

The sociopsychiatric pavilion wards in the Heidelberg Clinic were an exception in the 1960s because a sophisticated sociotherapeutic ward programme was practised and here, for the first time, a gradual path out of the clinic was organised and supervised. In contrast, in the other psychiatric departments until the end of the 1960s, after inpatient treatment, which in most cases took place on the same ward from beginning to end, patients were usually discharged home and handed over to the care of the attending, resident doctor. If the treatment was not successful, they were transferred to a psychiatric asylum. Follow-up care, if it occurred at all, was provided by the treatment ward or polyclinic.

Nevertheless, social psychiatric approaches were not limited to the Department of Social Psychiatry at the clinic in the 1960s. This was primarily due to the initiative of committed assistant doctors, who were given great freedom by the clinic director Baeyer. For example, in the late 1960s Christiane von Held and Uwe Genkel established a therapeutic community in the open men's ward, Männer Ruhe, with Baeyer's approval, and held daily ward meetings there (von Held and Genkel, 1974). Wolf Dieter Wiest, then assistant physician at the clinic, describes the spirit and the atmosphere of the 1960s in his memoirs:

> The Heidelberg Clinic was like a powder keg of ideas … At that time, the day and night clinics came into being, and every younger psychiatrist took psychotherapeutic care of schizophrenics who had been abandoned earlier. The time when psychopathological phenomena were merely observed and catalogued seemed to be gone forever. (Wiest, 2000: 91)

At the Psychiatric Polyclinic, new social-psychiatric services were introduced as early as 1964 and 1965 by the senior physicians Karl Peter Kisker and Dieter Spazier. They included group therapy as a new treatment method. Whereas until then the focus had been on diagnostics, psychiatric-neurological counselling and administration of medication to outpatients, individual psychotherapy and group therapy were now also offered. It is noteworthy that, in the polyclinic, social workers acted as co-therapists alongside psychiatrists. Furthermore, a patient club and social counselling were offered. Behind the reforms was the view that, as long as community-based treatment centres did not exist, the traditional polyclinics should fill the therapeutic gap between isolated hospital psychiatry and mental health practice (Kisker *et al.*,1967). These services were expanded by Spazier and his assistant doctor Wolfgang Huber, who launched the Socialist Patient Collective (Pross, 2017). After the SPK was thrown out of the clinic in 1970, the social-psychiatric services at the polyclinic were further developed by Helmut Kretz (Baeyer, 1977: 31).

It was essential for the spread of social psychiatric approaches at the Heidelberg Psychiatric University Clinic that Heinz Häfner and Walter Bräutigam offered psychotherapeutic training and supervision at the end of the 1960s, which all physicians and the social workers who conducted group therapy were required to undergo (Pross, 2017: 283). In addition, many Heidelberg physicians went to the US for several months to learn social psychiatric methods, and in doing so benefited from the close-knit, international network of the Heidelberg Clinic.[32]

Nevertheless, the importance of social psychiatry for the Heidelberg Psychiatric University Clinic, especially in the 1960s, should not be overestimated. In 1970, von Baeyer supervised a dissertation on the eighty-seven inpatient curative procedures carried out at the clinic from 1959 to 1965, which served to maintain or restore the patients' ability to work and earn a living and the costs of which were borne by the social insurance funds. The dissertation says about 'sociotherapy': 'Since its implementation was not one of the clinic's tasks, only corresponding suggestions could be recorded, but not the measures themselves' (Kemmerich, 1970: 5–6). A little later it is written that sociotherapeutic suggestions would have included changes in the housing situation, a change of job or retraining, for which the clinic physician would make recommendations in the final report. However, general practitioners, independent social workers, employment and housing offices, etc. were supposed to take care of their implementation. Altogether, sociotherapeutic suggestions were only made in fifteen of eighty-seven cases (Kemmerich, 1970: 73–4).

The significance of personnel changes, political events and the departure of the Department of Social Psychiatry in the 1970s

According to the narrative of the clinic psychiatrists of the time, at the beginning of the 1970s various personnel changes, political events and the departure of the Department of Social Psychiatry for Mannheim put an end to social psychiatry in Heidelberg (Häfner, 1979: 154; Pross, 2017: 50 with further references). Kisker was appointed to the Hanover Medical School in 1966 (Beyer, 2016). Since 1968, appointment negotiations had been underway for Häfner to become the chair of psychiatry at the Heidelberg University Medical Faculty in Mannheim, which had been founded in 1964. In this context, his Department of Social Psychiatry was split off from the main clinic and became part of the Faculty of Clinical Medicine in Mannheim. The wards and all research projects were moved to Mannheim in 1974, first to a temporary facility, then in 1975 to the newly opened Zentralinstitut für Seelische Gesundheit (Central Institute for Mental Health). This institute performed supraregional research and training tasks in the field of social psychiatry and organised psychiatric care for the Mannheim population according to the principles of a community mental health centre (Häfner and Martini, 2011: 92–4, 122–4).

The events surrounding the Socialist Patient Collective were also significant according to this narrative, as they influenced the mood in the clinic towards reform projects. The SPK, the first patient-organised body in Western Europe, was founded in 1970 by Wolfgang Huber at the Heidelberg Psychiatric Polyclinic and joined by several hundred patients before its dissolution in 1971. It was influenced by the student movement and anti-psychiatric ideas. It denounced the social psychiatric approaches at the psychiatric clinic as completely inadequate and acted particularly against Häfner and Baeyer. Nevertheless, many of the clinic's assistant doctors initially sympathised with the SPK, which saw itself also as a therapeutic community and wanted to make 'a weapon out of illness' with the goal of revolutionary change in society. After the conflict with Baeyer escalated and the SPK was expelled from the clinic, a small part of the group increasingly became violent and was put on trial as a criminal association (Pross, 2017: 173, 183, 399).

The change in the directorship from Baeyer to Werner Janzarik, who directed the clinic from 1973 to 1988, is described according to this narrative as the end of the reform era. Within the Heidelberg Clinic, classical psychopathology was seemingly once again the primary scientific interest (Mundt, 2001: 368–9; Bonah and Rotzoll, 2015: 283). Moreover, Janzarik himself declared his election to be politically motivated. The faculty had wanted clear structures and responsibilities to be reintroduced in the clinic, which had become 'unhinged' as a result of the anti-psychiatric excesses (Janzarik, 1979: 13). When he took over as director, he set himself the goal of reorganising the clinic. One of his measures was not to renew the contracts among the assistant and senior physicians of the reformist wing, about fifteen people, despite public protests by the assistant doctor committee (Pross, 2017: 152).

As a result, the social psychiatry built up by the reformers would apparently no longer play a role in Heidelberg. A contemporary witness who was an assistant doctor in the psychiatric clinic at the time described the subsequent period: 'The Heidelberg Clinic then continued to be exposed to the controversial discussions of anti-psychiatry without a social psychiatry that might have absorbed some of the concerns of antipsychiatry.'[33]

However, the processes described did not mean the death of social psychiatric care of Heidelberg patients in the 1970s. First, some of Heidelberg's social psychiatric facilities, which were spread throughout the city, did not close until much later, despite the relocation of the Department of Social Psychiatry to Mannheim in 1974; for example, the day clinic was not moved until 1982.[34] Second, there was close cooperation between the Heidelberg Clinic and the Central Institute for Mental Health in Mannheim in the 1970s, as the staff still knew each other personally and were aware of the respective specifics of the care structures, so that patients from Heidelberg were often referred to this institute and vice versa.[35]

Third, open wards continued to operate in the pavilion buildings after the move.[36] Here, a special emphasis was placed on psycho-therapy and group activities, which speaks for a certain continuity.

The frequent long stays, which can be detected up to the 1980s, point in the same direction. For example, a patient diagnosed with 'schizophrenic psychosis' stayed here for several months in 1975 and for more than a year in 1981.[37]

Fourth, in Heidelberg, the Psychosomatic Clinic compensated to some extent for the psychotherapeutic treatment in the Department of Social Psychiatry, in both inpatient and outpatient form. In 1968, Walter Bräutigam, who had previously worked closely with Heinz Häfner, had become director of Heidelberg's Psychosomatic Clinic. This clinic had already been established in 1950 as the first of its kind in Germany and was part of the university hospital, but it existed independently of the psychiatric clinic. From the beginning, both inpatient and outpatient psychoanalytic treatment was offered at the Psychosomatic Clinic, which was directed by Alexander Mitscherlich until 1968. While Mitscherlich saw the social psychiatric activities of Baeyer and his staff as competing with the Psychosomatic Clinic services and the relationships were not without conflict,[38] the cooperation between the Psychosomatic Clinic and the Department of Social Psychiatry intensified significantly under Walter Bräutigam. The Psychosomatic Clinic also received a new orientation. Not only did the number of beds increase from eight to twenty-four, the psychotherapeutic services also expanded. The infirmary was now organised as a therapeutic community, and therapies offered included classical psychoanalytic individual therapy, analytical group therapy and depth psychology-based individual and group therapy.[39] In addition, non-verbal group procedures such as concentrative movement and design therapy were offered. The inpatient individual and group therapies were subsequently continued on an outpatient basis (Bräutigam, 1986: 138–9).

Fifth, the split from Häfner's Department of Social Psychiatry was counterbalanced by the fact that social psychiatric ideas can be traced throughout the psychiatric clinic in the 1970s. Analysis of the medical records reveals that there was an uptake of psychotherapeutic methods and an increase in communal activities on all wards in the 1970s. For the first time, medical records from beyond the pavilion documented individual psychotherapies.[40] Even on the closed ward Frauen Wache, ward meetings were held in 1972.[41] And for 1975, there is evidence that even on the closed ward Frauen

Gartenhaus, sometimes no medication was given at all, and individual and group psychotherapy was carried out instead.[42]

On all wards, psychiatrists were increasingly concerned with the social needs of their patients. Nurses and social workers were given important roles in this area.[43] The importance attached to social rehabilitation and outpatient follow-up increased continuously throughout the 1970s. The medical records show that it was becoming more and more common for patients to be admitted first to a closed ward and then to an open ward, whereas previously patients had almost always stayed in one and the same ward from the beginning to the end of their hospitalisation. Thus, cooperation between the wards increased to a great extent. Moreover, transitional wards and outpatient aftercare services were expanded. For example, in 1972 there was outpatient group psychotherapy in the main clinic,[44] and in 1975 there were patient clubs on various wards, as well as several therapeutic residential homes that were directly related to the clinic.[45] An important role was played here by the 'Heidelberger Werkgemeinschaft' (Heidelberg Working Group), which was founded in 1973 to set up and expand 'night clinics, day clinics, residential homes, shared apartments, jobs protected from competition, occupational therapy workshops, lay help circles, training opportunities for caregivers and previously untrained personnel' in the Heidelberg area. This association was independent of the Heidelberg Psychiatric University Clinic, but many employees of the clinic were active on a voluntary basis.[46]

The fact that social psychiatric approaches continued to gain in importance and that no rollback can be detected in the Heidelberg Clinic can be explained on the one hand by the establishment of internal clinic routines which were continued. That the wards came into closer contact with each other helped spread these practices. On the other hand, since the 1970s at the latest, social psychiatric approaches were implemented in many places in the Federal Republic of Germany, more opportunities for exchange were created, and the will arose on a broad basis to advance social psychiatric reforms in psychiatry. The reform mood was shaped by a particular zeitgeist, embodied by the social-liberal government that Willy Brandt had launched in 1969 under the title 'Reforms dare'. The atmosphere was influenced by the social movements (student, women's, ecology and peace movements) with their anti-authoritarian critique of society, in which an increased awareness of 'the social' and of human and civil rights was immanent (Schmiedebach and Priebe, 2004: 469). Important books critical of psychiatry appeared in German during this period, notably Michel Foucault's *Madness and Society* (1969), Franco Basaglia's *L'istituzione negata* (The institution denied, 1971), R. D. Laing's *The Divided Self* (1972), and Erving Goffman's *Asylums* (1973). One of the best-known German works, which strongly influenced the public debate, was Frank Fischer's 1969 book *Irren-häuser: Kranke klagen an* (Lunatic asylums: Patients accuse) in which he denounced the miserable and inhumane everyday life in institutions that he, a Germanist and historian by training, had experienced for eight months as an auxiliary nurse in five psychiatric hospitals (Fischer, 1969).

In 1970, the Mannheim Circle and the German Society for Social Psychiatry (DGSP) were founded. It was not only psychiatrists who participated; nurses, caregivers, social workers, occupational therapists, physicians, psychologists and sociologists who worked in psychiatric clinics or connected institutions were also involved. The founding of the Aktion Psychisch Kranke (Action for the Mentally Ill) in 1971 by members of all parliamentary groups in the German Bundestag and committed professionals from the field of psychiatry was also an important vehicle for the formation and institutionalisation of the psychiatric reform movement. As early as 1972, 1,200 participants came to the social psychiatry conference in Bethel. The Mannheim Circle and the DGSP had become a kind of mass movement within psychiatry, whose credo was formulated by Klaus Dörner in 1972 in reference to a sentence by Max Fischer (1919) as follows: 'Psychiatry is social psychiatry or it is no psychiatry' (Dörner, 1972: 8).

Conclusion

The analysis of social psychiatric practices at the Heidelberg Clinic in the 1960s and 1970s on the basis of medical records, administrative files and records of the medical and nursing staff showed, on the one hand, the impressive achievement of the leading reformers Walter von Baeyer, Heinz Häfner and Karl Peter Kisker in creating a model institution of German social psychiatry in Heidelberg in the 1960s. On the other hand, in addition to the leading psychiatrists, the increasing relevance of other actors with their own ideas and interests and of routines and procedures, which did not coincide with the guidelines from above, came to the fore, whereby there were clear differences in their importance between the 1960s and 1970s.

In the 1960s, social psychiatric practices in Heidelberg were very much shaped by the senior doctors and the structural reforms they initiated. However, their scope within the Heidelberg Psychiatric University Clinic was largely limited to the Department of Social Psychiatry, with its transitional facilities, diverse forms of therapy (individual and group psychotherapy, work and occupational therapy) and intensive ward life with daily meetings and multiple leisure activities organised by the patients themselves. At that time, on most of the other wards of the clinic, the focus of treatment was primarily on medication and electroconvulsive therapies. Social psychiatric approaches were practised only on some other open wards and in the polyclinic from the 1960s.

The Heidelberg psychiatrists who initiated the social psychiatric reforms drew a large part of their assertiveness from the fact that they had clear objectives in mind through an orientation towards Anglo-Saxon models. They explicitly referred to the US model in their attempt to establish a Community Mental Health Centre and to give nurses a key position in social psychiatry. Great Britain served as a model for the therapeutic community and for 'industrial rehabilitation units'. For the important role of social workers in social psychiatry, the Heidelberg reformers cited the USA and Great Britain, but also Scandinavia and France as models.

Another finding regarding the 1960s is that the implementation of Heidelberg's social psychiatric reforms in everyday clinical practice often took longer than the publications of the senior physicians would suggest. In addition, the freedom that the reformers gave their employees allowed them to pursue and implement their own ideas. This led to reform initiatives by assistant doctors and, in the case of Wolfgang Huber, who founded the Socialist Patient Collective at the polyclinic in 1970, to his complete withdrawal from staff management at the end of the 1960s.

As far as the significance of the reformers for social psychiatry in Heidelberg is concerned, the situation in the 1970s is clearly different.

The medical records show that social psychiatry in Heidelberg had not lost its importance in everyday clinical life with the departure of Häfner, Kisker and the Department of Social Psychiatry, the events surrounding the Socialist Patient Collective and the change of director from Baeyer to Janzarik in the 1970s. There is no evidence of a break in the trend. The complaint of many doctors involved about the disappearance of social psychiatry was mainly about the lost spirit of reform in the clinic and the decline in social psychiatric research. In the 1970s, however, patient care at the Heidelberg Psychiatric University Clinic was even more influenced by social psychiatry than in the previous decade. On the one hand, this is due to the fact that the Department of Social Psychiatry was still being set up at the end of the 1960s and it was not until the 1970s that individualised therapies were increasingly described in the medical records. On the other hand, in the 1970s, patients in all departments of the psychiatric clinic increasingly benefited from psychotherapeutic services, a changed doctor–patient and nurse–patient relationship and continuously expanded support for reintegration into society. Heidelberg's transitional facilities increased overall in the 1970s. The day clinic did not move to Mannheim until 1982 and the residential homes and sheltered workplaces were mainly run and expanded by the Heidelberger Werkgemeinschaft, founded in 1973. This organisation was independent from the clinic, but, nonetheless, many employees of the psychiatric clinic were active in it.

In the 1970s, social psychiatric practices sometimes took place without normative guidelines – or in spite of them – and were strongly influenced by internal routines and by the spirit of the times. The analysis of the medical records shows that in this period, with regard to social psychiatric approaches, the dynamics of action within the psychiatric clinic were actor-bound, but not as hierarchically shaped as the institutional organisation envisaged, and the employees had a wide scope for action. Heidelberg social psychiatry of the 1970s is an example of a reform-oriented practice complex that shifted from the leading figures and representative structures to the lower levels through routinisation, where it developed and spread. This was favoured by the fact that within social psychiatry the scope for action of assistant doctors and non-medical staff was greater than in other areas of psychiatry.

Notes

1 The Psychiatry Enquete was a report on the situation of psychiatry in the Federal Republic of Germany, completed in 1975 by a commission of experts from all areas of psychiatry on behalf of the Bundestag.

2 Until 1969, the clinic was connected to the neurology department and was called the Psychiatric and Neurological University Clinic. In 1969, the Neurological and Psychiatric clinics became independent.

3 The quote comes from Kersting, who refers to innovative models in the Federal Republic of Germany before the Psychiatry Enquete (Kersting, 2004: 271).

4 One exception is Maike Rotzoll's study, which uses administrative files to trace the structure of social psychiatry in Heidelberg. Rotzoll (2012).

5 Cf. the section 'The significance of personnel changes, political events, and the departure of the Department of Social Psychiatry in the 1970s'.

6 See also the reflections by Marietta Meier in Chapter 8.

7 Bibliothek des Zentralinstituts für Seelische Gesundheit, Mannheim, Jahresberichte der Sozialpsychiatrischen Klinik am Klinikum der Universität Heidelberg [Annual reports of the social psychiatric clinic at the Heidelberg University Hospital], 1968–73 (henceforth Jahresbericht, Zweijahresbericht). Jahresbericht, 1968; Jahresbericht, 1970; Jahresbericht, 1971; Zweijahresbericht, 1973.

8 For example Psychiatrische Universitätsklinik Heidelberg, Aktenmanagement (henceforth referred to as PA), Heidelberg, Medical records from 1962, 1968, 1972, 1975, women 62/243, men 62/94.

9 Jahresbericht, 1969: 5.

10 Jahresbericht, 1969: 33; Jahresbericht, 1970: 15–16, 35–6.

11 Jahresbericht, 1969: 4.

12 Jahresbericht, 1969: 140–1.

13 The concept of the therapeutic community is also highly significant in the case studies by Despo Kritsotaki, Katariina Parhi and Henriette Voelker in Chapters 1, 5 and 10.

14 Cf. in particular PA women 62/217.

15 PA men 62/92; see also PA men 68/202.

16 Universitätsarchiv Heidelberg (henceforth UAH), Heidelberg, Rep. 49/367, Operation of the Psychiatric and Neurological Clinic, Day and night clinic 1962–68, Prof. Dr. W. v. Baeyer/PD Dr. Bräutigam on 27 September 1963 to the administration of the clinical university institutions.

17 See for example PA women 68/299.

18 See for example PA women 68/326.

19 PA men 68/133. See also PA men 68/219; PA women 68/411; PA women 68/417; PA women 68/440.
20 Early exceptions are PA men 68/167; PA men 68/211.
21 PA men 72/286. See also PA men 72/278; PA men 72/339; PA women 72/422.
22 PA men 75/281.
23 See, for example PA men 72/339.
24 This is particularly evident in PA women 68/474; PA women 68/326.
25 PA women 68/474.
26 Zweijahresbericht, 1973: 35–6.
27 PA women 72/335.
28 See for example PA women 68/268.
29 Jahresbericht, 1968: 8.
30 PA women 68/447.
31 See, for example, PA men 72/286.
32 Jahresbericht, 1969: 33; Jahresbericht, 1970: 12–13.
33 Eyewitness interview from 4 October 2012 by Christian Pross. Quoted in Pross, 2017: 50.
34 After the Heidelberg day clinic closed its doors, it took until the mid-1990s for a new day clinic to become operational in the city. Rotzoll, 2012: 144, 148.
35 See, for example, PA women 75/214. According to Maike Rotzoll, this changed in the following decades when the personal relationships no longer existed. Interview, 8 November 2021, with the Heidelberg psychiatrist and medical historian Maike Rotzoll, who had worked at the clinic since the 1980s.
36 These wards were now called 'Station Pavillon-West' and 'Station von Gebsattel'.
37 PA men 75/201.
38 Baeyer's annoyance at Mitscherlich's attempts to limit and question the scope of competence of Baeyer's staff with regard to psychotherapeutic topics is particularly evident in a letter from Baeyer to Mitscherlich in 1964. UAH, Rep. 63, Estate of Prof. Walter v. Baeyer, 15–17, Letter from Prof. v. Baeyer to colleague Mitscherlich, 4 November 1964.
39 While psychoanalysis comprehensively tries to uncover and change the foundations of neurotic conflicts in the imprints of childhood, depth psychology-based treatment primarily deals with currently effective conflicts in the patient and in his or her relationships.
40 PA men 72/341 is particularly detailed.
41 See, for example, PA women 72/336.
42 PA women 75/290.
43 PA men 75/203.

44 PA women 72/312.
45 PA men 75/218; PA men 75/225.
46 UAH, Rep. 63/103, Heidelberger Werkgemeinschaft, Flyer [undated, 1973].

References

Baeyer, Walter von, 1977, 'Walter Ritter von Baeyer', in Ludwig Jakob Pongratz (ed.), *Psychiatrie in Selbstdarstellungen* (Bern: Huber), pp. 9–33.

Beyer, Christof, 2016, '"Islands of reform": Early transformation of the mental health service in Lower Saxony, Germany in the 1960s', in Despo Kritsotaki, Vicky Long and Matthew Smith (eds), *Deinstitutionalisation and After: Post-War Psychiatry in the Western World* (Cham: Springer International Publishing), pp. 99–114.

Böker, Brigitte, 1966, 'Rehabilitationsaufgaben einer Sozialarbeiterin an der Psychiatrischen Universitätsklinik Heidelberg', *Moderne Krankenpflege unter besonderer Berücksichtigung der Nervenheilkunde*, 3:1, 13–15.

Bonah, Christian and Maike Rotzoll, 2015, 'Psychopathologie in Bewegung: Zur Geschichte der Psychiatriefilme in Straßburg und Heidelberg', in Philipp Osten, Gabriele Moser, Christian Bonah, Alexandre Sumpf, Tricia Close-Koenig and Joël Danet (eds), *Das Vorprogramm: Lehrfilm, Gebrauchsfilm, Propagandafilm, unveröffentlichter Film in Kinos und Archiven am Oberrhein, 1900–1970* (Heidelberg: A25 Rhinfilm), pp. 263–86.

Bräutigam, Walter, 1986, 'Psychosomatische Klinik', in Gotthard Schettler (ed.), *Das Klinikum der Universität Heidelberg und seine Institute* (Berlin: Springer), pp. 137–40.

Brückner, Burkhart and Franz-Werner Kersting (eds), 2021, *Eine vergessene Geschichte: Psychiatrische Sozialarbeit in Deutschland: Berichte, Dokumente und Analysen aus der Bundesrepublik und der DDR (1960–1990)* (Mönchengladbach: Hochschule Niederrhein).

Dörner, Klaus, 1972, 'Einleitung', in Klaus Dörner and Ursula Plog (eds), *Sozialpsychiatrie* (Neuwied: Luchterhand), pp. 7–20.

Dörner, Klaus and Ursula Plog, 1999, *Anfänge der Sozialpsychiatrie: Bericht über eine Reise durch die sozialpsychiatrischen Pioniereinrichtungen der Bundesrepublik im Jahre 1968 – Ein psychiatriegeschichtliches Dokument* (Bonn: Psychiatrie Verlag).

Fischer, Frank, 1969, *Irrenhäuser: Kranke klagen an* (Munich: Desch).

Häfner, Heinz, 1966, 'Ein sozialpsychologisch-psychodynamisches Modell als Grundlage für die Behandlung symptomarmer Prozeßschizophrenien', *Social Psychiatry*, 1, 88–96.

Häfner, Heinz, 1969, 'Resozialisierung bei psychischen Störungen', in Maria Blohmke (ed.), *Sozialpsychiatrie: Verhandlungsbericht der wissenschaftlichen Jahrestagung der Deutschen Gesellschaft für Sozialmedizin, Heidelberg, 1. und 2. Oktober 1968* (Stuttgart: Gentner), pp. 78–98.

Häfner, Heinz, 1979, 'Die Geschichte der Sozialpsychiatrie in Heidelberg', in Werner Janzarik (ed.), *Psychopathologie als Grundlagenwissenschaft* (Stuttgart: Enke), pp. 145–60.

Häfner, Heinz, 2003, 'Die Inquisition der psychisch Kranken geht ihrem Ende entgegen: Die Geschichte der Psychiatrie-Enquete und Psychiatriereform in Deutschland', in Franz-Werner Kersting (ed.), *Psychiatriereform als Gesellschaftsreform: Die Hypothek des Nationalsozialismus und der Aufbruch der sechziger Jahre* (Paderborn: Ferdinand Schöningh), pp. 113–40.

Häfner, Heinz and Hans Martini, 2011, *Das Zentralinstitut für Seelische Gesundheit: Gründungsgeschichte und Gegenwart* (Munich: C. H. Beck).

Häfner, Heinz, B. Vogt-Heyder and Detlev von Zerssen, 1965, 'Erfahrungen mit Schizophrenen in einem gleitenden klinischen Behandlungs- und Nachsorgesystem', *Zeitschrift für Psychotherapie und medizinische Psychologie*, 15, 97–116.

Häfner, Heinz, Walter von Baeyer and Karl Peter Kisker, 2011, 'Dringliche Reformen in der psychiatrischen Krankenversorgung in der Bundesrepublik (1965)', in Christfried Tögel and Peter Wellach (eds), *Dämonen und Neuronen: Quellen zur Entwicklung der Psychiatrie: Von der Antike bis zur Gegenwart* (Magdeburg: SALUS), pp. 192–215.

Häfner, Heinz and Detlev von Zerssen, 1964, 'Soziale Rehabilitation, ein integrierender Bestandteil psychiatrischer Therapie', *Der Nervenarzt*, 35, 242–7.

Held, Christiane von and Uwe Genkel, 1974, 'Die integrierte Station – Das Konzept einer therapeutischen Gemeinschaft', *Gruppenpsychotherapie und Gruppendynamik*, 8, 167–79.

Hemprich, Rolf D. and Karl P. Kisker, 1968, 'Die "Herren der Klinik" und die Patienten: Erfahrungen aus der teilnehmend-verdeckten Beobachtung einer psychiatrischen Station', *Der Nervenarzt*, 10, 433–41.

Janzarik, Werner, 1979, '100 Jahre Heidelberger Psychiatrie', in Werner Janzarik (ed.), *Psychopathologie als Grundlagenwissenschaft* (Stuttgart: Enke), pp. 1–18.

Jones, Maxwell, 1953, *The Therapeutic Community: A New Treatment Method in Psychiatry* (New York: Basic Books).

Kemmerich, Bernhard-Claudius, 1970, 'Zum Problem psychiatrischer Heilverfahren: Eine statistische Untersuchung der Heilverfahren, die im Zeitraum vom 1.11.1959 bis zum 31.10.1965 in der Psychiatrischen und Neurologischen Klinik der Universität Heidelberg durchgeführt wurden'. PhD Med. dissertation, Heidelberg University.

Kersting, Franz-Werner, 1998, 'Psychiatriereform und 68', *Westfälische Forschungen*, 48, 283–95.

Kersting, Franz-Werner, 2003, 'Vor Ernst Klee: Die Hypothek der NS-Medizinverbrechen als Reformimpuls', in Franz-Werner Kersting (ed.), *Psychiatriereform als Gesellschaftsreform: Die Hypothek des National-sozialismus und der Aufbruch der sechziger Jahre* (Paderborn: Ferdinand Schöningh), pp. 63–80.

Kersting, Franz-Werner, 2004, 'Abschied von der "totalen Institution"? Die Westdeutsche Anstaltpsychatrie zwischen Nationalsozialismus und den Siebzigerjahren', *Archiv für Sozialgeschichte*, 44, 267–92.

Kisker, Karl Peter, Aspasia Amsel-Kainarou and Dieter Spazier, 1967, 'Psychiatrie ohne Bett: Über eine zweijährige poliklinische Arbeit der Heidelberger Klinik', *Der Nervenarzt*, 38, 10–15.

Mundt, Christoph, 2001, 'Die Erinnerungskultur zur NS-"Euthanasie" an der Heidelberger Psychiatrischen Klinik: Ein persönlicher Rückblick', in Christoph Mundt, Gerrit Hohendorf and Maike Rotzoll (eds), *Psychiatrische Forschung und NS-'Euthanasie': Beiträge zu einer Gedenkveranstaltung an der Psychiatrischen Universitätsklinik Heidelberg* (Heidelberg: Wunderhorn), pp. 364–74.

Pross, Christian, 2017, *'Wir wollten ins Verderben rennen': Die Geschichte des Sozialistischen Patientenkollektivs Heidelberg 1970–1971* (Cologne: Psychiatrie Verlag).

Rave-Schwank, Maria and Dieter Kallinke, 1973, 'Das Rollenspiel in der Ausbildung von Schwestern und Pflegern: Einige lernpsychologische Aspekte', *Gruppendynamik: Forschung und Praxis*, 4, 35–41.

Rave-Schwank, Maria and Christa Winter-v. Lersner, 1974, *Psychiatrische Krankenpflege: Eine praktische Einführung für Schwestern und Pfleger* (Stuttgart: Fischer).

Rotzoll, Maike, 2012, 'Die Entstehung der "Sozialpsychiatrischen Klinik Heidelberg" in den 1960er Jahren: Sozialpsychiatrie in Heidelberg', *Heidelberg: Jahrbuch zur Geschichte der Stadt*, 17, 133–48.

Rotzoll, Maike, 2017, '"Fundamentally changed duties". The introduction of advanced training for nurses at the Psychiatric University Hospital Heidelberg as part of the early psychiatric reform in West Germany', in Sylvelyn Hähner-Rombach and Karen Nolte (eds), *Patients and Social Practice of Psychiatric Nursing in the 19th and 20th Century* (Stuttgart: Franz Steiner Verlag), pp. 185–98.

Rotzoll, Maike, 2021, Interview with Gundula Gahlen, Heidelberg, 8 November.

Schmiedebach, Heinz-Peter and Stefan Priebe, 2004, 'Social psychiatry in Germany in the twentieth century: Ideas and models', *Medical History*, 48:4, 449–72.

Schmuhl, Hans-Walter, 2003, 'Einführung', in Franz-Werner Kersting (ed.), *Psychiatriereform als Gesellschaftsreform: Die Hypothek des National-sozialismus und der Aufbruch der sechziger Jahre* (Paderborn: Ferdinand Schöningh), pp. 15–19.

Weick, Karl E., 1995, *Sensemaking in Organizations* (Thousand Oaks, CA: Sage).

Wiest, Wolf D., 2000, *Außer Mir* (Karlsfeld: Kaubisch).

4

'The general atmosphere of this admission unit is reassuring and optimistic': modernism, architectural research and evolving psychiatric reforms in post-war England

Christina Malathouni

The thirty years following World War II have been characterised 'as the age of reform in psychiatry' in Western countries (Henckes, 2011: 164). In the British context, major changes were manifested in a series of related legislation, policies and guidance, such as the launch of the National Health Service in 1948, the passing of the Mental Health Act in 1959 and the publication of 'The Hospital Plan for England and Wales' in 1962. The examples listed here suggest a bias towards approaches that relate to hospitals, and more broadly to overlaps with physical healthcare. These are indeed two key points of the discussion below, yet the primary focus of this chapter is the contribution, whether real or aspired, that architecture made to psychiatric reforms in post-war England.

The discussion below borrows Nicolas Henckes's (2011) proposition for a framework of analysis for reforms in psychiatric institutions in the mid-twentieth century that '[put] reform practices themselves at the centre of the analysis' (Henckes, 2011: 164). Within this context, Greg Eghigian (2011) highlights the expanding pool of new expertise that became directly relevant to the history of mental healthcare during the second half of the twentieth century. He points out 'the growing importance of psychologists, social workers, neuroscientists, drug manufacturers, nurses, pedagogues, self-help groups, counsellors, legislators, accountants and consumers since 1950' and the need to consider psychiatry 'as working within a complex ecology of sciences, technologies, policies and actors' (Eghigian, 2011: 205).

Both Eghigian and Henckes stress the multiplicity and diversification of actors in the post-war period and their critical role in reforms.

Despite this significant expansion of professionals associated with mental healthcare in the post-war period, architects are a professional group that is not automatically included in historiographic studies of post-war psychiatry. However, although an exclusive, or even 'proprietary', connection between architects and space has rightly been challenged by theorists such as Henri Lefebvre (1991, originally published in 1974), architectural practices can still influence spatial practices. Existing studies of mental healthcare spaces have firmly established the significance of asylum architecture (and more broadly of spatial arrangements) in the development of psychiatry and the social history of madness (see, for example, Scull, 1979; Topp, 2007), and the large scale and expansion of asylums in the nineteenth century have attracted extensive scholarship from an architectural history perspective (see, for example, Taylor, 1991; Richardson, 1998). However, scholarship on mental healthcare architecture in the twentieth century, although growing, remains largely fragmentary (see, for example, Soanes, 2011; Topp, 2017).

This chapter discusses how the architectural profession joined a larger pool of reformist actors in post-war psychiatry in England in the 1950s and to what extent architectural practices became, or envisioned becoming, reformist psychiatric practices in themselves.[1] It focuses on the admission and treatment unit for an existing psychiatric hospital for the mentally ill, Fair Mile Hospital[2] in Cholsey, near Wallingford, Berkshire (now Oxfordshire), England, commissioned before July 1954 and built by April 1956.[3] It explores a range of practices by its architects Philip Powell and Hidalgo Moya, from their design proposals and the building itself to their collaboration with specialist consultants and engagement with architectural research.

The full description of the building was 'Admission and Treatment Unit' and its cruciform plan comprised four wings on a single level: two separate male and female wings with thirty beds for women and twenty-three beds for men, a mixed-sex common room used for games and occupational therapy (*Architects' Journal*, 1956: 388), and a treatment wing for insulin and electroconvulsive therapy (ECT) that was to be open to inpatients as well as 'the ever-increasing number of outpatients requiring treatment' (*Architects' Journal*, 1956: 394).[4] The unit was to accommodate all new admissions,

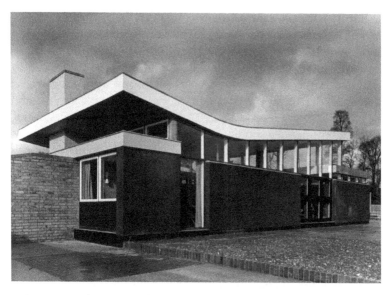

Figure 4.1 Admission and treatment unit, Fair Mile Hospital. Exterior (Common Room), 1956. Source: RIBA Architecture Image Library, RIBApix Ref. No. RIBA56469.

which were expected to stay for an average of seven weeks (*Architects' Journal*, 1956: 385).

Published in the *Architects' Journal* on 19 April 1956, an article on the newly completed building reveals the aspirations of the architectural profession to make its own mark in the field of mental healthcare. The building is hailed within as a most welcome architectural intervention as it embraces a departure from an 'institutional atmosphere', which is further linked to a positive perception of post-war mental healthcare as 'advancing', 'modern' and associated with (health and) illness, medicine and cure:

> The general atmosphere of this admission unit is reassuring and optimistic, to be in line with the modern conception of much mental illness as a curable condition. … It is fortunate that a building of this quality, without an institutional atmosphere, has been erected so early in the post-war mental health building programme; while medical work in this field has advanced greatly, architectural expression has not generally been of a very high order, and this building is therefore of particular significance (*Architects' Journal*, 1956: 385).

In line with the above, this chapter argues that the psychiatric reforms to which the architects of this 1950s unit envisioned giving expression were twofold. Firstly, they included the notion of deinstitutionalisation, by giving mental healthcare buildings a non-institutional character rather than by the actual abolition of institutional care; that is, closer to an early version of the movement's various and nuanced readings (Topp *et al.*, 2007; Eghigian, 2011; Henckes, 2011) and 'the ethos of deinstitutionalization' (Long, 2017: 125). Secondly, such reforms also included the medical model of mental health (Jones, 1993): both the overarching shift towards treatment (Hess and Majerus, 2011), and specifically the adoption of physical treatments and the aspiration to align mental and physical healthcare provision.

Architectural practices towards these two ends are also grouped into two areas. Firstly, through their principal architectural practice – that is, their active interpretation of a building programme into a material and spatial structure. The architects employed design principles of architectural modernism so as to give their buildings a non-institutional character.[5] Secondly, their practices expanded to embrace interdisciplinary research on hospital architecture so as to match the perception of mental health as a medical, curable condition, and to align it with physical healthcare provision. Overall, this chapter argues that the engagement with post-war psychiatry that envisioned new practices towards psychiatric reform came both from outside psychiatry, as discussed here with a snapshot of mid-1950s England, and from inside the mental health field.[6]

National policy context

The historical context of the British National Health Service (NHS), launched in 1948, is directly relevant to all post-war healthcare provision in England, including psychiatry. During its first administrative period (1948–73) its principal focus was the hospital, both as an organisational and as a spatial entity (Rivett, 2014). Under the NHS Act of 1946, the minister of health became the central authority for all health services and all hospitals were transferred to fourteen (later fifteen) new Regional Hospital Boards (Jones, 1993: 146). Under the boards' overview, Hospital Management Committees were 'the agents of the Boards' and mainly responsible for running their respective hospitals. Most power sat with the Regional Hospital Boards, as their regional functions included hospital capital works and the management of financial allocations to Hospital Management Committees (Rivett, 2014).

Whether mental hospitals should be 'included in the centralized NHS scheme, or left with the county authorities' had been questioned during the planning process of the National Health Service (Jones, 1993: 143–4). Eventually, mental hospitals were included within the NHS under their local Regional Hospital Boards, but under special conditions, as legislation at this point still kept mental health separate from physical health (RHB(47)1: §1). This absorption remained partial in other ways too, as mental hospitals were grouped separately under their own Hospital Management Committees (Rivett, 2014) and boards' medical officers for mental health were required to be psychiatrists (RHB(48)1: §62).

It would be more than a full decade before mental healthcare was fully integrated with the rest of the healthcare provided by the NHS – that is, following the appointment of the Royal Commission on the Law Relating to Mental Illness and Mental Deficiency in 1954, chaired by Lord Percy and completed in 1957, and the introduction of the Mental Health Act in July 1959. The Act brought about a complete overhaul of mental health services by 'replac[ing] much of the existing legislation on the provision of mental health services in England [and] bringing the provision of mental health services within the general administrative machinery of the NHS for the first time' (Rivett, 2014).

NHS hospital aspirations and constraints

The hospitals that the NHS inherited had previously been commissioned and administered under multiple separate systems, such as charitable, voluntary and municipal bodies (Rivett, 2014). In addition to the need to co-ordinate existing provision, there were also significant infrastructural shortcomings, both because of the advanced age of most hospital buildings, which were in need of maintenance and modernisation, and in terms of bed shortages that dictated the commission of new hospitals.

Despite these pressing needs, budgetary constraints and competing priorities meant it was not until the early 1960s that a commitment to substantial hospital rebuilding was actually undertaken. Nonetheless, limited activity was initiated in the 1950s. For the design of new buildings, tuberculosis initially came as first priority, but soon became less relevant, and mental healthcare came second (Harwood, 2015: 283). In 1950, Minister of Health Aneurin Bevan included mental hospitals among the top priorities set for hospitals (Jones, 1993: 143–4). However, as the enormous scale of the endeavour and state funding limitations were recognised, capital expenditure in 1954 worked out to be four hundred and thirty million pounds for housing, fifty-seven million for schools and only ten million for hospitals (Hughes, 1996: 39). Such delays in healthcare investment soon became alarming: by the mid-1950s there were fourteen new towns built but not one new hospital. A recommendation for a seven-year programme of capital investment followed (Hughes, 1996: 40–1). Most importantly for the discussion here, Minister of Health Iain Macleod allocated some 'meagre' funding for additional psychiatric facilities in 1954 and 1955: the so-called 'mental million' (Hughes, 1996: 41). To date there is no comprehensive survey of this period and it is not known how many buildings were commissioned under this scheme, nor how many were actually realised or survive at the date of this publication. However, preliminary research undertaken by the author suggests a number of admission and treatment units were commissioned in the mid-1950s as part of this scheme (see also *RIBA Journal*, 1957: 268). They were scattered across England and were, in fact, the effective continuation of a similar building programme started in the inter-war period.[7]

Fair Mile Hospital

Initially introduced in the architectural press as 'Berkshire, Reading, and Newbury Lunatic Asylum' (*Builder*, 1870), Fair Mile has been known under several different names during its lifetime. These mainly comprised variations on the following: 'Moulsford Asylum' (1870–97), 'Berkshire Lunatic Asylum' (1897–c.1915), 'Berkshire Mental Hospital' (c.1915–48) and 'Fair Mile Hospital' (1948–2010).[8] The original building for Fair Mile was purpose-designed and built as a 'lunatic asylum' in 1870, and further extended in 1878 by Charles Henry Howell, one of the 'key contributors to the design of asylums' during the 1870s (Taylor, 1991: 153).

The size of the institution varied significantly during its lifetime. Initially, it accommodated 133 male and 152 female patients (Wheeler, 2015: 13), but these numbers were far exceeded in subsequent decades. During World War II the hospital reached its greatest size, accommodating over 1,400 patients.[9] Overcrowding remained a problem following the war, with 1,202 beds recorded in 1947[10] and around one thousand beds in 1951 and 1959.[11] From the 1960s onwards, in line with new deinstitutionalisation policies, the hospital decreased in size, and by the end of the century it accommodated only 200 patients.[12] Following the regional administrative organisation of hospitals under the NHS, Fair Mile fell under the remit of the Oxford Regional Hospital Board and more specifically the Berkshire Mental Hospitals Management Committee, renamed 'St Birinus Group Hospital Management Committee' in 1957.

The new admission and treatment unit

The new admission unit was part of 'the first group of units to be sanctioned since the war by the Ministry of Health' (*RIBA Journal*, 1957: 268).[13] In local administrative documentation, the new admission unit was first reported in July 1954, found within the Hospital Inspectors' Reports, and was anticipated to 'assist in the better classification of patients, and ... provide good facilities for the clinical teaching of Student Nurses'.[14]

As was common practice in post-war England, under the oversight of the Oxford Regional Hospital Board and in collaboration with W. J. Jobson of its Architects' Department, the project was commissioned to a private architectural practice: Philip Powell and Hidalgo Moya, one of the most important post-war architectural firms in England. Such a commission for the new admission unit was particularly significant. Incremental building activity was carried out continuously in existing mental hospitals, whenever funds allowed it, yet this usually resulted in nondescript structures with no particular architectural merit. By contrast, upon its completion, the Admission Unit at Fair Mile was welcomed by the Commissioners of the Board of Control as a significant development in the history of the hospital and noted as original in design and appearing to be 'admirably suited to its purpose'.[15] The building was also widely published in the architectural press from January 1956 to May 1957, with dedicated reports appearing in the *Architect and Building News* (1956), *Architects' Journal* (1956), *The Builder* (1956) and *RIBA Journal* (1957), as well as a specialist journal, the *Hospital* (1956). In 1957 it was also awarded a Royal Institute of British Architects Bronze Medal.[16]

The above articles provide most of the factual information available about the admission unit as a built structure. The architectural vision and areas of interest are clearly highlighted, including detailed constructional information, as is common in similar publications for any type of building. In fact, the text across these articles is largely repetitive and one can assume a summary was provided by the architects themselves which closely reflected their priorities for the commissioned project. This is most noticeable in the article published in *The Hospital*, which is very similar to the rest, despite the journal otherwise having a more specialist character (*Hospital*, 1956).

Various individual design components are described and partly interpreted in the journal articles. First of all, good connections to external spaces and natural lighting dominate all accounts of the new building in the professional press. In addition, the cruciform plan is seen as serving to minimise the perceived size of the building and thus any institutional associations (*RIBA Journal*, 1957: 269), as well as allowing the creation of separate gardens for the male and female wings. Internally, the cruciform plan further created good connections between all four wings and allowed for efficient yet discreet supervision. The single-level design further minimised the perceived size of the unit and it was only the common room that stood out as a special space with its inverted 'butterfly' roof and extensive use of glazing (see Figure 4.1). In the rest of the building, the use of glass was also increased, as allowed by recently relaxed design requirements, and it is specifically noted that no windows had bars installed (*Architects' Journal*, 1956: 386). The single-storey design, we are told, was also enhanced by varying roof levels, clerestories and roof lights, which allowed for compact planning with short corridors (*Architects' Journal*, 1956: 388; *Builder*, 1956: 387).

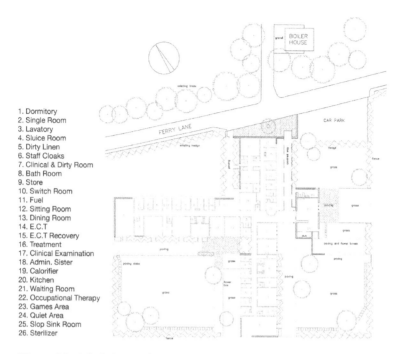

1. Dormitory
2. Single Room
3. Lavatory
4. Sluice Room
5. Dirty Linen
6. Staff Cloaks
7. Clinical & Dirty Room
8. Bath Room
9. Store
10. Switch Room
11. Fuel
12. Sitting Room
13. Dining Room
14. E.C.T
15. E.C.T Recovery
16. Treatment
17. Clinical Examination
18. Admin. Sister
19. Calorifier
20. Kitchen
21. Waiting Room
22. Occupational Therapy
23. Games Area
24. Quiet Area
25. Slop Sink Room
26. Sterilizer

Figure 4.2 Admission and treatment unit, Fair Mile Hospital. Floor plan (drawn by Alex Wood).

Even when not explicitly stated, these articles provide insights into some of the psychiatric reforms that its designers envisioned enacting or supporting through design: their principal architectural practice. Specifically, their application of modernist design principles is argued here to have aimed to materialise the pleasant atmosphere and non-institutional character mentioned in the quote from the *Architects' Journal* above. Such modernist design principles included: a functionalist design (that is, a design where 'form follows function'), an unadorned appearance, extensive openings and emphasis on the building's overall structure and mass composition. The functionalist interpretation of the wards, common room and treatment wing further aimed to give expression to the advances towards the treatment, or even cure, of mental illness – yet with a material outcome as complicated as the evolving psychiatric practices themselves, as will be discussed below. Other specific design elements of the building, such as its four- and six-bed wards, highlight the new architectural practices brought into the field in the post-war period – namely, the new practices of interdisciplinary research and collaborative practices between designers and researchers, also discussed below.

Along with the main text of those articles, the accompanying photographs and drawings allow for further insights. The impression that the unit is a separate, independent facility comes across very strongly and seems intentional. Although the addition of detached buildings within mental hospital grounds at that point already had a long history (see, for example, Richardson, 1998: 15, 177), several other features of the unit make the effort to hide its connections to the main hospital quite distinct. Telling in this respect is the placement of the new building, situated across a public road by the southern boundary of the hospital grounds, with trees screening the existing hospital from view, while the gentle slope from north-west to south-east and open views to the east, south and west further strengthen this visual separation (*RIBA Journal*, 1957: 268). Illustrations in all publicity material also omitted any images of the main hospital (*Architects' Journal*, 1956: 386, 394; *Architect and Building News*, 1956: 11).

However, this implied independence from the main asylum is contradicted by a key function that was omitted from the new unit: food service. Each ward wing had a day room and a dining room, but it is unlikely that the small kitchen near the junction of the four wings actually catered for these two dining rooms (see Figure 4.2). Its small size, as well as common practice in similar buildings,[17] suggest this was merely a distribution kitchen that was dependent on the central kitchen of the main hospital. Conversely, the inclusion of an area for occupational therapy in the common room strengthened the independence of the unit, but there is insufficient information as to what degree this was the case for other patient activities within the hospital grounds, or for extramural events.

A rare photograph showing the common room occupied was included in a nurse recruitment booklet published in 1959 (Figure 4.3).[18] Although this may have been staged, with staff posing as patients, the photograph supports the designers' intention for a non-institutional, almost domestic, character. Such an intention is further reflected in the unit's two sitting rooms, one in each single-sex

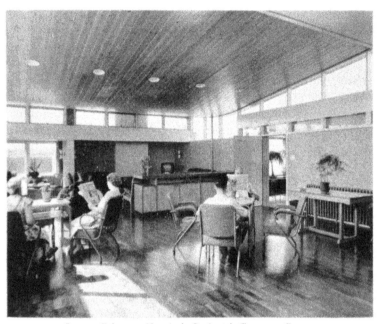

George Schuster Hospital, Patients' Common Room.

Figure 4.3 Admission and treatment unit, Fair Mile Hospital. Common room. Source: BRO, P/HA2/5/1, Fair Mile Hospital, 'Into the Light', staff recruitment booklet, 1959.

wing (see Figure 4.2), and can be traced back to the mid-nineteenth century.[19]

In this 1959 photograph, three pairs of people (two single-sex and one mixed-sex) are sitting in the games area of the common room, which is flooded with sunlight. One man and one woman, in each one of the two single-sex pairs seated around small tables, are reading newspapers. Well looked-after potted plants are noticeable throughout the otherwise scarcely decorated room, with one pot on each one of the room's tables as well as on the counter separating the games area from the 'quiet corner'. Three more pots can be seen on two console tables: one inside the common room and two on a second console table in the adjacent entrance hall, which can be seen through the open door. The room is tidy, clean and in good condition. The range of materials, including extensive use of timber and glazing, and exposed brick at the fireplace, make the space feel both warm and fresh. Apart from two books on two of the tables, however, the lack of other objects is striking. Whether a depiction of real patients or a staged photograph, the image reminds the viewer more of a hotel foyer or other type of communal living space, rather than a family home. The uniformity of some of the furniture further reinforces this impression, and so does the appearance of its occupants: neatly groomed, fully dressed and wearing shoes, they convey a message of care, but also diminish to a degree the implied domestic character of the space.

The open door of the room and the absence of staff are also interesting. Although not explicitly stated in any of the documentation identified so far, it is likely that an open-door policy was adopted in the unit. Not only had this become widespread practice in Britain in the 1950s (Hide, 2018), but moreover the floor plan of the unit and photographs also support such a conjecture: the entrance hall to the inpatient part of the building has no nurse station or reception controlling access (see Figure 4.2). In the external spaces, although the two yards outside the wards are fenced, those fences are transparent and suggest no intention to enforce confinement (*Architect and Building News*, 1956: 13).

The suggestion of a non-institutional character of the building as a whole and the implicit domestic character of the common room in particular are, however, challenged by various strongly clinical elements. Neither the intention for a domestic character nor the hybrid nature ('clinical, domestic, institutional, and in some respects carceral', as Hide (2020: 190) sums this up) of the building was a novelty. However, the conflict seems to be intensified in the admission unit, partly because of its condensed size, and therefore closer proximity between conflicting aspects, and partly because of certain additions of a clinical character: not only was one of the four wings devoted to a purely clinical purpose, it was also open to outpatients and bore the stamp of a highly technological nature in the form of ECT facilities. Moreover, the wards of the unit, in contrast to the common room, also have a strongly clinical atmosphere, rather than a domestic one.[20]

A number of photographs and drawings provide information on the wards. The plan demonstrates that these comprised single rooms, in addition to four-, six- and ten-bed wards (see Figure 4.2), while photographs demonstrate that due consideration was given to both natural and artificial lighting. The rooms are flooded with daylight through the extensive external glazing, including clerestories, and the individual wall-mounted light fittings at bedheads provide one opportunity for patient control over their personal space. However, the strongly clinical, even sterilised, character of these spaces is also conveyed in all images. This is the case in both a literal and a metaphorical sense: the spaces are unoccupied, with neither people nor personal belongings. There is no evidence of individual wardrobes, although a small side table or cabinet can be discerned next to each bed. Most strikingly, the beds, and the privacy curtains around them, strongly convey the character of a clinical environment. They have a similar but reverse effect to what Benoît Majerus has pointed out about the function of a bed changing when transposed from a standard room into an institutional setting (Majerus, 2017: 268): any domestic character is nullified and the hospital atmosphere becomes dominant.

Interestingly, no illustration of the actual treatment spaces features in any of the architectural articles. Only one photograph shows an insulin therapy dormitory, which looks like a starker version of the main wards (*Architect and Building News*, 1956: 16). Another photograph showing ECT treatment at Fair Mile was included in the 1959 nurse recruitment booklet 'Into the Light' (see Figure 4.4). The clerestory windows and wall-mounted light fittings indicate that this was taking place in the new admission unit. The room is sparsely furnished with a hospital bed and the necessary support for the technical equipment. A doctor in a white coat and a nurse in uniform strongly underline the clinical nature of the setting and the experience for the patient, while the presumably white[21] walls and sheets covering the patient further reinforce this tone.

The stark architectural space here seems to complement what Gawlich (2020) calls 'the concept of pushbutton psychiatry ... the uniform, disciplined, and disinterested treatment regimen, which therapeutically "shocked away" disorders as well as affective failures' (Gawlich, 2020: 215). The creation of a dedicated space further supported the development of 'concrete therapeutic action' through the push of a button by offering a second component: 'the availability

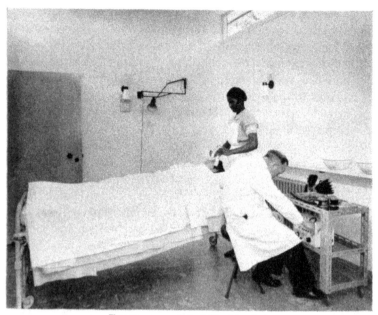

Treatment — Fair Mile Hospital.

Figure 4.4 ECT treatment at Fair Mile Hospital, *c.*1959. Source: BRO, P/HA2/5/1, Fair Mile Hospital, 'Into the Light', staff recruitment booklet, 1959.

of electroconvulsive therapy embedded into the room' (Gawlich, 2020: 217).

However, the omission of technological aspects of both the clinical and 'domestic' sides of the building in the published articles is intriguing. One wonders if this was perceived by the architects as threatening their imagined 'control' over their creation in adhering to the use of architectural symbols of domesticity. In the common room, one can notice the absence of a television set (see Figure 4.3), despite the device's increasing popularity both in mental hospitals and in domestic family life in the 1950s (Hide, 2020). Instead, 'patient' pairs pictured here at individual tables seem to suggest the intended encouragement of social interaction, even if no such interaction is actually captured in this instance. By contrast, a more traditional symbol of domesticity was emphatically introduced as part of the building design, namely fireplaces. These were included in the two sitting rooms and the 'quiet corner' of the common room. Notably, however, staff in a similar unit were reported to have expressed doubts as to whether the fireplaces would ever be used, 'as the heating system should be adequate, but these were regarded as contributing to the domestic character of the room' (*Architects' Journal*, 1959: 361).

Architectural practices in support of psychiatric reforms

Modernist architecture

Although rather late compared to certain other geographical regions,[22] the adoption of modernist design principles was relatively novel in post-war England. The Modern Movement barely took hold before the 1930s, and it was the Festival of Britain in 1951 that 'gave Britain modernist precincts at last' (Harwood, 2015: xii, xxv). Within this context, British modernist architecture was interlaced with post-war optimism and the welfare state. Powell and Moya were very much part of this important shift (Harwood, 2015: xii, xxv; Powell, 2009), and their admission unit at Fair Mile reflects this: entrenched in their roles as designers, Powell and Moya appear to have maintained a certain professional insularity as architects subscribing to the utopian and often limiting, even controlling, aspects of modernism. Nonetheless, through their associated design practices they managed to give the new unit a refreshing and uplifting appearance, which was perceived in the local community as 'ultra-modern' (Wheeler, 2015: 74). Leaving behind historical styles, monumental symmetrical elevations, masonry construction and pitched roofs, their design embraces a range of modern architectural features: an asymmetrical composition, large openings and extensive glazing, as well as both flat and 'butterfly' roofs, which matched the non-institutional aspirations of the evolving mental health field, despite the budgetary and building material supply constraints of the 1950s.

However, the functionalist side of the design leaves more to be desired: the 'hybrid' nature of the functions accommodated, both 'domestic' and medical, appears to remain unresolved. It is here that an expansion of architectural practices came into the picture as manifested by the introduction of the complementary role of architectural researchers, in parallel with the customary role of architectural designers. This expansion supported the evolving medical model of mental health, but also appears to have contributed to some of the unresolved issues with the dual atmosphere intended to be conveyed internally: both non-institutional and 'scientific'.

Research in hospital architecture

The increasing significance of research in hospital architecture during the period is strongly reflected in a study by the Nuffield Provincial Hospitals Trust (NPHT, 1955). It is argued here that this study had a direct influence on the new unit at Fair Mile. The Nuffield Provincial Hospitals Trust was founded in 1939 by Lord Nuffield, aiming to promote the co-ordination of hospital and ancillary services in the provinces, as a provincial equivalent of King Edward's Hospital Fund for London (McLachlan, 1992: 9). In 1949, the trust, with the co-operation of the University of Bristol, launched an investigation into the functions and design of hospitals (NPHT, 1955: xix). This was conducted by its Division for Architectural Studies under the direction of Richard Llewelyn Davies and a multidisciplinary team. In addition to architects and research and administrative assistants, other specialisms included: a statistician, a historian, a physician, a nurse and an accountant (NPHT, 1955: vi). Aside from the investigation, through co-operation with hospital authorities, two experimental hospital buildings were also built: a sixty-four bed medical ward unit added to Larkfield Hospital, Greenock, Scotland, and an eighty-bed surgical unit for Musgrave Park Hospital, Belfast, Northern Ireland (NPHT, 1955: xix).

Although there is no definitive evidence that Llewelyn Davies or his partner John Weeks had been directly involved at Fair Mile,[23] they had recommended Powell and Moya to the Oxford Regional Hospital Board in 1951 as 'the best young firm in the land' (Harwood, 2015: 285). What is more, the two men were consultants for other major hospitals designed by Powell and Moya, including the Princess Margaret Hospital at Swindon, Wiltshire, which was being designed in parallel with Fair Mile (Harwood, 2015: 285). Powell and Moya's involvement at Swindon began as early as 1951 (Powell, 2009: 87) and the hospital's eight forty-bed wards were based on the Nuffield layout developed at Musgrave Park (Hughes, 1996: 104).

Although the Nuffield study was limited to acute general hospitals, with mental hospitals specifically excluded, there are numerous design elements applied at Fair Mile that carry the stamp of that study. Two of these elements are briefly discussed below: the design of four- and six-bed wards, as applied at Musgrave Park, and the particular consideration given to both natural and artificial lighting.

The Nuffield report stresses the novelty of the wards' design, which would become widely influential:

> The arrangement of beds 3-deep parallel to the window-wall [as used in the 6-bed wards] is common on the Continent, and architecturally is valuable because it allows greater compactness in the building. This arrangement has yet to be fully accepted in Britain, but the Musgrave Park experimental ward units offer propitious conditions for testing the reactions of patients and staff to it (NPHT, 1955: 30).

As regards lighting, aiming simultaneously for maximum light and minimum glare made the design of hospital windows particularly challenging. Various possibilities were explored during the Nuffield studies and tested in the two experimental hospitals designed by Llewelyn Davies's team (NPHT, 1955: 91–9, figures 12, 76, 79–81, 83). These included what can be also seen applied in the wards at Fair Mile, namely the inclusion of 'a horizontal baffle to limit the view of the sky for patients in the beds nearest to the windows and thus reduce discomfort from glare' (NPHT, 1955: 99). Artificial lighting was also studied, again aiming at avoiding glare, and proposals for 'separately controlled local lighting at bed-head' bear close similarities to the fittings applied at Fair Mile (NPHT, 1955: 101–7, figure 88). Sun and daylight were also encouraged throughout hospitals for the benefit of patients as well as staff (NPHT, 1955: 148).[24]

Research in mental healthcare architecture: researchers and designers

Despite their exclusion from the 1955 Nuffield study, pleas for further studies that dealt with psychiatric hospitals were voiced by architects involved in designing similar admission units, as exemplified in an article appearing in the *Architects' Journal* in 1959 which discussed another admission unit, at St John's Hospital in Stone, Aylesbury, Buckinghamshire. Building of the facility began in November 1956 and was completed in April 1959. It was designed by Gollins, Melvin, Ward and Partners but, despite the different design teams, certain contributors took part in both the Fair Mile and St John's projects: both buildings were under the administrative remit of the Oxford Regional Hospital Board and as such the architect to the board, W. J. Jobson, was involved in both projects (*Architect & Building News*, 1957b: 761); moreover the work of the Nuffield study can be safely presumed to have influenced both projects.[25] In addition, there are some design similarities which make two points from the 1959 article on the St John's unit relevant to Fair Mile.

Firstly, the 1959 article comments on the distinct environmental needs that different mental health conditions may have, suggesting emerging knowledge in the field: 'With mental patients of certain types, awareness of certain aspects of the environment may be heightened, so the surroundings become more important than usual' (*Architects' Journal*, 1959: 360). Secondly, the article concludes by openly addressing the need for research into this particular area of hospital building and for such research to match advancements in treatment: 'So little building has been done in this field since new ideas of treatment for mentally sick developed that it will clearly be the job of the health authorities to establish research teams in mental hospital building similar to the Ministry of Education's' (*Architects' Journal*, 1959: 362).[26] Interestingly, a key such study appeared that same year in the form of a report for the World Health Organisation, led by Llewelyn Davies in collaboration with two psychiatrists, the French Paul Sivadon and the British Alex Baker, and titled *Architecture and Psychiatric Services* (Baker *et al.*, 1959).[27]

David Theodore's (2019) analysis of the connections between the work conducted at Nuffield and Llewelyn Davies's keen interest in architectural research is particularly enlightening here as it offers insights into two parallel architectural roles envisaged in the field: one for specialised research bodies and one for practising architects. Theodore points out that in 1960, as Llewelyn Davies was moving from his role at Nuffield to an academic job at the Bartlett School of Architecture at University College London, he organised a 'Hospitals

Course' at the Royal Institute of British Architects which demonstrated how he envisaged the interdisciplinary research on hospital design 'as a model for integrating specialist knowledge with design' (Theodore, 2019: 989). Notably, however, Llewelyn Davies also insisted that architects must remain architects, both when participating in multidisciplinary research teams and when practising architecture. The goal was the pursuit of *'specialist knowledge*, freely available, not *specialised men'* (emphasis in the original).[28]

Theodore's analysis throws light on the new division of labour applied in the admission units for the Oxford Regional Hospital Board as matching Llewelyn Davies's vision of 'a few specialist architects, engaged in research, and the majority of architects, engaged in practice' (Theodore, 2019: 991). Although prolific as architectural designers, neither Powell and Moya, nor Gollins, Melvin, Ward and Partners, ever became exclusively hospital architects, let alone dedicated to psychiatric buildings. In this respect, both the presumed role of the Nuffield study and the architects' pleas for further research in the area of mental healthcare architecture support the position put forward here that a new layer of research practices was introduced in the interface between architecture and psychiatry in post-war England.[29] This research element was added to design as the principal architectural practice, but also to known precedents in general hospital and asylum architecture, where architects specialised in such architecture and doctors or medical superintendents became experts in architectural design (see, for example: Adams, 2008: chapter 4; and discussion of G. T. Hine and Dr John Conolly in Taylor, 1991: 21–2, 25, 48, 135, 146).

Conclusion

The study here presents a snapshot of some of the architectural activity in 1950s England in relation to mental healthcare provision. The full scope of this activity remains to be established, yet evidence suggests this was widespread, varied, and had a degree of continuity with the inter-war period. The placement of importance on admission units in particular is not a novelty of the post-war period nor of the English context (see, for example, Topp, 2017). However, their inclusion in the restricted 'mental million' programme and the commissioning of distinguished private architectural practices further underline the role of the architectural profession as an actor in post-war psychiatric reforms.

At Fair Mile, the architects worked within the context of a former asylum, rebranded in the first half of the twentieth century as a mental hospital and in the post-war period simply as a hospital. The discussion above highlights how they aimed to give material and spatial expression to an early version of the notion of deinstitutionalisation. This related to a change in perceptions of institutions for long-term care, rather than a desire for their abolition, and was supported by an increase in voluntary admissions and outpatients. This type of deinstitutionalisation had already been implemented in the first half of the twentieth century both with attempts 'for lighter, more domestic designs', including looser planning and providing more accommodation in 'detached villas' (Taylor, 1991: 45), as well as with new spatial models of mental healthcare institutions (see, for example, Topp *et al.*, 2007). However, within the post-war British context, architects used their principal architectural practice, that is, design, to facilitate the expression of a non-institutional character, by engaging with principles of modernism, but also hospital design considerations, such as those included in the Nuffield study. Although research on other units of this period remains a work in progress, the building for Fair Mile stands out as an early example of this notion, designed by a notable modernist architectural practice and embracing several of the new trends put forward by the Nuffield study.[30]

In addition, the particular inclusion of a treatment hospital further stressed the shift towards the medical model of mental health, in line with the overarching reform of twentieth-century psychiatry towards treatment (Hess and Majerus, 2011). This was expressed at Fair Mile in a twofold manner: firstly, by the adoption and intensification of physical treatments in the treatment wing, and secondly by the implicit ambition to align mental and physical healthcare provision. Given the exclusion of mental hospitals from the Nuffield study, it is argued here that ongoing policy work towards the merging of mental and physical health services was seen as permissive towards, and even encouraging of, some permeability in architectural solutions between the two fields. Although the unit predated any political declarations of the abolition of mental hospitals as found in the Percy Report in 1957, the Mental Health Act in 1959 and 'The Hospital Plan for England and Wales' in 1962, the merging of physical and mental healthcare provision and psychiatry's 'parity of esteem with other medical specialisms' were being discussed for decades prior. Notable landmarks include the White Paper of 1944, which quoted the Macmillan Commission of 1924–26[31] on the interaction of mind and body, and an article published in the *British Medical Journal* in June 1945 (*British Medical Journal*, 1945; also cited in Jones, 1993: 143). During the 1950s the merging of psychiatric and physical health services was suggested by various publications, opining that the mentally ill would probably be accommodated in psychiatric units at general hospitals in future,[32] as well as more comprehensive propositions for the reorganisation of hospital services.[33] In this context, the engagement with Nuffield's research practices should not be seen as random, or even compromising. Instead, insider knowledge, probably through Regional Hospital Board officials and the Nuffield team, is most likely to have encouraged some reformist expansion of architectural practices by the architects involved, either in the form of design or research.

Notes

1 More broadly within this volume, questions relating to spatial and material aspects of psychiatric practices appear in several chapters, as Chapters 10, 11 and 12.

2 The name 'Fair Mile', rather than 'Fairmile', will be used here, as this version appears in most official records. 'Fairmile' will be used only in any exact quotes or titles where it appears in this form.

3 Following the hospital's decommissioning and closure in 2003, the admission and treatment unit was demolished. The Victorian asylum became a Grade II listed building in 1986 and has since been converted to housing.

4 The introduction of these treatments to Fair Mile predated the new unit. Electroconvulsive therapy was introduced by 1951 (The National Archives, Kew, General Nursing Council for England and Wales: Education, Hospital Inspectors' Reports and Papers, DT 33 (hereafter TNA, DT 33), file number DT 33/1243, 8 March 1951, p. 4) and insulin coma therapy by 1954 (TNA, DT 33/1243, 8 July 1954, p. 5).

5 This association with modern architecture is much more complex than what is briefly presented here. Leslie Topp (2017) has identified examples as early as the late nineteenth century, in Germany and Austria, in which the symbolic and representational role of architecture was used in the struggle for psychiatric legitimacy in order to improve the image of asylums. A comparison to the experimental work of the architect Kiyoshi (Joe) Izumi in Saskatchewan, Canada (also in the 1950s and whilst existing institutions were not being abolished) is equally fascinating (Dyck, 2010).

6 As discussed by Despo Kritsotaki, Marica Setaro and Gundula Gahlen in Chapters 1, 2 and 3.

7 A scoping exercise was started in early 2020 but interrupted by the Covid-19 pandemic. Although a full comparison with the inter-war period requires in-depth analysis, one immediately noticeable difference is the post-war shift towards architectural modernism.

8 Berkshire Record Office, Reading (hereafter BRO), Records of Fair Mile Hospital, Administrative History, D/H10 (hereafter BRO, Admin. Hist., D/H10), http://ww2.berkshirenclosure.org.uk/CalmView/TreeBrowse.aspx?src=CalmView.Catalog&field=RefNo&key=DH10 (accessed 6 July 2018). See also Wheeler, 2015: 18.

9 BRO, Admin. Hist., D/H10.

10 TNA, DT 33/1243, 13 November 1947, pp. 1, 3; 12 April 1962, p. 1.

11 BRO, St Birinus Hospital Group Management Committee (previously Berkshire County Mental Hospital Management Committee), P/HA2 (hereafter BRO, P/HA2), file number P/HA2/5/1, Fair Mile Hospital, 'Into the Light': 3; TNA, DT 33/1243, 8 March 1951, p. 6.

12 BRO, Admin. Hist., D/H10.

13 The unit is noted here as 'the second to be completed', which conflicts with later scholars naming this as the first NHS hospital to be completed in England. I mistakenly repeated this claim in an earlier article (Malathouni, 2020: 458).

14 TNA, DT 33/1243, 8 July 1954, p. 6.

15 TNA, General Nursing Council for England and Wales: Education, Nurse Training Schools, Correspondence and Papers, Parts I and II, DT 35 (hereafter TNA, DT 35), file number DT 35/194, Copy of the Report by the Commissioners of the Board of Control at their visit to Fair Mile and Hungerford Hospitals on the 12th and 13th of April, 1956.

16 BRO, P/HA2/1/1/3, 9 May 1957, p. 1160.

17 For example, this is known to be the case for an admission unit at Herrison Hospital, Dorset (*Architect & Building News*, 1957a: 764).

18 Also reproduced in Wheeler (2015: 76).

19 Hamlett (2015), as cited in Hide (2020: 190).

20 The discussion here regarding the domestic character of parts of the building naturally relates to newly admitted patients who stayed in the ward and not to patients of the main hospital or outpatients who only came for day treatment.

21 The colour scheme throughout the building cannot be seen in the photographs, as these are all printed in black and white. However, colour is mentioned in some detail in two articles (*Architect and Building News*, 1956: 16; *RIBA Journal*, 1957: 270).

22 International examples of mental healthcare facilities reflect a different timeline as regards stylistic evolution. See for example the very interesting analysis in Topp (2017).

23 Powell and Moya's professional papers survive only in part and are very limited in scope (Victoria and Albert Museum, London, RIBA British Architectural Library Drawings and Archives Collections, Sir Philip Powell's notebooks, illustrated lecture notes, and design feasibility reports for Powell & Moya, 1964–2000, PoP). Llewelyn Davies's papers, meanwhile, are considered lost.

24 For a much more nuanced and multilayered discussion on the role of light, see Sammet (2020). Sammet's article suggests further investigation into the origins and meaning of the title 'Into the Light', as used by Fair Mile for its 1959 staff recruitment booklet, may be a worthwhile future exercise.

25 Like Powell and Moya, Gollins, Melvin, Ward and Partners were also involved in further major hospital commissions, so their knowledge of the Nuffield work should likewise be assumed (Aldous, 1974).

26 This burgeoning realisation that there could be a correlation between distinctive characteristics of mental illness and associated care facilities was also strongly reflected in a 1961 memorandum of the Scottish Home and Health Department (Long, 2017: 118).

27 Notably, this report recommended that 'special admission units should be avoided' (Baker *et al.*, 1959: 50), yet the advantages of the number six (and to a lesser degree four) for the bed layouts of wards and other patient groupings was repeatedly recommended here too (Baker *et al.*, 1959: 25, 36, 42, 52, and figures 4–6).

28 Llewelyn Davies (1957: 189), as quoted in Theodore (2019: 990).

29 Close collaboration between mental health professionals and architects in the post-war period has been evidenced and discussed in other geographical settings too, both in terms of direct collaboration within individual projects and in terms of broader research in the field. Published scholarship to date includes studies in relation to 1950s and 1960s work in Saskatchewan, Canada (Dyck, 2010), in 1960s France, in relation to Nicole Sonolet's work as well as the research collective CERFI (Centre

d'etudes, de recherches et de formations institutionelles, or Centre for Institutional Studies, Research and Training) (TenHoor, 2019), and in the 1960s US, in relation to Community Mental Health Centers (Knoblauch, 2020: Chapter 2).

30 Articles concerning a small number of similar admission units have been published in the architectural press (for example, *Architect & Building News*, 1957a, 1957b; *Architects' Journal*, 1959). Several more units have been identified in the archival material of an English hospital historical survey conducted in the late 1990s (Richardson, 1998), held at the Historic England Archive in Swindon, Wiltshire.

31 The Macmillan Commission of 1924–26 had recommended the adoption of medical terminology ('hospital', 'nurse', 'patient' and so on) and voluntary treatment, and effectively led to the Mental Treatment Act 1930.

32 Godber (1958), as cited in Rivett (2014).

33 McKeown (1958), as cited in Rivett (2014).

References

Adams, Annmarie, 2008, *Medicine by Design: The Architect and the Modern Hospital, 1893–1943* (Minneapolis, MN: University of Minnesota Press).

Aldous, Tony, 1974, 'Introduction', in *Architecture of the Gollins Melvin Ward Partnership* (London: Lund Humphries), pp. 9–16.

Architect and Building News, 1956, 'Admission unit Fair Mile Hospital, Wallingford, Berks for the Oxford Regional Hospital Board', *Architect and Building News* (5 January), 11–18.

Architect & Building News, 1957a, 'New admission unit at the Herrison Hospital, Dorset', *Architect & Building News*, 212:23 (4 December), 763–4.

Architect & Building News, 1957b, 'St John's Hospital, Stone: Admission and treatment unit', *Architect & Building News*, 212:23 (4 December), 760–2.

Architects' Journal, 1956, 'Admission unit at the Fairmile Hospital, Wallingford, Berkshire', *Architects' Journal* (19 April), 385–98.

Architects' Journal, 1959, 'Hospital extension', *Architects' Journal* (15 October), 359–70.

Baker, Alex, Richard Llewelyn Davies and Paul Sivadon, 1959, *Psychiatric Services and Architecture* (Geneva: World Health Organization).

British Medical Journal, 1945, 'Future organization of the psychiatric services', *British Medical Journal*, 1:4406, 111–16.

Builder, 1870, 'Berkshire, Reading, and Newbury Lunatic Asylum', *Builder* (2 April), 264.

Builder, 1956, 'Admission unit at Fair Mile Hospital', *Builder* (27 April), 386–90.

Dyck, Erika, 2010, 'Spaced-out in Saskatchewan: Modernism, anti-psychiatry, and deinstitutionalization, 1950–1968', *Bulletin of the History of Medicine*, 84:4 (Winter), 640–66. doi: 10.1353/bhm.2010.0041.

Eghigian, Greg, 2011, 'Deinstitutionalizing the history of contemporary psychiatry', *History of Psychiatry*, 22:2, 201–14.

Gawlich, Max, 2020, 'Buttons and stimuli: The material basis of electro-convulsive therapy as a place of historical change', in Monika Ankele and Benoît Majerus (eds), *Material Cultures of Psychiatry* (Bielefeld: Transcript), pp. 201–22.

Godber, George E., 1958, 'Health services past, present and future', *Lancet*, 272:7036 (5 July), 1–6.

Hamlett, Jane, 2015, *At Home in the Institution: Material Life in Asylums, Lodging Houses and Schools in Victorian and Edwardian England* (Basingstoke: Palgrave Macmillan).

Harwood, Elain, 2015, *Space, Hope and Brutalism: English Architecture, 1945–1975* (New Haven, CT: Yale University Press).

Henckes, Nicolas, 2011, 'Reforming psychiatric institutions in the mid-twentieth century: A framework for analysis', *History of Psychiatry*, 22:2, 164–81.

Hess, Volker and Benoît Majerus, 2011, 'Writing the history of psychiatry in the 20th century', *History of Psychiatry*, 22:2, 139–45.

Hide, Louise, 2018, 'In plain sight: Open doors, mixed-sex wards and sexual abuse in English psychiatric hospitals, 1950s–early 1990s', *Social History of Medicine*, 31:4 (November), 732–53. doi: 10.1093/shm/hky091.

Hide, Louise, 2020, 'The uses and misuses of television in long-stay psychiatric and "mental handicap" wards, 1950s–1980s', in Monika Ankele and Benoît Majerus (eds), *Material Cultures of Psychiatry* (Bielefeld: Transcript), pp. 186–201.

Hospital, 'Fair Mile Hospital, Wallingford: New admission unit', *Hospital* (January), 9–16.

Hughes, Jonathan Frederick Allan, 1996, 'The Brutal Hospital: Efficiency, Identity and Form in the National Health Service'. PhD thesis, Courtauld Institute of Art, University of London.

Jones, Kathleen, 1993, *Asylums and After: A Revised History of the Mental Health Services from the Early 18th Century to the 1990s* (London: Athlone Press).

Knoblauch, Joy, 2020, *The Architecture of Good Behavior: Psychology and Modern Institutional Design in Postwar America* (Pittsburgh, PA: University of Pittsburgh Press).

Lefebvre, Henri, 1991, *The Production of Space* (Malden, MA: Blackwell).

Llewelyn Davies, Richard, 1957, 'Deeper knowledge: Better design', *Architectural Record*, 121:4, 184–91.

Long, Vicky, 2017, '"Heading up a blind alley"? Scottish psychiatric hospitals in the era of deinstitutionalization', *History of Psychiatry*, 28:1 (March), 115–28. doi: 10.1177/0957154X16673025.

Majerus, Benoît, 2017, 'The straitjacket, the bed, and the pill: Material culture and madness', in Greg Eghigian (ed.), *The Routledge History of Madness and Mental Health* (London: Routledge), pp. 263–76.

Malathouni, Christina, 2020, 'Beyond the asylum and before the "care in the community" model: Exploring an overlooked early NHS mental health facility', *History of Psychiatry*, 31:4 (December), 455–69. doi: 10.1177/0957154X20945974.

McKeown, Thomas, 1958, 'The concept of a balanced hospital community', *Lancet*, 271:7023 (5 April), 701–4.

McLachlan, Gordon, 1992, *A History of the Nuffield Provincial Hospitals Trust 1940–1990* (London: Nuffield Trust).

Nuffield Provincial Hospitals Trust and the University of Bristol (NPHT), 1955, *Studies in the Functions and Design of Hospitals: Report of an Investigation* (London: Oxford University Press).

Powell, Kenneth, 2009, *Powell & Moya* (London: RIBA Publishing).

RHB(47)1, 1947, 'National Health Service: Regional Hospital Boards: General scope of their work and relationship to the Minister and others' [ministerial guidance circular], www.nuffieldtrust.org.uk/sites/default/files/2019-11/rhb-47-1.pdf (accessed 22 September 2023).

RHB(48)1, 1948, 'National Health Service: The development of specialist services (1948)' [ministerial circular: early planning document in the NHS], VIII: Mental Health Service, www.nuffieldtrust.org.uk/sites/default/files/2019-11/nhs-history-book/48-57/rhb481.html (accessed 22 September 2023).

RIBA Journal, 1957, 'New admission unit: Fair Mile Hospital, near Wallingford, Berkshire', *RIBA Journal* (May), 268–71.

Richardson, Harriet (ed.), 1998, *English Hospitals 1660–1948: A Survey of their Architecture and Design* (Swindon: Royal Commission on the Historical Monuments of England).

Rivett, Geoffrey, 2014, *From Cradle to Grave: The History of the NHS 1948–1987* (London: King's Fund). www.nuffieldtrust.org.uk/health-and-social-care-explained/the-history-of-the-nhs/ (accessed 7 August 2023).

Sammet, Kai, 2000, 'Silent "night of madness"? Light, voice, sounds and space in the Illenau Asylum in Baden between 1842 and 1910', in Monika Ankele and Benoît Majerus (eds), *Material Cultures of Psychiatry* (Bielefeld: Transcript), pp. 44–73.

Scull, Andrew, 1979, *Museums of Madness: The Social Organization of Insanity in Nineteenth Century England* (London: Allen Lane).

Soanes, Stephen, 2011, 'Rest and Restitution: Convalescence and the Mental Hospital in England, 1919–1939'. PhD thesis, University of Warwick.

Taylor, Jeremy, 1991, *Hospital and Asylum Architecture in England 1840–1914: Building for Health Care* (London: Mansell).

TenHoor, Meredith, 2019, 'State funded militant infrastructure? CERFI's *équipements collectifs* in the intellectual history of architecture', *Journal of Architecture*, 24:7, 999–1019. doi: 10.1080/13602365.2019.1698638.

Theodore, David, 2019, 'Treating architectural research: The Nuffield Trust and the post-war hospital', *Journal of Architecture*, 24:7, 982–98. doi: 10.1080/13602365.2019.1698640.

Topp, Leslie, 2007, 'The modern mental hospital in late nineteenth-century Germany and Austria: Psychiatric space and images of freedom and control', in Leslie Topp, James E. Moran and Jonathan Andrews (eds), *Madness, Architecture and the Built Environment: Psychiatric Spaces in Historical Context* (New York: Routledge), pp. 241–61.

Topp, Leslie, 2017, *Freedom and the Cage: Modern Architecture and Psychiatry in Central Europe, 1890–1914* (University Park, PA: Pennsylvania State University Press).

Topp, Leslie, James E. Moran and Jonathan Andrews (eds), 2007, *Madness, Architecture and the Built Environment: Psychiatric Spaces in Historical Context* (New York: Routledge).

Wheeler, Ian, 2015, *Fair Mile: A Victorian Asylum* (Stroud: The History Press).

II

Experimentation

5

Non-hierarchical experimentation: the outpatient treatment of drug-using young people in Finland, 1969–75

Katariina Parhi

In 1966, the social physician Lenni Lehtimäki described the drug scene in the capital city Helsinki by concluding that 'narcomania' in Finland was of 'luckily modest proportions', although he emphasised that it was important to monitor this phenomenon, which was also referred to as an 'epidemic disease' (Lehtimäki, 1966: 128). In the latter half of the 1960s, the extent of drug use in Finland changed significantly. The new drug scene was primarily young and experimental, emphasising psychoactive drugs, particularly cannabis (Hakkarainen, 1992; Salasuo, 2003). However, there was also a user segment that took drugs on a more regular basis (Kainulainen *et al.*, 2017; Parhi, 2021), and fear among the public that the phenomenon would spread was evident.

This chapter analyses the development of expertise in treating drug-using young people in the metropolitan area of Finland. The focus is on the role of psy-sciences[1] in new forms of outpatient care, which were situated on the border between social work and medicine. The main argument is that the psy-sciences exerted a major influence on drug treatment, but not directly. Instead, they were embedded in practices that stemmed from various sources, such as folk healing, the Mental Research Institute in the United States and therapeutic communities. The influence was also reciprocal; the subculture that influenced drug use internationally also influenced psy-sciences (e.g. Halliwell, 2013: 260–87; Richert, 2019).

Drug use in Helsinki proliferated earlier than in the provinces, which explains why it was also the main location for new treatment experiments. At the time, the drugs varied significantly; for example, according to a list collected by medical students in 1969–70, 156 different 'misused drugs' were found, grouped into analgesics, antihistamines, psychostimulants, antipsychotics, muscle relaxants, sedatives, cough medicines and others (Parhi, 2023). This chapter introduces two significant facilities: Arkadian (poli)klinikka (henceforth the Arkadia Clinic) and Nuorisoasema (henceforth the Youth Station), set up in 1969 and 1970 respectively. Both were popular among young people. For example, in 1970 alone, 1,207 clients attended the Arkadia Clinic, and the Youth Station reported 484 visits (*Tietoa huumausaineongelmaan*, 1972: 6). In 1976, these facilities were merged into one due to Arkadia's financial problems (Ahonen, 2005: 192–3). Around the same time, the number of drug-using people dropped. Finnish drug policy scholars refer to waves of drugs; the second wave emerged only in the latter half of the 1990s (Hakkarainen, 1992: 58–72; Partanen and Metso, 1999: 143–9).

This chapter builds on oral history sources, supported by archival data, research reports and published sources. The oral material consists of three semi-structured interviews with experts who witnessed and took part in developing treatment for young people aged between 13 and 25 in the 1960s and 1970s. Their own experiences have a focal role in the analysis – without trying to find the 'historical truth', these personal understandings of the past (see Haapala, 2021) are tied into a commentary on expertise and its formation through experimental practice. The interviewees would possibly not call themselves experts; they typically had their own ideological ways of defining their roles in drug treatment. In defining expert position, I follow the sociologists Michael Meuser and Ulrike Nagel, who define expertise as active participation. The status of an expert goes beyond the professional role and includes actors who acquire special knowledge through their actions because they have privileged access to information. The information is derived from structures of relevance – insider groups and networks (Meuser and Nagel, 2009: 18–31). The interpretation of expertise is rendered flexible by this definition, which is crucial in understanding drug treatment at the time. It also helps in rethinking drug treatment historiography, which tends to focus more on political and academic debates than on those working in the field and on the practices there.

The historian Johan Edman has characterised Swedish drug treatment from 1968 until 1981 as heterogeneous and as primarily an ideological rather than a therapeutic project (Edman, 2013). While this characterisation also relates to neighbouring Finland, the following sections exemplify how experimentality characterises Finnish drug treatment far more accurately. The first section introduces the facilities, the three interviewees and their professional positions. The second section analyses the variety of approaches in treating drug-using young people in the facilities. The third section focuses on the development of expertise through experience and sums up the perspectives adopted by the interviewees as most suitable for their work. Overall, the sections demonstrate processes of professionalisation and discuss expertise based on actions.

The original principles

Both facilities, the Youth Station and the Arkadia Clinic, were established as alternatives to traditional institutions, such as prisons, reform schools and mental hospitals, and were experimental from the outset. The idea was in line with the international process of deinstitutionalisation which assumed many forms (for Finland, see Korkeila, 1988), and applied to young people in particular as it was believed that those in need of the new services had been institutionalised earlier in their lives. The new services should thus be positive experiences in comparison to institutions, i.e. non-hierarchical. Medical expertise was needed in both facilities, but it was to be offered in a non-hierarchical way.

Despite the experimental nature of the facilities, establishing new forms of outpatient treatment was in line with state policies. From a legislative point of view, developing outpatient care was seen in a positive light, as both the Act on Public Welfare (Huoltoapulaki 116, 1956) and the Act on the Treatment and Care of Abusers of Intoxicating Substances (Laki päihdyttävien aineiden väärinkäyttäjien huollosta 96, 1961) encouraged the use of outpatient services. Since the 1930s, the national treatment of alcohol abuse had been based on social work. The operations can be characterised as strict social control (Rosenqvist and Stenius, 2014: 552). The Finnish 1961 Act on the Treatment and Care of Abusers of Intoxicating Substances used the term 'intoxication' to refer to the treatment of alcohol and drug problems. Drug users, who had had very few treatment options prior to the passing of the Act, were thus included under the same category as alcohol abusers. Even after the change, the number of treatment facilities for drug users was still scarce. Some experts by experience have confirmed this in interviews about their experiences in the 1960s and 1970s (Rönkä, 2017: 175–6). None of the existing facilities were geared specifically to young people, which is not surprising given that use among young people was rare. Before World War II, drug abuse in Finland had been uncommon in general (Ylikangas, 2009). Until the mid-1960s the total number of users remained low.

Throughout the 1960s, drug use increased internationally (e.g. Stephens, 2003; Marquis, 2005; Marchant, 2014), and the situation in Finland, too, gave rise to concern. On 14 April 1968, the Finnish government set up a committee to gather information about drugs and to find means for treatment and prevention. The committee believed that voluntary care would be more successful than 'official' forms of care in reaching drug-using young people and achieving results in their treatment, so it recommended increasing the voluntary treatment options and experimenting with novel methods. Among other suggestions, the committee recommended that the A-Clinic Foundation establish a youth station and a care home for recovering drug users (Committee on Narcotic Drugs, 1969: preface, 180–1). The A-Clinic changed the foundation's regulations to include young drug users, who were characterised as 'intoxicant abusers' (Ahonen, 2005: 185). The A-Clinic Foundation, founded in 1955, was and remains a non-profit, non-governmental organisation for the prevention of substance abuse. It differed from the strict social control characteristic of Finnish alcohol abuse treatment at the time, and instead it laid the foundation for therapeutic social work (Toikko, 2005: 183). The foundation's outpatient care was progressive and can be characterised as psychosocial, which meant focusing on the individual's psychological and social issues (Kuusisto and Ranta, 2020: 122–5). In 1970, the A-Clinic Foundation opened youth stations in various cities. The Helsinki Youth Station was an outpatient unit with sixteen beds for inhouse treatment.

One of the interviewees, Tapani Ahola, is a social psychologist who worked at and led the Youth Station from its beginning until the 1980s, initially while still a university student. Among the most important principles of the Youth Station Ahola mentioned was that it was not led by physicians – 'it was not medicalised in that sense' (Ahola, 2019). The Youth Station clients had the option to remain anonymous, and the station contacted family members or officials only with the client's consent. The aim in interaction between staff and clients was to create trusting relationships and provide information (*Medisiinari*, 1970: 5). According to the A-Clinic Foundation, young drug users perceived other existing services as 'alienating and undemocratic' (Mattila, 1970: 8–9). Dr Katriina Kuusi, the second interviewee from the Youth Station, was recruited to work as its physician in 1969. At the time, she was in her twenties and had qualified as a general practitioner. The Youth Station preferred general practitioners to psychiatrists (Sirén, 1977: 27–8).

Similarly to the Youth Station, the Arkadia Clinic, named after the street Arkadiankatu, where the first premises were located, was founded after alarmed discussions: the city officials in Helsinki had raised concerns about young people and their use of drugs. The Mannerheim League for Child Welfare, which was and remains an NGO promoting the wellbeing of children and their families, suggested organising first aid services for young drug users. The league recruited one of the interviewees, Aulis Junes, described in the clinic documents as a deacon and a social worker, to lead and plan the operations of the Arkadia Clinic. The Clinic was characterised by the league in 1969 as 'the first and unique experiment to help drug-abusing children and young people', up to twenty-five years of age. Among the early treatment strategies were training former substance users to work at the clinic, and operating as a 'non-hierarchical care community' that learned from experiences in the field.[2]

The Arkadia Clinic staff consisted of social workers, a psychiatrist, a general practitioner, a psychologist, and medical and psychology undergraduates. Despite the availability of medical expertise, no medical procedures were conducted at the clinic. If there was no risk of unconsciousness so hospitalisation was not necessary, the clients could sleep at Arkadia for one night, and the following day they got a chance to talk. The staff helped in contacting parents or officials, if needed.[3] The psychiatrist Dr Pekka Sävy characterised the role of the psy-sciences: 'The therapeutic work is done almost entirely by social workers and psychology undergraduates – the psychiatrist and psychologist acting only as consultants' (*sic*).[4] While leading the Arkadia Clinic, Aulis Junes opposed prescribing medicine: 'I did not want to medicalise the place', he recalled, and positioned himself in opposition to biological psychiatry. 'I said we don't write prescriptions, we heal people with the mind, not with drugs' (Junes, 2019).

Chaotic beginnings

Both facilities experienced a disorganised beginning. The problems concerned a lack of experience. According to a research report on the first year of the Youth Station, the staff were 'young and open-minded, but inexperienced', and got 'the opportunity for quite some time to independently, by trial and error, search for guidelines' (Sirén, 1977: 7). The staff felt that the situation was not entirely under control (Ahonen, 2005: 187–8). The interviewees Ahola and Kuusi confirmed this in their interviews: 'We had no fucking clue ... We took in everyone off the streets and then we started wondering [what to do]. It was total chaos', Ahola reminisced. He remembered a night shift when out of sixteen people staying in the care home of the Youth Station, twelve were tripping (Ahola, 2019). Kuusi elaborated the feeling of an uncontrolled beginning: 'We were too gullible.' Someone stole her expensive suede jacket and Kuusi believed it was sold or traded for drugs. Many people came by and, according to Kuusi, the staff did not know who was there for treatment and who was just hanging out. The open doors operated on a 'low threshold' basis so that it would be easy for anyone who came to ask for help. The staff did not test the clients for drugs enough. And some of the Youth Station inhabitants would suddenly disappear. The constant surprises sapped most of Kuusi's energy.

According to Kuusi, the group meetings, inspired by Maxwell Jones's idea of therapeutic communities, were chaotic. The rules at the Youth Station had been made together with the clients, and Kuusi thought in retrospect they were cruel. For example, others wanted to eject inhabitants who relapsed (Kuusi, 2019). According to the psychiatrist Matti Isohanni, therapeutic communities had been increasingly accepted in Finland since the 1960s after the psychiatrist Veikko Tähkä adopted ideas about therapeutic milieus from Austen Riggs in the United States at the beginning of that decade (Isohanni, 1983: 32–3), and since then they have continued as a form of drug treatment (e.g. Selin, 2010a). The Youth Station, however, was only learning how therapeutic communities worked.

The new staff received professional training before the Youth Station opened. According to Kuusi, at the time the ideology was that young people understand other young people (Kuusi, 2019). The average age of the employees was 24 (Sirén, 1977: 32). Initially there were thirteen employees, and the number grew to seventeen by the end of 1970. It is noteworthy that twelve people resigned during the first year (Sirén, 1977: 32–3). The theoretical training included lectures by experts in different fields, study visits, seminars, studying literature and introductions to various treatment models. The training also included practical training in existing institutions and organisations such as A-Clinics, the Arkadia Clinic and the Hesperia Hospital (Mattila, 1970: 8–9). According to Kuusi, she was trained for the job before the Youth Station was established, but in her opinion no one knew how young drug users should be treated. She recalled a demonstration of a therapy session as part of her training: 'It was pseudoanalysis, playing analytic therapy without proper training.' She remembered criticising how one should also talk about the drugs. Kuusi argued that the only thing she remembers from the training was how skilfully the patient in the demonstration, not even a drug user but a person with a history of alcoholism, spoke 'psy-language' (Kuusi, 2019). The expertise available in the form of professional guidance was of high quality, 'the best that was available in the country', Kuusi said, but in her view the problem was that even the experts – the psychoanalyst Pirkko Siltala and group and family therapist Heimo Salminen – did not know how to treat young drug users (Kuusi, 2019).

The use of prescribed drugs in the Youth Station was modest; some were used when the client was suffering from withdrawal symptoms or if the symptoms were psychotic. Mostly, the staff organised group meetings and private discussions. Kuusi remembered ideological differences. At first, the A-Clinic, which was responsible for the personnel training, was in favour of a psychotherapeutic approach. 'We tried to do family work, but no one at the time was trained for family therapy … We should have had firm structures for implementing it', she said (Kuusi, 2019). Family therapy was developed in the United States in the 1950s and 1960s. The core idea was to search for the source of pathology in family interaction (Weinstein, 2013: 2). According to the interviewee Tapani Ahola, the Youth Station initially tried to adopt the idea of homeostasis, which referred to the family dynamic in coping with addiction: when one family member got clean, another fell ill (Ahola, 2019). Originally, the concept of homeostasis had been used in connection with the ability of an organism to self-regulate, but the idea was used as a way to explain the family's internal environment, an inner capacity to register and counteract deviations (Weinstein, 2013: 52, 59–60). Ahola did not look back fondly on his memories about their homeostatic interpretations: 'It was awful. If I ask, why does your son take drugs, there is an indirect accusation in the question. Asking "why" produces an explanation that includes accusations – in practice' (Ahola, 2019). Ahola remembered how attempts were made to separate young people from their drug-taking peers, but he thought this should not be done by force: 'I quickly realised that their most important relationships were, well, they had families, but many of them came from broken homes. Their peer group is important at a certain age' (Ahola, 2019). In addition to paying attention to the importance of their peers, Ahola realised that daily routines were crucial: studying and working were efficient forms of social control. Some of the clients travelled in big Nordic cities such as Gothenburg or Copenhagen: 'They started living outside society, there was no control in a positive or negative way. It became absolutely crazy', Ahola recalled (Ahola, 2019).

During the first days of the Arkadia Clinic in April 1969, no one showed up; but when a local gang heard about it and spread the word, the facility soon became crowded. According to Arkadia Clinic reports, the operations were initially 'informal' and the employees hosted callers and served them tea and beef broth. Problems followed when the gang members started using the clinic as their regular base, and during the first summer there was also drug use on the premises. Some clients used the clinic as their base at night, borrowed money and drugs during the day, loitered on the beach, and then returned to the Clinic. In November the same year the staff made new, tighter rules, which significantly reduced the number of clients.[5]

The interviewee Aulis Junes saw himself as a folk healer and his approach at the Arkadia Clinic was what he understood to be folk healing. 'Folk healing' is the term Junes used at the time I interviewed him in 2019. His idea of folk healing, however, is in line with his views presented in the Arkadia Clinic records in the 1960s and 1970s: he emphasised a critical approach toward the psy-sciences, preferring presence, warmth and respect, which he associated with folk healers. The sociologists Meuser and Nagel refer to new forms of knowledge production that loosen the link between expert knowledge and the professional role. They refer to a development that has occurred since the 1960s, heading towards a growing scepticism regarding science (Meuser and Nagel, 2009: 20). Aulis Junes had a leading role in this perspective as he took an active part in public and among drug-using young people and was portrayed as an expert on problem youth. This expertise was also criticised. According to Junes, for many, he was too 'unorthodox' in his work (Junes, 2019). In the interview, Junes saw himself as antiauthoritarian – besides referring to himself as a folk healer, he also considered himself an anarchist. Junes's antiauthoritarian attitude was evident in the way he educated the clients. He compared himself to Socrates in Plato's park academy as he let the young people read psychiatric, psychoanalytic and cognitive literature. His idea was to avoid 'outsider consultants' and to work with other employees as a group. Junes emphasised how he wanted to avoid leadership. As an anarchist, as he underlined, he was inspired by Erich Fromm's interpretation of a strong ego. 'I did not want to be an authority at the clinic. If someone with a powerful ego like myself, a narcissist, is an opinion leader, he will soon be wearing jackboots, jodhpurs and a cheesecutter cap, and raising his arm in salute' (Junes, 2019). Junes thought that his recruits – former alcoholics and drug users – were experts in interacting with the young people. He juxtaposed medical expertise and expertise through experience: 'I took an old skid row alcoholic to work as a janitor … He had been sober for two years already. He was extremely good, like a grandfather there … He was so calm. An outsider asked if he was the clinic doctor? I said yes, kind of' (Junes, 2019).

In the course of time, the Arkadia Clinic introduced new activities, including summer camps, peer counsellors in schools as a preventative measure, an outpatient centre for clients and their families, guidance on finding accommodation, a group home, and field social work for young people who needed help but did not come to the clinic.[6]

In addition, the Arkadia Clinic had a sobering up or detoxification station. Although some of the Arkadia Clinic experiments were less successful than others, the Clinic psychiatrist Pekka Sävy did not perceive the experimental method in a negative light in 1970: 'Nobody had any experiences of treating these young abusers of new drugs in Finland. Old methods were inadequate. Models of functioning in other countries were probably not valid in Finland. The personnel had to start experimenting without prejudice by using flexibly the trial and error method' (*sic*). Even more so, Sävy deemed it a necessity: 'The experimental aspect is important because it gives us fresh and direct information about the out-patient treatment of drug abusers. Maybe private institutions are best: they are allowed to make mistakes and learn from them whereas government authorities don't even know that such process exists, mistakes are not allowed, that is admitted' (*sic*).[7]

Learning by doing

As the staff gained more experience of young people and gathered more information about ways to help them, they found new approaches which worked well for them. Katriina Kuusi's experience at the Youth Station may have been troubling for her, but around the same time she became increasingly interested in democratic communities, which were inspired by antipsychiatry. Already in 1970, Kuusi started to work part-time in Veikkola, which was a private psychiatric hospital that was also known for taking in drug-using young people. After a while, Kuusi was offered a full-time job there, and she left the Youth Station in 1971. Based on her article on youth in treatment, published in 1972, it seems that Kuusi preferred Veikkola's heterogeneous sample of patients, as she criticised communities with patients based on one symptom or characteristic: 'No one is just "young" or an "alcoholic". Instead, there are a lot more important common characteristics between individuals' (Kuusi, 1972: 122).

Kuusi admitted retrospectively that she escaped from the Youth Station when she got a chance to work full time in Veikkola. The Youth Station left its mark: 'For some years after the Youth Station experience, when I passed the place on the bus, I felt uneasy in my

stomach. It was rough' (Kuusi, 2019). Kuusi compared the inexperi-
ence of the Youth Station to the more experienced staff in Veikkola.
According to her, some social workers in the Youth Station came
straight from university with no experience of working life. Moreover,
she thinks that Veikkola also had more authority than the newly
founded Youth Station because it was a private hospital, and hospitals
as such were organisations with long, respected traditions. 'Health
care enjoys a much higher status in our society than social care, it
makes no sense to claim otherwise!' Kuusi concluded (Kuusi, 2019).

For Katriina Kuusi, her work experience in Veikkola sanatorium
was a significant phase in her life: 'We felt we were part of an
international reform movement, that gave us more energy, that we
have to do something about hospital democracy in Finland' (Kuusi,
2019). Veikkola sanatorium evoked interest in international spheres
and Kuusi remembered visitors such as Thomas Szasz, the Italian
psychiatrist Franco Basaglia and David Cooper. According to Kuusi,
Basaglia's work in the Gorizia asylum[8] was of particular inspiration
to her and the physician-in-chief Claes Andersson. The main idea
in Veikkola was to have a democratic community. The treatment
included compulsory meetings, groups and family meetings. Kuusi
was particularly proud that the first patient association was established
in Veikkola (Kuusi, 2019). Since the 1970s, Kuusi has had a long
career as a psychiatrist and family therapist (Kuusi, 2019).

Tapani Ahola continued working in the Youth Station, but he
adopted the principles of brief therapy, an approach that focuses
on the present. Frykman was close to Milton H. Erickson, an
influential psychiatrist and psychologist, referred to as the father of
modern clinical hypnosis and known to have influenced brief therapy,
solution-focused brief therapy and neurolinguistic programming
(Gorton, 2005). Frykman had been the founding director of the
drug treatment programme in Haight Ashbury Free Clinic in San
Francisco, California. During his visit to Helsinki, Frykman described
his methods and thus introduced Ahola to brief therapy (Ahola and
Furman, 2014: 21–2). This is how Ahola learned more about the
Mental Research Institute and its form of family therapy, which
differed from homeostasis. Ahola was fascinated by the Institute's
take on problems: 'They studied what people do when they successfully solve problems. Not what causes them' (Ahola, 2019).
Brief therapy training began in the 1980s and Ahola was one of its

significant advocates. His brief therapy institute Lyhytterapiainstitu-utti, founded in 1986, has also published a version of *Uncommon Therapy: The Psychiatric Techniques of Milton H. Erickson, M.D.* (Haley, 2016) translated into Finnish.

Ahola perceived brief therapy as an alternative to psychodynamic therapy: 'The most common model to solve problems has been causal-linear thinking: problems have been explained by other problems. If you take drugs, they study what other problems you have. In the 1960s, we had this psychoanalytic, psychodynamic thinking.' Brief therapy did not focus on problems: 'They never ask, if you go to their appointment ... "what is your problem?". They ask, "what would be a good result from this conversation?" There is a wish to change built into every problem.' And life could be good without long-term therapy, which could help some people, but not enough: 'Even when people do stupid things, there is the goal of a good life in the background, and they have the right to it' (Ahola, 2019).

Ahola was critical in the interview of psychiatric treatment of drug problems: 'Traditional psychiatry cannot cope with substance users and asocial ones. The system, the psychiatric hospital system, does not work, it breaks down.' He characterised psychoanalytic psychotherapy as a pessimistic way of thinking, which he associated with incompetence: 'When I started doing brief therapy, I bragged about it at the psychiatric clinic. When they said there are hopeless cases, I said bullshit, there are no hopeless cases, only hopeless employees. They said they have such clients and I said, send them to me, I'll take care of them' (Ahola, 2019).

The Arkadia Clinic legacy as the pioneer of youth drug treatment is evident because various city and child guidance officials recognised its importance in documents preserved among the Arkadia Clinic records. At the same time, Junes's contrary character seems to have hampered the reputation. In December 1975, Aulis Junes defended the Arkadia model. He characterised it at that time as a 'treatment chain including a detoxification station and an outpatient clinic, attached to the contact centre, group spaces, operations for acquiring a home, and to the youth hotel'.[9] According to Junes, the most important aspect of the treatment chain was that there were employees acting at different stages of the chain, creating long-lasting relation-ships. Junes characterised young drug users as people with many problems. These people had experienced setbacks in their social and emotional lives, and they had often had short-term relationships, exacerbated by periods of institutionalisation. Yet Junes proclaimed that drug treatment should not be seen as psychiatric or clinical. 'Drug use is not an artificially induced drive that is so powerful it overcomes the sexual drive, as some doctors claim. It is not an independent and separate problem or a contagious illness that anyone can get'.[10] Despite his criticism, Junes perceived the psychiatric guidance of work to be necessary because it offered the 'needed theoretical ground for the outpatient clinic'. Polyclinic procedures without coercion and fear of punishment were essential in drug treatment.[11]

In his interview, Junes stated that his method was to ask what the person wanted to talk about. He believed that solving problems in therapy was a mistake. 'When they started telling me I have this kind of problem, I used to say, that is not a problem. What you have deep down in your childhood and youth rises to the surface over time, for either good or ill.' He wanted to save children from their parents, teachers and professional helpers, and be a sensible adult in finding the right way. When the child found the right path, it was his turn to step back. 'In folk healing, the human being is seen as a whole. Instead of diagnosing the client, it is crucial to listen which concepts the client uses, and what the client thinks about life and its troubles, and his or her family, mother, and father', Junes explained. He was reluctant to 'rummage in people's mouldy cellars', by which he meant going over past events: 'There is no yesterday, no one knows about tomorrow, we only have this day' (Junes, 2019). Junes referred to the healing persona of the therapist, by which he meant a warm and humane ability to care for others, which was based on the parents' and grandparents' care in childhood (Junes, 2019).

The Mannerheim League for Child Welfare ceased to fund the Arkadia Clinic in 1976. The primary reason was financial, as the clinic had originally been designed as an experiment, and it became much more expensive than the Mannerheim League for Child Welfare had planned. However, the Clinic records also contain some hints of disputes. For example, the city of Helsinki criticised the Clinic for not having sufficient control over its operations, and there were challenges in collaboration between the various officials providing help for young people.[12] In another meeting, the staff talked about different collaboration options. A willingness to do so was reported among the employees, but 'the differences of opinion among the directors and their desire to stay at the forefront were detrimental to co-operation in the field'.[13] Tapani Ahola recalled Junes as an uncooperative character (Ahola, 2019). Junes was unwilling to compromise, and he admitted it: 'In this unorthodox work of mine, I am a hate individual, I do not hate anyone, but I am Socrates' soulmate. I do not want to adjust in this civilisation in any way, and yet I will not drink the poisoned chalice' (Junes, 2019). Junes dedicated his life to working with young people – for example, he was one of the founders of Aseman Lapset (Children of the Station), a non-profit organisation aimed at promoting the well-being of children and young people.

Conclusion

This chapter has been a case study about two new and experimental outpatient facilities that focused on young people, a new user segment that emerged in Finland in the latter half of the 1960s. Influenced by the process of deinstitutionalisation, the new Finnish substance use-related legislation and international approaches, these facilities sought new ways to deal with the new drug user segment. The approaches in both facilities, the Youth Station and the Arkadia Clinic, were influenced by the psy-sciences. On the one hand, both facilities exemplify processes in which psychiatry was embedded in social work. On the other hand, the role of psychiatry in Finnish treatment of young drug users in the 1960s and 1970s was limited in daily practice.

The reminiscences of the interviewees extend and challenge the history of Finnish drug treatment by bringing to the fore three aspects about expertise in this field. First, if the definition of expertise in the field was based on expert appearances in public, the role of medical expertise would seem more influential and straightforward, as certain medical experts were active and significant in public debates, including disputes in the Finnish parliament (Hakkarainen, 1990: 294–8; Putkonen and Parhi, 2019: 636–7). As this chapter demonstrates, the role of medical expertise was more diffuse in daily work, and social work had a significant role. The psy-sciences were, however, more significant in the social services field than is apparent in contemporary Finnish journals of social work and social care (see Rosenqvist and Stenius, 2014). Rather than seeing the history of drug treatment expertise as a competition for power between the two, my interpretation is closer to what the historian Greg Eghigian has termed a 'collaborative enterprise' (Eghigian, 2011: 210).

Second, if expertise was based on publications, the treatment of drug-using young people would look different. The sociologist Jani Selin has researched theories about drug use in Finnish medical publications in the 1960s and 1970s. According to Selin, psychodynamic psychiatry had a focal role in explaining drug use and addiction, and the emphasis was on the role of the family and childhood trauma as the main causes for use (Selin, 2010b: 253–5). This perspective is far from everyday treatment practice. The facilities did not focus on ascertaining the causes of drug use. On the contrary, they developed and adopted treatment methods that were based on the present moment, not the past. The interviewees all referred to the pervasive influence of the psychodynamic approach in treatment for drug addiction at the time, but in practice, not many young people encountered psychodynamic treatment. One of the interviewees, Tapani Ahola, characterised the situation as follows: 'These asocial young people, only a fraction of them is in the hands of youth psychiatry. They are in institutions!' (Ahola, 2019). By institutions, Ahola meant prisons, children's homes, and former reform schools – the very places that were seen to create the need for something different and new.

Third, the definition of expertise changed in the 1960s and 1970s. For example, Finnish physicians started discussing their hierarchical position, and the attitude toward patients gradually changed from authoritarian to more empathetic. The change was in general slow, but the field of drug addiction treatment appealed to the so-called radicals. The discussion was led by a small but vociferous minority (Aalto, 2010a, 2010b), which was also interested in the treatment of marginal groups (see Parhi and Myllykangas, 2019). The definition of expertise was in flux and the change paved the way to different kinds of professional roles. There were also structural predispositions that enabled the gaining of expertise through experimentation. Welfare scholars Pia Rosenqvist and Kerstin Stenius have commented on the increased role of the medical perspective in understanding the drug problem since the 1990s. They compare the small Finnish welfare system of the 1960s to the mature version in the 1990s: in the 1960s, there was a general social and political mobilisation, which was conducive to open debate. By the 1990s, the welfare system had become conservative and difficult to change. This, among more obvious causes such as the medical expertise needed in opioid substitution treatment, strengthened the weight of medical expertise (Rosenqvist and Stenius 2014: 565). Another aspect that enabled experimental methods in the 1960s and 1970s was related, as Johan Edman and Kerstin Stenius have pointed out, to the social democratic welfare state: there was a general belief in structural solutions to social problems (Edman and Stenius 2013). Drug-related expertise was and is political. The sociologist Tuukka Tammi has problematised expertise in drug policy because different professions and interest groups aim to increase their power to promote the drug policies they support – Tammi refers to the 'ownership' of drug problems (Tammi, 2005). There are many layers of expertise in connection with the treatment of drug use: more recently, users have also been recognised as experts (Tammi, 2006; Mold and Berridge, 2008).

Overall, this chapter has shown that the Arkadia Clinic and the Youth Station in the 1960s and 1970s were both significant pioneers in the development of new treatment methods, and their approaches were unprecedented in the era. The experimental nature of the facilities was both a strength and a weakness: they experienced chaos, but at the same time seem to have thrived on it, as they managed to develop methods and practices that the interviewees were pleased with and have since then used in their work with children and young people.

Notes

1 Psychiatry, psychology, psychotherapy and psychoanalysis.
2 The National Archives of Finland, Helsinki, Mannerheimin Lastensuo-jeluliiton arkisto II, Arkadian poliklinikka (hereafter NA), S23/274, Perustamisvaiheet, 22 October 1969, pp. 1–4.
3 NA, S23/276, Arkadian poliklinikan toimintasuunnitelma, 30 April 1969, pp. 1–2.
4 NA, S23/276, Memo by Pekka Sävy, Arkadia Clinic for young drug abusers in Finland, 13 April 1970, p. 3.

5   NA, S23/274, Memo by Eeva Kaivamo, Kartoitus Arkadian poliklinikan asiakkaista klinikan raporttien pohjalta vuonna 1969, 25 March 1970, pp. 1–4.
6   NA, S23/274, Toimintakertomus v. 1974, n.d., pp. 1–7.
7   NA, S23/276, Memo by Pekka Sävy, 'Arkadia Clinic for young drug abusers in Finland', 13 April 1970, p. 5.
8   Cf. the contribution by Marica Setaro in Chapter 2.
9   NA, S23/274, Memo by Aulis Junes, Unnamed document, 1 December 1975, p. 1.
10 *Ibid.*
11 NA, S23/276, Memo by Aulis Junes, Lasten ja nuorten avohoitoklinikkatoiminta / Arkadian nuorisoklinikka, 1 August 1972, p. 2.
12 NA, S23/275, Arkadian nuorisoklinikan johtokunnan kokous, 11 September 1974, p. 4.
13 NA, S23/275, Pöytäkirja n:o 1/74 Mannerheimin lastensuojeluliiton Arkadian nuorisoklinikan johtokunnan kokouksesta, 11 September 1974, 9 §, p. 2.

References

Aalto, Sari, 2010a, 'Lääketieteen opiskelijayhteisö ja radikaalit medisiinarit', in Samu Nyström (ed.), *Vapaus, terveys, toveruus: Lääkärit Suomessa 1910–2010* (Hämeenlinna: Suomen Lääkäriliitto ry.), pp. 103–9.

Aalto, Sari, 2010b, 'Lääkärikunnan yhtenäisyys lujilla: Murroksen ja politisoitumisen vuodet', in Samu Nyström (ed.), *Vapaus, terveys, toveruus: Lääkärit Suomessa 1910–2010* (Hämeenlinna: Suomen Lääkäriliitto ry.), pp. 110–18.

Ahola, Tapani, 2019, Interview by Katariina Parhi, Helsinki, 14 August (author's translation from Finnish to English).

Ahola, Tapani and Ben Furman, 2014, *Juonia juopoille: Ratkaisukeskeinen lähestymistapa päihdeongelmiin* (Helsinki: Lyhytterapiainstituutti).

Ahonen, Jukka, 2005, *Päihdehuoltoa rakentamassa: A-klinikkasäätiö 1955–2005* (Jyväskylä: A-klinikkasäätiön julkaisusarja nro 51).

Committee on Narcotic Drugs, 1969, *Huumausainekomitean mietintö*, Komiteanmietintö, B 53 (Helsinki: Sosiaali- ja terveysministeriö).

Edman, Johan, 2013, 'Red cottages and Swedish virtues: Swedish institutional drug treatment as an ideological project 1968–1981', *Social History of Medicine*, 26:3, 510–31.

Edman, Johan and Kerstin Stenius, 2013, 'Conceptual carpentry as problemhandling: The case of drugs and coercive treatment in social democratic welfare regimes', *International Journal of Drug Policy*, 25:2, 320–8.

Eghigian, Greg, 2011, 'Deinstitutionalizing the history of contemporary psychiatry', *History of Psychiatry*, 22:2, 201–14.

Gorton, Gregg E., 2005, 'Milton Hyland Erickson, 1901–1980', *American Journal of Psychiatry*, 162:7, 1255.

Haapala, Pertti, 2021, 'Lived historiography: National history as a script to the past', in Ville Kivimäki, Sami Suodenjoki and Tanja Vahtikari (eds), *Lived Nation as the History of Experiences and Emotions in Finland, 1800–2000* (Cham: Palgrave Macmillan), pp. 29–57. https://doi.org/10.1007/978-3-030-69882-9_2.

Hakkarainen, Pekka, 1990, 'Hoito vai rangaistus?: Käytön kriminalisointikeskustelu vuoden 1972 huumausainelain eduskuntakäsittelyssä', in Osmo Kivinen (ed.), *Muutoksen pysyvyys: Sosiologisia näkökulmia yhteiskuntaan* (Turku: Turun yliopisto), pp. 277–301.

Hakkarainen, Pekka, 1992, *Suomalainen huumekysymys: Huumausaineiden yhteiskunnallinen paikka Suomessa toisen maailmansodan jälkeen* (Helsinki: Alkoholitutkimussäätiö).

Haley, Jay, 2016, *Lyhytterapian lähteillä: Milton H. Ericksonin terapeuttiset menetelmät* (Espoo: Lyhytterapiainstituutti).

Halliwell, Martin, 2013, *Therapeutic Revolutions: Medicine, Psychiatry, and American Culture, 1945–1970* (New Brunswick, NJ: Rutgers University Press).

Isohanni, Matti, 1983, *The Psychiatric Ward as a Therapeutic Community* (Oulu: University of Oulu).

Junes, Aulis, 2019, Interview by Katariina Parhi, Helsinki, 14 August (author's translation from Finnish to English).

Kainulainen, Heini, Jenni Savonen and Sanna Rönkä (eds), 2017, *Vanha liitto: Kovien huumeiden käyttäjät 1960–1970-lukujen Helsingistä* (Helsinki: SKS).

Korkeila, Jyrki, 1988, *Perspectives on the Public Psychiatric Services in Finland: Evaluating the Deinstitutionalisation Process* (Helsinki: Stakes).

Kuusi, Katriina, 1972, 'Nuoret hoidossa', in *Psykoterapeuttinen Aikakauskirja* 2 (Helsinki: Therapeia-säätiö), pp. 120–40.

Kuusi, Katriina, 2019, Interview by Katariina Parhi, Helsinki, 22 March (author's translation from Finnish to English).

Kuusisto, Katja and Johanna Ranta, 2020, 'Psykososiaalisen päihdetyön asema Suomessa 1900-luvulta nykypäivään', in Johanna Moilanen, Johanna Annola and Mirja Satka (eds), *Sosiaalityön käänteet* (Jyväskylä: SoPhi), pp. 112–40.

Lehtimäki, Lenni, 1966, 'Narkomaniasta Suomessa', *Alkoholikysymys*, 34:3, 119–28.

Marchant, Alexandre, 2014, 'When "drugs" become "drugs": Issues of pharmaceutical abuse in France from the 1960s to the 1990s', *Medicina nei secoli arte e scienza*, 26:2, 557–96.

Marquis, Greg, 2005, 'From beverage to drug: Alcohol and other drugs in 1960s and 1970s Canada', *Journal of Canadian Studies*, 39:2, 57–79.

Mattila, Pirkko, 1970, 'Nuorisoasemien henkilökunnan koulutus', *Tiimi*, 6:1, 8–9.

Medisiinari, 'Nuorisoasemat toimivat', 1970, *Medisiinari*, 1, 5.

Meuser, Michael and Ulrike Nagel, 2009, 'The expert interview and changes in knowledge production', in Alexander Bogner, Beate Littig and Wolfgang Menz (eds), *Interviewing Experts* (Basingstoke: Palgrave Macmillan), pp. 17–42.

Mold, Alex and Victoria Berridge, 2008, '"The rise of the user?": Voluntary organizations, the state and illegal drugs in England since the 1960s', *Drugs: Education, Prevention, and Policy*, 15:5, 451–61.

Parhi, Katariina, 2021, 'No coming back to sick society: The emergence of new drug user segment in the Järvenpää Social Hospital in Finland, 1965–1975', *Journal of the History of Medicine and Allied Sciences*, 76:4, 417–39.

Parhi, Katariina, 2023, *Saadaan vähän kamaa: Suomen ensimmäinen huumeaalto ja hoidon pioneerit* (Helsinki: Gaudeamus).

Parhi, Katariina and Mikko Myllykangas, 2019, 'Liberating the deviants: How to change the politics of social control – a case study from Finland, 1967–1971', in Petteri Pietikäinen and Jesper Vaczy Kragh (eds), *Social Class and Mental Illness in Northern Europe* (London: Routledge), pp. 194–213.

Partanen, Juha and Leena Metso, 1999, 'Suomen toinen huumeaalto', *Yhteiskuntapolitiikka*, 64:2, 143–9.

Putkonen, Hanna and Katariina Parhi, 2019, 'Lääkärit ja puoli vuosisataa suomalaista huumepolitiikkaa', *Yhteiskuntapolitiikka*, 84:5–6, 635–9.

Richert, Lucas, 2019, *Break on Through: Radical Psychiatry and the American Counterculture* (Cambridge, MA: MIT Press).

Rönkä, Sanna, 2017, '"Kaikki oli ihan keltasii": Pistämisestä ja yliannostuksista', in Heini Kainulainen, Jenni Savonen and Sanna Rönkä (eds), *Vanha liitto: Kovien huumeiden käyttäjät 1960–1970-lukujen Helsingistä* (Helsinki: SKS), pp. 159–78.

Rosenqvist, Pia and Kerstin Stenius, 2014, 'Medicalisation of the social perspective: Changing conceptualisations of drug problems in Finnish social care and substance abuse treatment', *Nordic Studies on Alcohol and Drugs*, 31:5–6, 551–68.

Salasuo, Mikko, 2003, 'Tajunnan kumous: Ensimmäinen huumeaalto', in Matti Peltonen, Vesa Kurkela and Visa Heinonen (eds), *Arkinen kumous: Suomalaisen 60-luvun toinen kuva* (Helsinki: Suomalaisen Kirjallisuuden Seura), pp. 84–109.

Selin, Jani, 2010a, 'Kansalaisuuden tuottaminen yhteisöllisissä huumehoidoissa', in Jani Kaisto and Miikka Pyykkönen (eds), *Hallintavalta: Sosiaalisen, politiikan ja talouden kysymyksiä* (Helsinki: Gaudeamus), pp. 213–29.

Selin, Jani, 2010b, 'Lääketiede, huumeriippuvuus ja huumeriippuvuuden hoito Suomessa 1965–2005', *Sosiaalilääketieteellinen Aikakauslehti*, 47, 250–67.

Sirén, Pirkko, 1977, *Nuorisoasema päihteitä käyttävien nuorten hoitoyhteisönä*, Alkoholipoliittisen tutkimuslaitoksen tutkimusseloste n:o 111 (Helsinki: Alkoholipoliittisen tutkimuslaitoksen).

Stephens, Robert, 2003, 'Drug use and youth consumption in West Germany during the 1960s', *Journal for Cultural Research*, 7:2, 107–24.

Tammi, Tuukka, 2005, 'Diffusion of public health views on drug policy: The case of needle-exchange in Finland', in Tommi Hoikkala, Pekka Hakkarainen and Sofia Laine (eds), *Beyond Health Literacy: Youth Cultures, Prevention and Policy* (Helsinki: Finnish Youth Research Network), pp. 185–99.

Tammi, Tuukka, 2006, 'Who is the expert? Patient groups and Finnish substitution treatment policy', in Jørgen Anker, Vibeke Asmussen, Petra Kouvonen and Dolf Tops (eds), *Drug Users and Spaces for Legitimate Action* (Helsinki: NAD Publications), pp. 23–35.

Tietoa huumausaineongelmaan: Lapsiraportti A6, 1972 (Helsinki: Mannerheimin Lastensuojeluliitto).

Toikko, Timo, 2005, *Sosiaalityön ideat: Johdatus sosiaalityön historiaan* (Jyväskylä: Vastapaino).

Weinstein, Deborah, 2013, *The Pathological Family: Postwar America and the Rise of Family Therapy* (Ithaca, NY: Cornell University Press).

Ylikangas, Mikko, 2009, *Unileipää, kuolonvettä, spiidiä: Huumeet Suomessa 1800–1950* (Jyväskylä: Atena).

6

Last resort or early intervention: discourse and practice of psychosurgery in Strasbourg (late 1940s to early 1960s)

Florent Serina

As of 2024, almost ninety years have passed since the foundational experiences of modern psychosurgery, and seventy-five years from the peak of these practices, which led to some of the the most lively controversies in the history of psychiatry.[1] The surgical treatment of mental pathologies is often considered a highly problematic method, mostly because of its side effects, generally irreversible, on the cognitive capacities or personality of the treated individuals, the lack of clarity of its results, and the questionable value of the arguments and scientific data supporting the interventions. Although it has been seen as a prime symbol of punitive psychiatry and has been outlawed for several decades in many countries such as Germany and Japan, and several USA states, psychosurgery is not formally prohibited by law in some European countries such as Sweden, Great Britain, Spain and France.[2] Moreover, it seems to have benefitted from the resurgence of interest in neurosurgery, sometimes described as 'spectacular', since the advent of deep brain stimulation (Lévêque, 2014; Lévêque and Cabut, 2017). The apparent exhaustion of the postulates and hopes initially raised by psychopharmacology, the decline of psychoanalysis, the continuous development of neurosciences, the highlighting of brain connections and the emergence of neo-localisationist conceptions seem to support the notion of new brain interventions. As the current context seems more favourable than ever to a re-emergence of invasive practices, though not without provoking heated debates (Bottéro, 2005; Benabid, 2006; Parada,

2016), the development of historical studies on the topic seems particularly welcome. This applies especially to the Francophone context, where historians have until this point shown relatively little interest in this contentious and thorny topic.[3]

The present chapter aims to give an overall account of the history of psychosurgical practices at the Strasbourg Psychiatric University Clinic, regarded as the central university hospital service in the mental healthcare system of north-eastern France. This case study traces the modalities of its introduction after an initial period of reluctance, its progressive routinisation, the spectrum of its indications and contraindications, as well as its gradual abandonment. Methodologically, this research first consisted of collecting all the medical records of the patients concerned in order to form a database allowing a detailed reconstruction of the range of psychosurgical practices implemented. The results were obtained by comparing this database with the content of all the publications of the practitioners of Strasbourg psychosurgery in order to highlight possible divergences, paradoxes, and even contradictions between their discourse and their practices (Risse and Warner, 1992). In other words, this chapter intends to uncover and report on the history of the surgical treatment of mental pathologies, at a time when it was regarded as revolutionary and potentially effective, by providing solid numerical data as well as a critical account of the main principles, whether explicit or implicit, guiding its practical implementation for just over a decade.

A progressive lifting of reticence

Unlike in neighbouring Italy (Kotowicz, 2008), the idea that mental illnesses were due to an organic cause, located in the brain, which could be eliminated by surgery, did not provoke immediate euphoria within the French medical community. In 1936, Egas Moniz (1874–1955), who supervised the first twenty 'leukotomies'[4] in Lisbon, went to Paris to present the results of his experiments before the Académie nationale de médecine (Moniz, 1936a). The Portuguese neurologist, who had done part of his studies at the Salpêtrière, was no doubt hoping for support from his peers. Although the majority gave a cold welcome to his presentation (Parada, 2016: 31–7), some Strasbourg physicians seem to have paid favourable attention to it, as Moniz was invited to publish his paper in the *Strasbourg Médical* (Moniz, 1936b), the main Alsatian medical journal. This publication certainly owes more to René Leriche (1877–1955), the inventor of the concept of non-aggressive surgery, thanks to which the Strasbourg surgical clinic gained an international reputation,[5] than to the director of the psychiatric clinic at that time, Charles Pfersdorff (1875–1953) who arguably remained refractory towards psychosurgery.

At first, only Gaston Ferdière (1907–90), medical director of the agricultural colony of Chezal-Benoît for chronic psychiatric patients, tried to replicate Moniz's experiment, at the Issoudun hospital in central France on a case of 'catatonic schizophrenia' (Vernet *et al.*, 2021), though not without incurring the wrath of his colleagues. This intervention remained the only psychosurgical operation made public in France until the mid-1940s. It was only after World War II, and quite gradually, that several other French teams tried to reproduce Moniz's experiments, which by that point were increasingly being practised in North and Central America (Parada, 2016: 41–8). At that time, the hope of being able to heal mentally ill people was more prevalent than ever. The thesis of incurability had been questioned since the appearance of malaria therapy for the treatment of progressive paralysis and the development of other shock therapies. However, while electroshock therapy was becoming prominent at that time, the perceived potential of cardiazol and insulin therapies began to wane markedly. Against this background, psychosurgery aroused a renewed general optimism despite its potential dangers. Strasbourg could not remain cautious for long in the face of what appeared to be a major trend and groundswell spreading throughout the Western world and beyond. Despite its controversial character, the Strasbourg psychiatrists were forced to ask themselves whether all or part of the future of the treatment of mental illness might not lie in the mastery of this practice.

Maintain one's rank

Exhausted by the war years, Pfersdorff resigned in 1945, shortly after his return to Strasbourg.[6] Eugène Gelma (1882–1953) succeeded him as director, carrying out a series of remarkable transformations.

Whereas diagnoses were previously based primarily on Kraepelinian nosology, the new director, formerly trained in Paris, made a breakthrough by introducing the diagnostic categories promoted by his French counterparts (such as the 'brief delusional disorder' of Magnan, the 'chronic hallucinatory psychosis' of Ballet, the 'interpretative delusions' of Sérieux and Capgras, and the 'psychasthenia' of Janet).[7] And despite his advanced age, Gelma was more open to therapeutic innovations than his predecessor. He immediately advocated the use of insulin therapy and made electroshock therapy routine practice. Gelma felt that the clinic had to keep up with the times and had no interest in ignoring the potential of the 'surgery of madness'. Thus, his establishment would not miss the boat by rejecting these rapidly expanding techniques at the cutting edge of scientific modernity. Indeed, in his view the prestige of academia, drawn in part from research and experiments, may have also depended in part on the mastery of psychosurgery and the recognition of their excellence in the field.

First, Gelma suggested that a student devote her thesis to 'leukotomy' (Gross-Offenstein, 1949). However, this work, based on the observation of patients operated on at the hospital in Rouffach (Haut-Rhin), was somewhat cautious and refrained from arguing in favour of, or making generalisations about the efficacy of, the operation. Gelma also reached an agreement with René Fontaine (1899–1979), director of the surgical clinic and former student of Leriche, to allow patients to undergo this treatment in Strasbourg as well. Gelma and Fontaine chose Demetre Philippidès (1907–99) and Adrien Dany (1918–2008) as surgeons. To this end, the latter was sent to Lyon to be introduced to psychosurgical techniques by Pierre Wertheimer (1892–1982), another student of Leriche, trained by the two leading figures of American psychosurgery, James W. Watts and Walter Freeman. Gelma also solicited one of his most promising interns, Léonard Singer (1923–2009), a former extern of Fontaine's department, to prepare a thesis on the interventions carried out within the clinic (Singer, 1951).[8] Strasbourg's first 'leukotomy' appears to have been performed in January 1948 on a 28-year-old woman diagnosed with 'schizophrenia'.[9] A few months later, Gelma's team, often in collaboration with colleagues from the Lorquin hospital (Moselle), began to take part in more talks and publish more articles on the topic. Within three years, they published a dozen papers in their in-house journal *Cahiers de Psychiatrie* and in nationwide journals, in which they praised the advantages of the treatment method.[10] Patients once considered incurable and condemned to confinement for the rest of their lives could now leave hospital to reintegrate with their families, parents could care for their children, women could care for their households, and men could return to work or find gainful employment for the first time. This was at least the earnest belief shared by Gelma and his team, who still asserted emphatically in 1953 that the rejection of psychosurgery would be 'an anti-medical stance' undermining the successes they had achieved to that point (Dany *et al.*, 1953: 553).

Diagnostic and technical assessment

In May 1953, Dany, Singer and Boittelle put forward the figure of 163 patients operated on before the end of 1952 (Dany *et al.*, 1953: 551). If one subtracts six cases of 'cancer patients with pains', and adds four other patients operated on before Kammerer took charge of the clinic, the total number of patients operated on during Gelma's directorship comes to 161. This makes up 3 per cent of the total number of patients admitted between 1948 and 1953. This first group of patients was mainly composed of individuals of French nationality living in the region. Among them, males made up a majority (59.5 per cent male and 40.5 per cent female). The youngest was a 6-year-old boy; the oldest was a man aged 65. Thirteen of them were underage, of which two were girls; nine were diagnosed with 'schizophrenia', one with 'epilepsy', one with 'depression', one with 'hysteria' and one with 'psychological retardation'. The vast majority of adult patients were single, divorced or widowed (70 per cent). One man was apparently 'without family',[11] and another a baker's apprentice who was admitted through public assistance.[12] Others were geographically distant from their families, mostly of immigrant origin, such as a 36-year-old 'former head trauma victim' diagnosed with 'nervous breakdown', described as an 'Italian with no family'.[13]

With a good reputation among the population in comparison to other psychiatric hospitals in the region (in particular Hoerdt, which then housed a high-security ward for dangerous criminals), the clinic received patients from a variety of social backgrounds. However, most patients operated on were of modest social rank; only one patient, the son of an industrialist, benefitted from a 'special regime' including a stay in a single room.[14] Thirty-nine per cent of patients were 'without profession', including a majority of women (85 per cent), whose overall employment rate was still much lower than that of men at that time. Among the workers, most were in low status and socially undervalued occupations (the most qualified was an engineer, the others were farmers, domestic servants, craftsmen, railwaymen, blue-collar workers, etc.). In addition, three patients were physically disabled, including a World War I veteran.[15] The last patient to be operated on under Gelma's supervision, a woman charged with theft, breach of trust and fraud, was presented as a 'stallholder': homeless, and belonging to 'a very special environment, similar to that of the gypsies, where lies, duplicity, amorality, fraud, trickery are common conduct', and who, although married, would not hesitate to 'run wild with several Algerians',[16] suggesting a racist bias on the part of the record taker towards the Traveller community and North African immigrants.

Although the majority of patients were considered 'schizophrenic', the diagnostic spectrum went far beyond this single category, reflecting a willingness to experiment on a broad spectrum. According to Dany and Singer's assessment, eighty-five were diagnosed with 'schizophrenia' (54.5 per cent); nineteen with 'epilepsy' (12.2 per cent); thirteen with 'obsessional neuroses' (8.5 per cent); eleven with 'chronic mania and melancholia' (7 per cent); ten with 'chronic delusions' (6.5 per cent); seven with 'constitutional psychopathy' (4.5 per cent); five with 'psychalgia' (3.2 per cent); two with 'chronic psychasthenia' (1.3 per cent); two with 'hypochondria' (1.3 per cent); one with 'hysteria'; and one with 'oligophrenia' (0.5 per cent). The last, a 6-year-old 'deaf-mute' diagnosed with 'psychological retardation, agitation syndrome, aggressiveness',[17] appears undoubtedly among the most atypical cases, especially since the 'topectomy' undertaken remained 'without effect'. Another rare case was a 21-year-old left-handed girl with tics. She underwent a 'lobotomy' whose results were also quickly judged 'null'.[18]

Initially, the Strasbourg team seem to have preferred topectomy over lobotomy. In a letter dated March 1950 to Gelma's assistant, Roland Lanter, Gelma stated that the latter technique had not brought anything conclusive.[19] A few months later, Singer and Dany differed from Gelma's view by pointing out the limits of topectomy, and expressing their preference for lobotomy (Gelma *et al.*, 1951: 527). Singer even concluded in his thesis that it was 'clearly superior to topectomy' (Singer, 1951: 95). Singer and Dany stated that they decided to abandon topectomy in favour of lobotomy, using Poppen's technique, and that the last topectomy was performed in May 1950. Two reasons led to this rejection, the first of which was 'some osteitis of the flap'. In fact, the records reveal six cases of bone inflammation, of which three patients had to undergo a second operation,[20] and one, three operations.[21] The second motive was the 'less valid' results of topectomy compared to those obtained by lobotomy (Boittelle *et al.*, 1952: 461–2). While the records attest that Poppen's technique was indeed favoured, especially to treat 'schizophrenics', they also show that the practice of topectomy continued for a little over a year. Fourteen operations of this type were performed between June 1950 and July 1951, mostly on 'schizophrenics', as well as on two cases of 'manic-depressive psychosis', one 'psychasthenic', and one 'epileptic'.

Institutional routine and patients' trajectories

One can distinguish patients sent to the clinic by a physician, generally a specialist from Strasbourg or its region (approximately sixty patients, or 39 per cent) and patients from other sections of the Strasbourg hospital (neurological, surgical, dermatological, or outpatient clinics, making up 6 per cent), or from the various other facilities in the region. Other psychiatric establishments in the east of France (Colmar, Rouffach, Nancy and Maréville) already performed psychosurgery and therefore did not send any of their patients to the Alsatian capital. The Lorquin hospital appears to have been the largest provider of patients with sixty-six inmates transferred (44 per cent). However, these transfers ceased when Lorquin set up its own surgical department, where within two years around fifty operations were carried out (Diligent, 1997: 179). The number of patients sent from other hospitals was much smaller: eight from Ravenel (5.5 per cent); seven from Notre-Dame-du-Bon-Secours Hospital (5 per cent); and seven from Hoerdt. Stéphansfeld, the largest psychiatric hospital in the

Bas-Rhin region, whose post-war staff were known to be reluctant about shock therapies (in reaction to its tragic past during the German occupation), sent only three patients (2 per cent). In a letter to one of his Strasbourg colleagues, a Stéphansfeld psychiatrist stated that the patient's husband had 'begged' them 'to submit her to psychosurgical intervention and it was only at his insistence and under his responsibility that she was proposed for this treatment'.[22] Unlike Hoerdt, Lorquin did not share records with their Strasbourg colleagues, but provided a summary of the transferred patient's history. This summary could take the form of a letter of a few lines, occasionally handwritten or as short typed reports, where the state of the patients before their transfer is described succinctly. Lorquin also organised simultaneous transfers of inmates, diagnosed by different diagnostic criteria, on whom Dany was called upon to operate in series.

Regardless of the modalities of their transfer, and following their admission to one of the clinic's four services (two for the 'agitated', and two others for the 'calm' of each sex), each patient underwent a battery of routine examinations, except for a few from other institutions. In addition to somatic tests, the first constant was the determination of the patient's blood type in the emergency blood transfusion laboratory. Depending on their condition, radiological, ophthalmological and electroencephalographic examinations were performed. Some patients underwent psychological tests, especially the Rorschach test, most often performed before the operation. However, no report found reflects the research carried out by Robert Durand de Bousingen during his thesis, carried out between 1950 and 1952 (Durand de Bousingen, 1955).

The decision to operate, taken after repeated admissions and several months of hospitalisation, was most often made before the patients were transferred from another establishment. Then, before intervening, psychiatrists sought the agreement of the patients or their family, regardless of whether they were underage. This procedure was specific to psychosurgery. The implementation of shock therapy, in contrast, does not seem to have required the slightest consent. Psychosurgery and the risks involved seem to have led the physicians to adopt a more cautious attitude, and to obviate, in case of failure, any objection. This authorisation, always handwritten by a caregiver, could be endorsed by the patients, a sign that the physicians considered them to have a sufficient capacity to consent, or otherwise one of the patient's parents, a sibling, the husband or spouse, or the legal guardian. The text is always succinct: it stipulates that the patient or the solicited relative 'authorises the surgeons' to intervene. The exact name of the operation is sometimes given, but the terms are often imprecise. It is also worth noting that many records do not contain any such document, although the patient was clearly not living in isolation. In fact, one record suggests that operations may have been carried out without authorisation. The sister of a patient of Italian origin wrote to the clinic to find out why her brother was transferred from Lorquin to Strasbourg. Singer replied laconically that he had 'the honour of letting [her] know that this patient had undergone brain surgery'.[23] However, there is no record suggesting that the doctors would have decided to override the opposition of a patient or of his family.

All operating reports are brief. The first ones from 1949 are limited to indicating the patient's name, their age, date of admission, health insurance company, department where they stayed, diagnosis, type of operation performed, date of the operation and the surgeon's name. A second type of report appears from 1950 onwards. The above information was accompanied by details of the type of anaesthesia used, a brief description of the technique implemented, how the operation was carried out, the weighing of the brain 'pieces' extracted, and the means used to plug the holes made with the trepan. The expression 'operation without incident' usually concludes the report on the successful completion of the procedure. A few reports contain observations on the patient's brain, such as that of a 'hebephrenic' described as 'a distinctly pathological brain with small lesions in the form of whitish placards'.[24] Over time, these reports became gradually shorter, indicating that this procedure had become routine. Thus, for an 'epileptic', the report simply states: 'Bilateral prefrontal lobotomy following Poppen's technique. Galley closure and silk skin';[25] or for a 'depressive' woman: 'The lobotomy is done according to the usual Poppen technique. It is total. Operation without incident.'[26]

Records reveal the occurrence of seven deaths between 1948 and 1953, making up almost 4.5 per cent of documented operations during the peak of Strasbourg psychosurgery. Among them were six men and one woman, aged between 23 and 53 years, diagnosed with 'schizophrenia', 'neurasthenia', 'depression', 'mental debility' and 'hypochondriac delirium'. All of them underwent a 'lobotomy using Poppen's technique', except for a former head trauma patient with mild brain atrophy and 'nervous breakdown', who underwent a 'topectomy'.[27] When a patient died from the intervention, the operating surgeon formally requested an autopsy via a form to determine the exact cause of death. At least one patient's brain was subsequently preserved in formalin as a result of this autopsy process.[28]

The stay in the surgical clinic rarely exceeded one week. Patients were then sent back to the previous psychiatric department for observation and post-operative psychotherapy, about which little is known due to a lack of recorded data. According to Singer, of 'all the hypotheses concerning the mechanism of the transformation of symptoms following psychosurgical intervention', the preference was for the idea of Jacksonian inspiration that the operation 'would produce a uniform dissolution of the psyche, followed by a revolution' which 'was not always complete'. It was then up to post-operative psychotherapy 'to perfect it: it had to use replacement in a favourable family environment, and, for the schizophrenics, a resumption of insulin treatment combined with re-education; rehabilitation in hospital if the family environment proved to be of poor help, with individual and group' (Singer, 1981: 66). In Lorquin, this rehabilitation took the form of:

> an extremely rapid start to work on jobs requiring a certain precision: unclogging intravenous needles, cleaning syringes, trays, rolling up bandages (work obviously taken over by the nursing staff). Around the tenth day of the return, those whose even slight improvement allowed it were taken out into the gardens for most of the day, entrusting them to other so-called serious patients in order to break the monotony of the neighbourhoods as much as possible ... Finally, they were put to real work, in a branch corresponding to their previous profession (most of our patients are manual workers) ... The start of work coincided with the passage to a semi-liberty service, which led to the granting of free discharge in the village. (Boittelle *et al.*, 1951b: 547)

As Singer mentioned, some patients underwent insulin therapy for 'consolidation', in order to reinforce the effects of the operation. According to the director of Lorquin psychiatric hospital, Georges

Boittelle (1916–66) and his wife and collaborator, Claudine Boittelle-Lentulo (1919–77), 'the improvements obtained' were often 'only temporary, but the insulin therapy which had given no results before the operation "proved" to be otherwise effective after the operation. Of this, we cannot give an explanation other than that of experience' (Boittelle *et al.*, 1951b: 547). Apart from a man diagnosed with 'chronic psychasthenic depression', this consolidation therapy only targeted 'schizophrenics' (about a quarter of the patients). In light of the records collected in Strasbourg, the effects of this treatment were not especially impressive, since out of twenty patients, twelve had results listed as 'null', six as 'excellent', and four as 'improved' or 'mixed'.

Lastly, the records do not show post-operative follow-up in the medium or long term. Nevertheless, while working on his thesis, Singer endeavoured to gather information on the progress of patients by sending a questionnaire to each of them. Thanks to this he concluded in his thesis that 48 per cent of the patients' results were 'excellent', 14 per cent were 'moderate', 34 per cent 'failed', and 4 per cent resulted in death (Singer, 1951: 111). Beyond 1951, in the vast majority of the cases, the clinic ceased to follow patients from the moment they were discharged. These patients were probably monitored or taken in charge, either by their attending physician (possibly by a member of the clinic – these for the most part also practised in private practice, including Gelma and Singer), or in another institution. However, it also happened that patients spontaneously wrote to their 'saviours' to give them news, such as the 'topectomised schizophrenic' who sent several letters to her 'dear and devoted benefactors' in the months following her operation.[29]

The evolution of recommendations

At first sight, psychosurgery was presented as a treatment of last resort, reserved for the most 'agitated' patients and the 'incurables'. Selection seems to have been based on their symptomatology rather than on strict diagnostic considerations. One argument that repeatedly arose was that the patients could not be worse off after the operation than they already were. Nevertheless, it seemed essential to question the criteria established in this respect, in light of the fact that psychiatrists argued that these operations should only be reserved for incurables and individuals who had been ill for an average of two years and who presented a serious clinical picture (Porot, 1947). But as we shall see, the standard of chronicity gradually moved over time.

Certainly, in the early days, Strasbourg treated mostly patients who had long since fallen into chronicity. If one considers only patients operated on in 1948 and 1949, there are only five patients out of twenty-six whose onset of the disease was estimated at less than two years prior. The oldest patient was regularly followed for more than thirty years,[30] the most recent ones for one year,[31] and the average was about six and a half years. As a result, among the patients operated on, twenty individuals were hospitalised during World War II, and experienced difficult, even disastrous internment conditions.[32] The most striking case is undoubtedly the woman who began to show serious disorders after her husband's enlistment in 1939, and her evacuation to Vichy and to the Dordogne.[33] Hospitalised in Clairvivre, Strasbourg and Philadelphia between 1944 and 1950, she underwent a 'prefrontal lobotomy' in Strasbourg as a patient diagnosed with 'chronic mania' in 1951. Singer asserted in a medical certificate that 'the anti-Semitic persecutions to which the patient was subjected may to some extent have triggered her mental disorders.' Others were direct or indirect victims of the German occupation, such as the 26-year-old woman diagnosed as 'schizophrenic', whose troubles dated back to her return from the Reich Labour Service in 1944, and who underwent a 'topectomy' in 1950.[34] This case appears all the more tragic as she was one of the fifteen thousand girls from eastern France who were forcibly incorporated into different Nazi structures during the war, known today as the *malgré-elles* (see Anstett, 2015).

Singer insisted on the following point: just as this type of operation could only be envisaged for 'schizophrenics' after 'exhausting all other therapies', so 'there is no point in delaying either, because when the disease has already been evolving for some time ... the chances of spontaneous remission have diminished'. Thus, even if 'excellent results' had been recorded in patients 'whose schizophrenic process was long-standing', 'the duration of the preoperative morbid evolution' should 'not be too long' (Singer, 1951: 44–5). He came to a similar conclusion about patients diagnosed with 'obsessions', while simultaneously criticising the effectiveness of the Freudian method:

> it is questionable whether patients should be allowed to suffer for long periods of time while waiting for the problematic results of expensive, lengthy psychotherapy reserved for the privileged few. It is true that obsessional neurosis is seen above all in the rich classes, but it is also true that this condition exists both in the poor classes and in those who are excluded from psychoanalysis because of a lack of resources (Singer, 1951: 50).[35]

The following year, Strasbourg and Lorquin finally began to exclude the chronic nature of schizophrenia from their selection criteria. The chronicity of the disease, coupled with a very pronounced distancing from social life, was retained only for the treatment of epilepsy, neuroses, pains and severe depression. Boittelle, Singer and Dany noted that all the failures had 'occurred in patients whose conditions had been evolving for many years, with uninterrupted hospital stays, or who had been hospitalised on several occasions, the discharges were only more or less brief remissions', and that, on the other hand, 'good results' were only obtained in patients who had been 'troubled for scarcely more than two years, but who were on the path to chronicity'. They also formulated three criteria which were to be checked before a psychosurgical intervention: the first two consisted of tossing aside patients with 'a marked schizophrenic family heredity', or suffering from tuberculosis, 'for fear of post-operative reactions'; the last criterion was to consider the operation only after having attempted all other possible treatments, and foremost insulin shock therapy, generally practised twice. In conclusion, they stressed the importance of an early intervention:

> It is better to intervene quickly, before the transition to chronicity. Beyond four or five years of evolution, the prognosis seems very poor to us, our best results are around the second year of evolution. Sometimes, we had to intervene much earlier, when the dissociative process was evolving rapidly in a 'flash in the pan' (Boittelle *et al.*, 1952: 462).

An examination of 'schizophrenia' records affirms these assertions. Nevertheless, there is no evidence of the exclusion of chronically ill older patients or a significant increase in non-chronic patients. In fact, the surgeons continued to operate on both older and younger individuals. For example, in 1951, Dany operated on a man who had been sick for at least eleven years prior to surgery,[36] and on a woman sick for ten years prior.[37] In 1953, Dany was still operating on a woman of Polish origin, hospitalised in Hoerdt for 'delusional schizophrenia', who had been sick for sixteen years at that point.[38] Conversely, some patients were operated on very soon after the onset of disease.[39] But the effects of these operations were inconclusive, as evidenced by their subsequent readmissions.

Gradually, the Strasbourg psychiatrists came to believe that it was necessary to intervene before the illness could definitively take hold and flourish, and not only for those diagnosed with 'schizophrenia'. Records show that young patients diagnosed with 'neuroses' were operated on, although their disease had manifested only a few months before.[40] The priority was therefore to operate on cases that were insensitive to other treatments, but which had not yet become chronic. Although the objectives put forward by the doctors were similar, a careful examination of the records clearly shows that between 1950 and 1952 there was a noticeable shift both in the selection of patients and in the arguments used to justify the intervention.

A more reasoned practice?

Questioned by a mainstream journal on the future of his discipline, a Swiss neurosurgeon declared with optimism in 1950: 'Psychosurgery is only a stopgap measure while waiting for the progress of psychoanalysis or other medications. In ten years, leukotomy will be an outdated method, I hope, and then it will be banned. But without forgetting the services it has rendered' (Caloz, 1950: 14). Finally, it was not in any way Freud's exponents who put a stop to psychosurgery (in fact, some even defended it), but rather its mixed results, and the introduction of the first neuroleptics, with their apparent reversibility.[41]

It was under Gelma's direction that the very first patients were treated with Largactil, as shown in several records from 1953. A few patients, who would otherwise have been operated on, were spared thanks to these new medications. This was notable in the case of a man admitted for 'hypochondriac depression'.[42] An operation was initially envisaged, as shown in a letter from Gelma, who wavered between recommending a long psychotherapy programme and a lobotomy. The patient was at last administered chlorpromazine, as well as electric shocks, and left the establishment after two months without having been operated on. Although it is impossible to say whether his condition improved consistently over the long term, the patient in question was never rehospitalised in a psychiatric ward, at least in Strasbourg.

Théophile Kammerer (1916–2005) officially took over the directorship of the clinic in October 1953. While not making it one of his areas of specialisation, this former extern in Leriche's department had put his faith in psychosurgery (Gelma and Kammerer, 1951; Kammerer, 1951). Although he had built up an image as a reformer and a humanist practitioner, especially because of his psychoanalytical orientation (Serina, 2022), his arrival at the head of the establishment did not immediately put a definite end to psychosurgery. Kammerer, like other psychiatrists of his generation, never set Freudianism in opposition to psychosurgery, as one might be tempted to think from a modern-day perspective. Nevertheless, his appointment was undeniably followed by a very sharp decline in the number of interventions, especially due to the spread of the pharmacological innovations.

The profile of the group of patients who underwent psychosurgery during Kammerer's directorship differed markedly from the patients who were operated on during the previous period. Selection became much more limited, as it was only reserved for individuals who were resistant to all other therapies, including neuroleptics, antipsychotics and antidepressants. Only eight cases were recorded in the space of six years – i.e. about 0.1 per cent of total admissions between 1954 and 1959.[43] The last psychosurgical operation was apparently performed by Marcel David (1898–1986) from the Sainte-Anne hospital in Paris, called to Strasbourg to intervene. David performed a 'leukotomy' on a single beekeeper diagnosed with 'obsessional neurosis with the onset of schizophrenisation', whose results were quickly judged as 'null' and 'disappointing'. Unlike during the last months of Gelma's era, it was no longer possible to hope to counter the chronicity of the disease by operating rapidly, since most cases were chronic or very long term in nature.

Each patient presented a rather particular profile. Among them were three women, including a 'neurotic' nun,[44] and five men, including a 13-year-old epileptic boy.[45] One was a 'delinquent' diagnosed with 'constitutional psychopathy',[46] who was the only patient transferred from a hospital in the region. The others were sent by their attending physician, notably by Kammerer.[47] With four cases, 'obsessive neuroses' formed the largest part, including one with 'latent homosexuality',[48] and another with 'the onset of schizophrenisation'.[49] Two were diagnosed with 'melancholia',[50] and the last two with 'epilepsy' and 'constitutional psychopathy, mental debility and delinquency'. We have also identified at least one case of a woman being treated for 'obsessive neurosis' for whom Kammerer recommended a lobotomy.[51] Nevertheless, her husband refused and took her away against the advice of the doctors, who considered the operation 'necessary'. This assessment shows that psychosurgery had not proved its worth in the treatment of 'schizophrenics' to the general public, although a few years earlier they were considered the main target group. No operation undertaken during Kammerer's tenure resulted in the death of a patient.

A few records explicitly testify to the abandonment of psychosurgery. In 1960, a 36-year-old man was referred to the clinic at the request of a doctor from the small town of Meurthe-et-Moselle for a 'lobotomy'.[52] His records indicate that he was suffering from a 'character neurosis with obsessive elements' that had been evolving for several years, and that he was already undergoing all kinds of treatment (including electroshock and sleep therapy) without improvement. Even though a psychosurgical operation might have seemed appropriate, Kammerer voiced his opposition after an interview with the patient and treated him with an antidepressant. Nevertheless, in 1961, the patient's wife, lamenting the lack of improvement in her husband's condition and his 'inability to return to work full time and be productive', asked an intern about the advisability of a 'new treatment', namely lobotomy. The latter replied a few days later: 'Lobotomy is an intervention that we know well, but that we have practically abandoned for a few years', and ended up proposing an outpatient treatment in the policlinic. It is also worth mentioning that in the records of a 'schizophrenic', admitted the same year, who was convinced that she was going to undergo a lobotomy, is an attestation by Kammerer in which he formally guarantees the patient that 'there is no question of performing a surgical operation on her'.[53]

Contrary to other French facilities (such as the Salpêtrière), Kammerer and his team stayed away from all international psychosurgery conferences, and Singer decided to reorient himself towards psychopharmacological therapeutic research, the epidemiology of mental illness, and criminology. There is no doubt that the disappointing results of many interventions as well as the apparent effectiveness of the new drug treatments contributed in large part to the abandonment of psychosurgery. However, it seems that Dany's departure for Limoges in 1959, where he performed one or two operations per year until the late 1970s (Hanon, 1979), can be seen as the main practical reason for psychosurgery losing importance in Strasbourg. This end came before many other French institutions, including other hospitals in the region which continued the practice and study of the effects of these kind of operations for many years. This was notable in the case in Colmar, but also in Nancy, where psychosurgery was practised until the end of the 1960s, and where three theses on this topic were defended (Poiré, 1960; Lamarche, 1961; Mabille, 1961).

Finally, it should be noted that, except for Durand de Bousingen's thesis (summarised in an article co-authored with Kammerer and Singer (Kammerer et al., 1956)), no study on the effects and after-effects of long-term psychosurgery was conducted in Strasbourg.[54] This absence is perplexing for at least two reasons. Firstly, because some patients treated in this way had subsequently been readmitted and treated in the establishment again (most often with insulin therapy, neuroleptics, and to a lesser extent with shock therapy, before being transferred elsewhere), sometimes nearly ten, twenty, even thirty years after having been operated on. Secondly, many studies on long-term results of psychosurgery have been carried out in other French institutions since the early 1950s: first in Paris (Bartier, 1952; Ferrieu, 1952; Nguyen-Tuan, 1960; Dachary, 1963), then in the provinces (Roullet, 1960; Simon, 1960; Lamarche, 1961; Guillou, 1963; Souet, 1965; Zemmour, 1970). Thus, Strasbourg clearly stood on the fringes of the French medical community with respect to this research trend, even though some lobotomised patients were likely to have received outpatient care in the polyclinic. A thesis defended in Strasbourg in 1979 before a jury chaired by Singer could have been an exception. In fact, the thesis only concerned patients operated on in the Paris region and Colmar (Foucrier, 1979).

Conclusion

In total, about 169 patients were operated on in Strasbourg in the space of just over a decade – i.e. about 1.1 per cent of patients admitted between 1948 and 1959. The majority of them were men (60 per cent). This result might appear questionable as it contrasts with the claim that psychosurgery was more targeted at women (Terrier *et al.*, 2017). [55] However, this can be explained by the fact that the clinic admitted more men overall at the time, whereas women were more numerous among the patients admitted in all French hospitals until 1953 and were the majority of the interned population until 1968 (von Bueltzingsloewen, 2007b: 100). More broadly, and on the basis of the few known statistics (Jaubert, 1975–76), the total number of patients operated on in Strasbourg seems rather low compared to national figures. It is higher than in Le Mans, with 115 operations between 1949 and 1962 (Guillemain, 2010: 77), or in Bourg-en-Bresse, where 153 operations were performed between 1949 and 1958. On the other hand, this total is much lower than the 500 operations carried out at the Salpêtrière, or the 485 operations in Nancy (1947–68). Finally, if the figure of 1,344 lobotomies performed in French-speaking Europe between 1935 and 1985 is taken as reliable (Terrier *et al.*, 2017), it can be concluded that 13 per cent of them were performed in Strasbourg.

In addition to providing a fairly accurate numerical estimate, this research has shown that the extensive use of patient records can counterbalance an internalist narrative solely based on the publications and memory of physicians. In a kind of balance sheet of his career published in 2000, Singer devoted only a few lines to psychosurgery, saying that 'from 1949 to 1954 a number of prefrontal lobotomies were performed in a surgical department. Psychosurgery was only practised on schizophrenics hospitalised for decades or had completely disabling obsessional neuroses. It was abandoned as soon as chlorpromazine was introduced' (Singer, 2000: 60). The study of the medical records shows, on the contrary, that the first operations were carried out long before 1949 and Moniz's Nobel Prize. If psychosurgery was indeed, and obviously without much success, mainly applied to people diagnosed with 'schizophrenia', it also targeted many other pathologies. While this treatment was initially aimed at patients with long-standing disease, the Alsatian psychiatrists gradually considered that psychosurgery could be used before patients' conditions became chronic. Psychosurgery was therefore used not only as a last resort, but also as a means of halting the progression of the disease, and as such could be used early in the treatment of certain patients. Moreover, the advent of psychopharmacology did not lead to its immediate stop. In the absence of data on the lives of those operated on in the medium or long term, it must be added that any attempt at retrospective evaluation of long-term results seems impossible to envisage. Finally, it should be noted that while psychosurgery may have been considered during the post-war years as one of the most innovative, if not one of the most effective, techniques for the treatment of mental illness, it is striking to note, through the study of the records, the extent to which this method was, in practice, more a kind of bricolage based on a series of beliefs, assumptions and risky speculations than the rigorous implementation of a truly scientific method.

Notes

1 See especially Pressman, 2002; El-Hai, 2005; Raz, 2013; and Meier, 2015.

2 In France, a report by the Inspectorate General of Social Affairs reported thirty-two lobotomies out of thirty patients between 1980 and 1986. Its authors also admitted that they did not know the reality of the figures at the time they were writing their conclusions. See CCNE, 2002.

3 For an internalist perspective, see M. Zanello *et al.*, 2017. Parada's (2016) essay deals with the history of the controversy in a documented way, but its argumentation is never based on the examination of medical records. Recently, Guillemain has examined the effects of psychosurgery from the archives of the hospital of Le Mans, but only for 'schizophrenics' (Guillemain, 2021). On Wallonia, see Missa, 2006: 195–244.

4 Among the most used techniques, one distinguishes 'leucotomy' or 'lobotomy', which consists in the incision, inside a lobe, of the nerve fibres, from 'topectomy' whose goal is an ablation or excision of one or both sides (unilateral or bilateral) of certain zones of the cerebral crust (a layer of grey cells covering the brain, specifically cortical areas). The reader will find more details in the set of references mentioned in footnote 1.

5 On this preeminent figure of French surgery, see Rey, 1994.

6 It should be noted that the Germans who controlled the clinic between June 1940 and November 1944 do not seem to have practised psychosurgery during this period (personal communication from Lea Münch, author of the PhD thesis in development *Von Straßburg nach Hadamar: Patient*innen-biographien und Alltagsgeschichte der NS-Psychiatrie im annektierten Elsass, 1941–1944*).

7 For an overview of this topic, see Ey, 1954: 11–34.

8 Singer's thesis was rewarded with the Herpin prize of the National Academy of Metz. A few months later came a greater honour: a favourable review by Walter Freeman himself (Freeman, 1952). Singer became a psychiatrist by default, and reluctantly at first. He admitted that he initially felt a deep uneasiness when he saw himself surrounded by patients dressed as concentration camp inmates. A few years earlier, Singer, who was of Jewish origin, contributed to the identification of the remains of the Struthof camp prisoners. See Singer, 1993.

9 Patient records of the University Psychiatric Clinic of Strasbourg, Département d'Histoire des sciences de la Vie et de la Santé, Strasbourg (hereafter DHVS), file number 48–0442, 1948.

10 In July 1950, at the French Congress of Alienist Physicians and Neurologists, Gelma, Singer, Dany and Kammerer, in cooperation with colleagues from the hospital of Lorquin, gave a series of presentations on this topic (Gelma *et al.*, 1951; Boittelle *et al.*, 1951a; Boittelle *et al.*, 1951b). In December 1950, Dany and Singer presented an initial assessment of their practice before the French Society of Neurology, prior to presenting a case study in collaboration with Fontaine (Dany *et al.*, 1951). In November 1951, Gelma and Kammerer jointly presented a case at a session of the Eastern Psychiatric Meetings (Gelma and Kammerer, 1951).

11 DHVS, File number 49-0055, 1949.

12 DHVS, File number 51-0048, 1950–51.

13 DHVS, File number 49-0344, 1949.

14 DHVS, File number 52-1090, 1952.

15 DHVS, File number 55-0810, 1939–55.

16 DHVS, File number 53-0813, 1952–53.

17 DHVS, File number 50-0228, 1950.

18 DHVS, File number 52-0785, 1952.

19 DHVS, File number 50-0694, 1950.

20 DHVS, File number 50-0742, 1950; and 50-1079, 1950.

21 DHVS, File number 50-0244, 1948–50.

22 DHVS, File number 50-0662, 1940–50.

23 DHVS, File number 51-0223, 1951.

24 DHVS, File number 50-0014, 1950.

25 DHVS, File number 51-0315, 1951.

26 DHVS, File number 51-0762, 1951.

27 DHVS, File number 49-0344, 1949.

28 DHVS, File number 49-0248, 1949.

29 DHVS, File number 50-1079, 1950.

30 DHVS, File number 49-0344, 1949.

31 DHVS, File number 49-0055, 1949; and 49-0692, 1949.

32 On the conditions of internment during World War II in France, see von Bueltzingsloewen, 2007a.

33 DHVS, File number 51-0912, 1945–51.

34 DHVS, File number 64-0945, 1944–64.

35 Singer followed up on the effects of a 'topectomy' on a former patient of René Allendy, one of the founders of the Société Psychanalytique de Paris (DHVS, 50-0159, 1950). He maintained strong reservations about psychoanalysis throughout his life. See Serina, 2022.

36 DHVS, File number 51-0221, 1951

37 DHVS, File number 58-1283, 1941–58.

38 DHVS, File number 53-0852, 1953.

39 DHVS, File number 54-0476, 1952–54; and 53-0485, 1952–53.

40 DHVS, File number 51-0311, 1951; and 52-0785, 1952.

41 Some French psychiatrists curiously used the image of 'chemical lobotomy' to talk about the effect produced by neuroleptics on their patients' minds (see Parada, 2016: 3).

42 DHVS, File number 53-0007, 1953.

43 Among the clinic's records is that of a patient who was initially treated in the neurology clinic where it was decided to perform a lobotomy to remove a right frontotemporal tumour. The woman was then transferred to the psychiatric ward due to a 'confusional syndrome'. A few months later, she was admitted again to psychiatry because of 'severe behavioural disorders with clastic attacks' (DHVS, 64-0655, 1964). Thus, it is not impossible that other psychosurgical operations took place in Strasbourg, not at the request of the psychiatric clinic, but that of the neurological clinic.

44 DHVS, File number 55-1150, 1955.

45 DHVS, File number 56-0435, 1956–77.

46 DHVS, File number 54-0293, 1954.

47 DHVS, File number 59-1189, 1959; 61-0786, 1954–61.

48 DHVS, File number 59-1052, 1959.

49 DHVS, File number 59-1189, 1959.

50 DHVS, File number 57-0159, 1955–57; 57-1710, 1957–58.

51 DHVS, File number 58-1095, 1958.

52 DHVS, File number 60-0556, 1960.

53 DHVS, File number 61-1057, 1961.

54 The production of scientific research related to psychosurgery significantly decreased from the mid-1950s. In addition to Durand de Bousingen's thesis, one finds a short paper on a case of 'chronic melancholia' lobotomised (Kammerer *et al.*, 1958).

55 It should also be noted that the result put forward by Terrier is not based on the study of patient records, but only on the scientific literature, which constitutes a significant methodological bias.

References

Anstett, Marlène, 2015, *Gommées de l'histoire: Des Françaises incorporées de force dans le service du travail féminin du IIIe Reich* (Strasbourg: Editions du Signe).

Bartier, Jean-Marie, 1952, 'À propos de l'évolution de quelques schizophrènes traités par la lobotomie'. PhD dissertation, University of Paris.

Benabid, Alim-Louis, 2006, 'Attention, la psychochirurgie est de retour!', *Revue neurologique*, 162:8–9, 797–9.

Boittelle, Georges, Claudine Boittelle-Lentulo and Adrien Dany, 1951b, 'Récupération sociale des malades après leucotomie', in *Congrès des médecins aliénistes et neurologistes de France* (Paris: Masson), pp. 546–55.

Boittelle, Georges, Claudine Boittelle-Lentulo, Adrien Dany and Jean Houcard, 1951a, 'Lobotomie et épilepsie', in *Congrès des médecins aliénistes et neurologistes de France* (Paris: Masson), pp. 542–5.

Boittelle, Georges, Léonard Singer and Adrien Dany, 1952, 'Indications et résultats de la lobotomie dans les schizophrénies', *Annales médico-psychologiques*, 110:1, 461–4.

Bottéro, Alain, 2005, 'L'éthique au secours de la psychochirurgie?', *L'Évolution psychiatrique*, 70:3, 557–76.

Bueltzingsloewen, Isabelle von, 2007a, *L'Hécatombe des fous: La famine dans les hôpitaux psychiatriques français sous l'Occupation* (Paris: Flammarion).

Bueltzingsloewen, Isabelle von, 2007b, 'À propos de Henriette D.: Les femmes et l'enfermement psychiatrique dans la France du XXe siècle', *Clio: Femmes, Genre, Histoire*, 26:2, 89–106.

Caloz, René, 1950, 'Le bistouri contre la folie', *L'Illustré*, 44:2, 11–14.

Comité consultatif national d'éthique (CCNE), 2002, 'La neurochirurgie fonctionnelle d'affections psychiatriques sévères', *Cahiers du CCNE*, 32, 3–21.

Dachary, Jean-Maurice, 1963, 'Réflexions sur la lobotomie préfrontale: Étude des résultats thérapeutiques après 14 ans d'expérience'. PhD dissertation, University of Paris.

Dany, Adrien, Léonard Singer, Georges Boittelle and Claudine Boittelle-Lentulo, 1953, 'Résultats cliniques de la psychochirurgie. Statistiques personnelles', *Revue neurologique*, 88:6, 551–3.

Dany, Adrien, Léonard Singer and René Fontaine, 1951, 'Leucotomie bilatérale pour psychalgies anciennes chez un malade atteint depuis 3 mois d'une section indolore du nerf médian au poignet', *Revue neurologique*, 85:6, 566–9.

Diligent, Marie-Bernard, 1997, 'Histoire contemporaine de la psychiatrie en Moselle', *Mémoires de l'Académie nationale de Metz*, 159, 159–95.

Durand de Bousingen, René, 1955, 'Le test de Rorschach avant et après intervention psychochirurgicale. Intérêt pronostic'. PhD dissertation, University of Strasbourg.

El-Hai, Jack, 2005, *The Lobotomist* (Hoboken: Wiley & Sons).

Ey, Henri, 1954, *Études psychiatriques 3: Structure des psychoses aigues et déstructuration de la conscience* (Paris: Desclée de Brouwer & Cie).

Ferrieu, François, 1952, 'Contribution à l'étude des résultats éloignés de la leucotomie préfrontale'. PhD dissertation, University of Paris.

Foucrier, Yves, 1979, 'Résultats à long terme de l'expérience psychochirurgicale'. PhD dissertation, University of Strasbourg.

Freeman, Walter, 1952, 'Review of Singer, L., *La psychochirurgie des névroses et des psychoses*', *American Journal of Psychiatry*, 108:11, 866.

Gelma, Eugène and Théophile Kammerer, 1951, 'Schizophrénie de type paranoïde et extinction post-opératoire des idées délirantes après leucotomie', *Annales médico-psychologiques*, 109:2, 607.

Gelma, Eugène, Léonard Singer and Adrien Dany, 1951, 'Résultats obtenus après lobotomies et topectomies', in *Congrès des médecins aliénistes et neurologistes de France* (Paris: Masson), pp. 524–7.

Gross-Offenstein, Yvette, 1949, 'Contribution à l'étude de la leucotomie: Cas traités à l'hôpital psychiatrique de Rouffach'. PhD dissertation, University of Strasbourg.

Guillemain, Hervé, 2010, *Chronique de la psychiatrie ordinaire: Patients, soignants et institutions en Sarthe du XIXe au XXIe siècle* (Le Mans: La Reinette).

Guillemain, Hervé, 2021, 'Une histoire de la lobotomie du point de vue des patients et des archives hospitalières', *Les Cahiers du Comité pour l'histoire de l'INSERM*, 2:2, 35–41.

Guillou, Nicole, 1963, 'Résultat de la lobotomie préfrontale à l'hôpital psychiatrique de Rennes'. PhD dissertation, University of Rennes.

Hanon, Jean-Noël, 1979, 'La psychochirurgie en 1978: Marchepied ou chausse-trape?'. PhD dissertation, University of Limoges.

Jaubert, Alain, 1975–76, 'L'excision de la pierre de folie', *Autrement*, 4, 22–63.

Kammerer, Théophile, 1951, 'Leucotomie préfrontale dans un cas de psychonévrose obsessionnelle', in *Congrès des médecins aliénistes et neurologistes de France* (Paris: Masson), pp. 561–5.

Kammerer, Théophile, René Ebtinger, Roland Lanter and Demetre Philippidès, 1958, 'Mélancolie chronique déclenchée par une affection somatique: Guérison par lobotomie', *Annales médico-psychologiques*, 116:1, 157.

Kammerer, Théophile, Léonard Singer and René Durand, 1956, 'Intérêt pronostic des tests de Rorschach comparatifs avant et après intervention psychochirurgicale', *L'Évolution psychiatrique*, 1, 207–4.

Kotowicz, Zbigniew, 2008, 'Psychosurgery in Italy, 1936–39', *History of Psychiatry*, 19:4, 476–89.

Lamarche, Jean-Marie, 1961, 'Contribution à l'étude des résultats éloignés de la lobotomie préfrontale'. PhD dissertation, University of Nancy.

Lévêque, Marc, 2014, *Psychosurgery* (Berlin: Springer).

Lévêque, Marc and Sandrine Cabut, 2017, *La chirurgie de l'âme* (Paris: Lattès).

Mabille, Philippe, 1961, 'Une forme d'épilepsie traumatique: Séquelles convulsives de la lobotomie préfrontale'. PhD dissertation, University of Nancy.

Meier, Marietta, 2015, *Spannungsherde: Psychochirurgie nach dem Zweiten Weltkrieg* (Göttingen: Wallstein).

Missa, Jean-Noël, 2006, *Naissance de la psychiatrie biologique* (Paris: Presses Universitaires de France).

Moniz, Egas, 1936a, 'Essai d'un traitement chirurgical de certaines psychoses', *Bulletin de l'Académie de Médecine*, 115, 385–93.

Moniz, Egas, 1936b, 'Essai d'un traitement chirurgical de certaines psychoses', *Strasbourg médical*, 9, 113–16.

Nguyen-Tuan, Anh, 1960, 'Résultats d'une enquête sur 54 cas de lobotomie préfrontale avec un recul de 6 à 10 ans'. PhD dissertation, University of Paris.

Parada, Carlos, 2016, *Toucher le cerveau, changer l'esprit* (Paris: Presses Universitaires de France).

Poiré, Roger, 1960, 'Évolution électroencéphalographique après lobotomie préfrontale'. PhD dissertation, University of Nancy.

Porot, Antoine, 1947, 'La leucotomie préfrontale en psychiatrie', *Annales médico-psychologiques*, 105:2, 121–42.

Pressman, Jack D., 2002, *Last Resort: Psychosurgery and the Limits of Medicine* (Cambridge: Cambridge University Press).

Raz, Mical, 2013, *The Lobotomy Letters* (Rochester, NY: University of Rochester Press).

Rey, Roselyne, 1994, *René Leriche: Une œuvre controversée* (Paris: CNRS Editions).

Risse, Guenter B. and John Harley Warner, 1992, 'Reconstructing clinical activities: Patient records in medical history', *Social History of Medicine*, 5:2, 183–205.

Roullet, Alain, 1960, 'Résultats lointains de l'expérience psychochirurgicale d'un service psychiatrique'. PhD dissertation, University of Lyon.

Serina, Florent, 2022, 'From anti-Freudianism to a bastion of psychoanalysis: History of psychoanalysis at the University Psychiatric Clinic of Strasbourg in the twentieth century', *Psychoanalysis and History*, 24:2, 181–203.

Simon, Michel, 1960, 'Contribution à l'étude des résultats éloignés de la leucotomie préfrontale'. PhD dissertation, University of Lyon.

Singer, Léonard, 1951, *La psychochirurgie des névroses et des psychoses: Bilan de deux années à la Clinique psychiatrique de Strasbourg* (Strasbourg: Imprimerie des Dernières Nouvelles d'Alsace).

Singer, Léonard, 1981, *Titres et travaux scientifiques* (Strasbourg: n.p.).

Singer, Léonard, 1993, 'Pourquoi suis-je psychiatre?', *Psychiatrie internationale*, special issue, 55–6.

Singer, Léonard, 2000, '50 ans d'évolution de la psychiatrie et de son image', *Revue française de psychiatrie et de psychologie médicale*, 36, 59–63.

Souet, Michel, 1965, 'Résultats éloignés de 47 lobotomies pratiquées à l'hôpital psychiatrique de Léhon'. PhD dissertation, University of Rennes.

Terrier, Louis-Marie, Marc Levêque and Aymeric Amelot, 2017, 'Most lobotomies were done on women', *Nature*, 548, 523.

Vernet, Alain, Nadine Fresquet, Benoist Fauville and Cyril Boutet, 2021, 'La première intervention de lobotomie documentée en France. 2 décembre 1939 – Docteur Gaston Ferdière', *Annales médico-psychologiques*, 179:9, 857–65.

Zanello, Marc, Johan Pallud, Nicolas Baup, Sophie Peeters, Baris Turak, Marie Odile Krebs, Catherine Oppenheim, Raphael Gaillard and Bertrand Devaux, 2017, 'History of psychosurgery at Sainte-Anne Hospital', *Neurosurgical Focus*, 43:3, E9. doi: 10.3171/2017.6.FOCUS17250.

Zemmour, Geneviève, 1970, 'Contribution à l'étude des indications actuelles de la lobotomie préfrontale à partir de ses résultats éloignés'. PhD dissertation, University of Montpellier.

7

Treating mutism in Hungarian child psychiatry, 1957–60

Gábor Csikós

In April 1957, a teenage boy was admitted to Országos Ideg- és Elmegyógyintézet (National Institute of Neurology and Psychiatry). Also known as Lipótmező, this was the only child psychiatry ward in operation in Hungary at that time. The castle-like hospital was surrounded by a twenty-eight-acre park and located at the outer edge of Budapest. The boy had not spoken since 1950, when certain events caused him to have a nervous breakdown. The mother explained that her son had been an open-minded and energetic child beforehand, who began to speak fluently after his third birthday: 'He was a calm kid, he attended kindergarten where he even recited poems.'[1]

At Lipótmező, the boy, now fourteen, was diagnosed with elective mutism. The uncommon syndrome was interpreted as a manifestation of an anxiety disorder, in which the person remained silent in social situations. He was treated by the most renowned Hungarian expert of mutism, Blanka Lóránd (1891–1974), who was the head of the child psychiatry department. She described the case in detail in her basic study on elective mutism, which appeared in 1961. In this study, she summarised her decade-long experience in the therapy of elective mutism. She described the syndrome as a neurotic speech disorder that could have a significant impact on the child's subsequent mental development, social relations, and even their 'whole future life', as speech disorders raise the question of fitting into society. Moreover, she highlighted that the disorder always has a history and included the boy's case in her review (Lóránd, 1961).[2]

Although she was a highly influential expert of her time, even called 'the mother of child psychiatry' (Vekerdi, 1984), Blanka Lóránd's biography has not yet been written, and the information about her scientific career is fragmentary and scattered. Lóránd's special interest in this case was certainly an important reason why the boy's medical history is exceptionally detailed in its description of the antecedents and the therapeutic process. His medical history, apart from the previously mentioned study, is preserved within the collection of the National Institute of Neurology and Psychiatry. These documents otherwise rarely contain a detailed description of the therapeutic process. Generally, only the behaviour of the children within the institution was recorded, and notes can be found on the (side)effects of their medication or their interactions with peers and the hospital staff.

The exceptionally rich source material in this instance makes it possible to write a detailed case study of the boy's diagnosis and treatment, in order to gain insight into the contemporary practice of Hungarian child psychiatry in the late 1950s. This case study is contextualised by an outline of the life paths of the boy and his doctor Blanka Lóránd, as well as by an outline of the institutional development of Hungarian child psychiatry, contemporary academic discourses within the discipline, and Hungarian political history in the 1950s.

Before analysing the case study, it is important to provide some general information on the specific situation of psychiatry in Hungary in the 1950s. From the end of the 1940s, academic discourse was characterised by the communist political line of implementing Pavlovian theory in the sciences. In 1897, the Russian physiologist Ivan Petrovich Pavlov had demonstrated the effect of reinforcement and aversion in modifying animal behaviour. His views were warmly welcomed in Marxist-Leninist scientific circles, which saw these experiments as proof of the human ability to change. His teachings were widely adopted in Soviet science and made binding on other socialist states as part of the Pavlov campaign in the 1950s (Leuenberger, 2007). In psychiatry, especially in the first half of the 1950s, a biologistic perspective based on the stimulus-response pattern, conditioned reflexes, and the theory of higher neural activity prevailed.

In 1956, Hungary witnessed a popular uprising. The revolutionaries demanded democratic changes, but the movement was violently repressed with Soviet support. The new government under János Kádár was aware of the lack of popular support and assumed political apathy to be the key to staying in power (Feinberg, 2021: 109–10). This political context also had repercussions for the scientific field. In the psy-sciences, the Pavlovian approach became less and less dominant after 1956. As psychiatric practices could differ from academic discourse, this case study will examine the relevance of Pavlovianism to treatment practice in Lipótmező in the second half of the 1950s, by focusing on electrotherapy and hypnotherapy as treatment methods.

Muted people, politicised science

The period from the boy's birth to his silencing (1944–50) was a turbulent phase in Hungarian history. Several doctors had fallen victim to the devastations of World War II and the Holocaust. One of them was Pál Ranschburg (1870–1945), a pioneer of Hungarian child psychiatry and a former student of Wilhelm Wundt, who starved to death during the siege of Budapest. The post-war period did not bring balanced democratic development for the country, which belonged to the Soviet-dominated zone. Communist rule became increasingly manifest and in 1949 they seized all political power. Their ambitious social project was characterised by a high level of voluntarism and utopian salvationism (Bottoni, 2017; Kovács, 2014). Communist theorists believed that creating a new society would free people from alienation. However, this utopian objective had to be adapted to economic and political realities over time (Janos, 1996).

The boy's family was deeply affected by the events of these years as the 'maternal grandfather became epileptic due to war injuries … and the father has been feeling ill since the war' (OPNI, 0161–004053.335). The accelerated industrialisation of the post-war years offered industrial work for unskilled labourers like the family father. He started to work as a mine-labourer in Tatabánya, a larger industrial town 250 km from their home village near the Romanian border. His average salary only allowed the family of six to live in poverty. By the time of their move to the border, the boy was mute as in 1950 'a great shock caused him a nervous breakdown and from that time he was in complete lethargy and talked to no one' (OPNI, 0161–004053.335). The circumstances that caused his silence only became clear to his doctor in the course of his treatment in Budapest.

The year 1950 also opened an important chapter in the life of doctor Blanka Lóránd. She was offered a position as head physician in the newly founded child psychiatry ward in Lipótmező. Regarding her career, this offer was reasonable in terms of both political and scientific standards. She had received her diploma in 1916, nearly twenty years after the first female physician's Swiss diploma had been naturalised in Hungary. When she started to work, associations focusing on child psychiatry were already operating. The Gyógy-pedagógiai és Pszichológiai Magyar Királyi Laboratórium (Hungarian Royal Laboratory of Psychology and Special Education) was founded by Pál Ranschburg in 1899. Despite constant struggles with financial issues, this institution contributed significantly to child psychopathology research. From 1932, Lóránd worked as a neurologist at the Research Institute of Child Psychology, a successor of Ranschburg's institute that examined questions of child psychotherapy in a positivist manner. She conducted neuropsychiatric research inspired by the Viennese Pötzl school and focused on aphasia and the pathology of speech development. She also developed criteria for differential diagnosis in mentally disabled people (Vetró, 1999).

Her scientific views and neuropsychiatric framework fitted in well with Pavlovian theory, which became binding in psychiatry in the socialist states under the influence of the Soviet Union after 1945. Pavlovian doctrines were not necessarily ideology-driven, but they easily met the expectations of communist policymakers after their seizure of power. They articulated views on human functioning that were in line with Stalinist expectations in social planning. In contrast, psychoanalytic associations were dissolved partly because their concept of irrational motives threatened the project of fully conscious social engineering (Frosh, 2019; Lászlófi, 2019).[3] Instead, reductionist versions of Pavlovian reflexology flourished. Pavlov soon became the cultic representative of 'authentically' Soviet science that promised the explanation and cure of mental problems by conditioning (Doboş, 2015).

Since it was not possible that Pavlovian scientists could be trained in masses in a short period, scientific policy had to rely on those who had worked within a similar theoretical framework before. This particularly applied to representatives of the 'organic school' with a biological orientation, which followed the Wundtian tradition of experimental psychology. They mainly investigated basic elementary psychic processes with the methodology of the natural sciences and excluded philosophical approaches. Concentrating solely on the organs, these experts could not be blamed for psychologization (Laine-Frigren, 2016: 44–52). Blanka Lóránd belonged to this tradition: her scientific status based on her publications on neuropsychiatric disorders in the late 1930s and her neurological approach fitted in well with the Pavlovian framework.

For Lóránd, Lipótmező was an attractive workplace. Her job at the Research Institute of Child Psychology had ended. The institution had been subordinated to the Hungarian Academy of Sciences as communist health policy favoured specialist centres. State control of people working in the same field was an important element of social and economic planning, which can be seen in the cases of the nationalisation of industrial companies, collectivisation of agriculture (Kovács, 2014) and centralisation of health care. Following this concept, the prestigious institution of Lipótmező became the centre of psychiatry.

Since its foundation in 1868 as 'Buda Asylum', this hospital had remained the largest psychiatric institute and received constant support from post-war governments. Public servant status was given to the formerly freelance psychiatric professionals (Bakonyi, 1984; Szokolszky, 2016; Kovai, 2019) and there was a significant expansion of staff. From 14 doctors in the pre-war period, their number grew to 43 in 1952 and 70 in 1958. The number of nurses increased from 150 to 282, and in the late 1950s, 5 special education teachers were hired. Material improvement was visible as well. Nevertheless, it was noticeable in Lipótmező that psychiatry as a whole remained an underfinanced sector within the healthcare system. The fact that Lipótmező was commonly led by powerful political lobbyists, whose connections could have more weight in decision-making than the patients' actual needs, did not help (Kovai, 2015). The general scientific spirit of the place facilitated it becoming a central institution. Although there had been some important psychoanalytic initiatives before,[4] the dominant approach in Lipótmező was organic and thus easily harmonised with Pavlovian principles. This applied to Lóránd, too: in 1955, she was celebrated as a physician who brilliantly used Pavlovian nervism in the assessment and cure of childhood mental diseases (Gegesi Kiss, 1955).

The establishment of child psychiatry followed European specialisation trends. István Tariska (1915–89) was the director of Lipótmező and the former head of the Health Protection Department of the Ministry of Health. In 1950, he visited Maudsley Hospital in London, where insulin and electroshock therapy dominated the therapeutic design (Varga, 1964). Eventually, Tariska decided to 'make something similar' in Hungary (Ferenczy, 2014). At first glance it might be surprising that a communist country imported know-how from capitalist Great Britain. However, there were striking therapeutic similarities. The head of the psychology department at Maudsley, Hans Eysenck, preferred suggestion and conditioning over psychoanalysis. Although he had some critical remarks on Marxism (Eysenck, 1954), the ideological gap between Western behaviourism and Pavlovism did not hinder knowledge transfer.

In Hungary, the field of child psychiatry had received little scientific attention until then: even the first post-war comprehensive psychiatry textbook paid little attention to childhood mental problems. Only ten out of seven hundred pages discussed this scientific subfield, and they drew attention to the importance of the specialisation (Nyírő, 1962: 655). However, it was to be a long time before child psychiatry was established as an independent subdiscipline in Hungary. A qualifying exam for child psychiatrists was only introduced in 1965 (Herczeg, 1993; Vetró, 1999). The high workload of those working in this field and organisational difficulties hindered child psychiatry in becoming an independent discipline. Members of the Lipótmező ward staff in the 1950s were not necessarily trained psychiatrists or paediatricians.[5]

The department had complex and divergent tasks. In 1961, the following was written about the first decade: 'The 50-bed child psychiatry department, established in 1950, has already greatly facilitated the widening of the healing, research, and prevention work carried out in the field of mental and nerve diseases in childhood' (Fekete, 1961: 60). This assessment of the situation was optimistic as it was rather a beginning than an expansion of child psychiatric work in Hungary. Beside the limited possibilities of the district clinics in Budapest, Lipótmező was the only place to treat mentally ill children. Furthermore, this remained the only institute where wards were operating. Only in 1960 was another ward for child psychiatry, with fourteen beds, established at the Clinic of Neuropsychiatry of the Medical University in Szeged in southern Hungary.

The limitations of child psychiatry provision are visible in the boy's medical history. After his nervous breakdown in 1950 the family sought support at the Institute for the Deaf and Dumb in Szeged as well as the Centre of Special Education in Budapest. Finally, in another hospital, the boy was diagnosed with epilepsy. He showed symptoms of this disorder, such as grimacing, but they disappeared when he turned eight. The only treatment for his persistent muteness was to prescribe tranquillisers. Even though he did not speak, the boy was integrated into the school community. The school community accepted him, and the teacher replaced oral exams with written ones. The medical history of 1957 reads:

> He is open, he reads novels and does his homework. Based on his written performance he could finish three classes, but the teachers constantly suggested special education for him. He received tranquilizers that reduced his stress, but he did not start speaking. He used his left hand, which was tied down. He did not get food if he used the left hand, so for now, left-handedness is not a problem.

Only when the boy had not spoken to anyone except his mother for eight years did he receive explicit child psychiatric treatment. In 1957, he came to Lipótmező where Blanka Lóránd became his doctor. Because of his response to environmental harm, a psychological trauma, with passive resistance, he seemed to be an ideal case for research and treatment by an expert who followed Pavlovian principles.

Diagnostic methods for elective mutism

Lóránd herself pointed out in her study on infantile mutism that the differential diagnosis of mutism was difficult. On the one hand, the child's silence, passivity, and oppositional defiance could mask mental disability. On the other hand, contact opportunities were rare because most children had not yet acquired literacy. These problems appear in the boy's medical history before his treatment in Lipótmező due to uncertainties over adequate diagnosis and treatment. So, Lóránd recommended caution in the diagnosis and treatment of mutism: 'The prognosis without any longitudinal observations is insecure since the modern diagnostic tools – e.g. electroencephalographic or the arsenal of psychological tests – can often fail ... During the child's development constant surprises, both positives and negatives might occur' (Lóránd, 1961: 16).

In a way, Lóránd's circumspect sentences contradicted the prevailing optimism, especially in regard to Pavlovian-inspired psychiatry in the early 1950s. This can partly be explained by the fact that the Pavlovian approach lost some of its scientific dominance at the end of the 1950s. The aforementioned psychiatry textbook by Gyula Nyírő shows more permissive attitudes towards the non-Pavlovian approaches, including psychoanalysis: 'Psychoanalysis taught the neurologist that they must listen to their patient ... Some diagnostic significance of the analytical method cannot be denied, but it has no healing importance' (Nyírő, 1962: 329).

At the same time, the fact that child psychiatry had been using psychoanalytical methods in diagnostics long before this official acceptance certainly had an effect. While psychodiagnostics ceased in adult wards in the 1950s, they persisted in child psychiatry. However, these had the flaw that with the elimination of psychological training and psychoanalytic workshops, interpretations of projective tests like the Rorschach or Thematic Apperception Test showed great variance. Children were commonly tested by neurologists, who were untrained in the method and produced less reliable interpretations. Psychologists in the institute were in marginal positions and were listed under the term 'other professions'.

The fact that psychoanalytic diagnostic methods were not taboo in Lipótmező was related to the specific structure of this institution, which could modify political power. As the historian of the institute, Melinda Kovai, points out, this was a place of 'strong professional solidarity, an inner hierarchy tainted with patriarchalism, and a very heterogeneous milieu, both institutionally and professionally' (Kovai, 2015: 130). Because the hospital was not linked to university education, it could apply a wide range of diagnostic methods, and these were less determined by ideological influences than in university clinics. Moreover, it is likely that projective methods were a better fit with the play and free-associative games of childhood. Finally, methodological eclecticism was also promoted by the fact that child psychiatry was still emerging. The practice was characterised by a small team of specialists and, as in this case, they typically (but not exclusively) had a neurological focus (Brunecker, 1968; Szakács and Bagdy, 1993).

However, in her case study of the boy in the context of her 1961 study, Lóránd does not reflect this eclecticism in terms of diagnostics: 'In a left-handed child who had a neurological illness and was violently accustomed to right-handedness, great scare caused hysterical mutism. The fixation of infantile reaction mode – fear of strangers – resulted in elective mutism' (Lóránd, 1961: 18).

In her summary, Lóránd stressed three circumstances that characterised the case. Highlighted here were firstly his former left-handedness, then his writing skills that made the patient contactable, and finally that the patient experienced stormy panic reactions during the treatment. These viewpoints prioritised biological and situational features and paid relatively little attention to social factors. Lóránd's study briefly referred to the mental health history of the family (epilepsy of the grandfather and stomach complaints of the father) but left several details unelaborated. It mentioned that the mother was neurotic and 'was hospitalized after the burn injuries of her daughter' (Lóránd, 1961: 17–18). Only the health report reveals that these burn injuries led to the death of the 14-year-old girl. It is also noted here that five other siblings – including four twins – died shortly after their birth.

It is noticeable that in the case of the adolescent boy, views of the organic school continued to dominate the diagnostic work. This also applies to Lóránd's study in general: divergent diagnostics cannot be detected in the central hospital. In the case study of the boy, however, the eclecticism mentioned is evident in the therapies.

Electroshock treatment in child psychiatry

Lóránd suggested the following design for the treatment of elective mutism in her 1961 study. First sedatives and drugs with euphoric effects (caffeine, codeine) should reduce the child's anxiety caused by the new environment. If the child became calm, electroconvulsive therapy and psychotherapy should be used. It is worth noting that in Lóránd's study the politically optimistic premise that socialism would prevent mental disorders[6] was replaced by the optimistic premise that medication would remedy the mental disorder.

The subsequent therapy was electroshock treatment, which was administered without anaesthesia and was primarily intended to have a behavioural therapeutic effect. Here, too, Hungary relied on Western European experiences. The first reports on applying electroconvulsive therapy to children were published in 1941, on the Bristol City and County Mental Hospital, and in 1942, on the Hôpital des Enfants-Malades in Paris. The application in children appears to have been carried out not with awareness, but rather with indifference to the patients' age. In Paris, electroshock therapy was typically used to treat childhood schizophrenia – only one Parisian boy was diagnosed with elective mutism (Shorter, 2013). The first Hungarian reports, which also date from the 1940s, reveal the same pattern (Angyal and Juba, 1943). For example, Pál Ranschburg reported in 1943 on his experiences with the outpatient treatment of 'intelligent' schizophrenic patients aged 17 to 65 (Ranschburg, 1943). Later, electroconvulsive therapy became widespread in Europe and the United States in the treatment of tic, melancholia, and other mental disorders. Its popularity declined notably with the raise of pharmacotherapies and the critique of Swedish child psychiatrist Anna-Lisa Annell in the second half of the twentieth century (Shorter, 2013).

Although it was not Soviet science that brought electroshock treatment to Hungary, it was undoubtedly a good fit with the Pavlovian ideas on conditioning. Electric shocks could be applied in a behavioural manner, in which undesirable behaviours were to be eliminated by repeated unpleasant stimuli (Davison, 2021). This aversive approach combined healing with punishment, and was, as already mentioned, commonly used in the Maudsley Hospital in 1950, which inspired Tariska in organising the Hungarian child psychiatry ward.

Lóránd reported in her 1961 study on the electrotherapy of a 7-year-old girl and a pair of siblings from 1954. No neurological abnormality was identified behind the elective mutism of the 8- and 10-year-old boys: initially, the staff tried glutamic acid therapy in vain. The older boy became attached to one of the nurses and wrote about his motivation to help her. However, he displayed panic reactions to all interventions and only accepted electrotherapy after watching his brother's treatment. The 1959 follow-up showed that a partial cure had been achieved. There were no complaints about his behaviour as he was working in the fields, but he spoke only to the cemetery watchman, apart from his family (Lóránd, 1961).

Although the behavioural use of electroshock had declined somewhat with the spread of drugs, the institute's documentation shows that it remained the standard therapy for children with elective mutism in later years. In 1960, a 7-year-old boy was treated for anxiety and feelings of inferiority. His muteness was explained by inappropriate coddling which made starting school traumatic. According to the institute's diary, his initial dysphoria turned into euphoria after treatments with tranquillisers and electric shocks.

Lóránd found that electric shocks were effective in treating mutism. This is even more surprising since, in her summary study, she writes that the child's development might present the doctor with constant surprises, both positive and negative. Based on pre-war German literature, she stated that those affected by mutism were generally 'anxious, gentle, good-natured, affectionate children who have great difficulty in adapting to new surroundings and become mute in all such situations' (Lóránd, 1961: 16). It is noticeable that despite this description, she nevertheless advocated aversive methods that increased anxiety. One reason for this was certainly that Lóránd was convinced of the empirical results. She writes in her summary that in seven of sixteen cases presented, a persistent cure was achieved.

The boy's first treatment started in April 1957. Lóránd noted:

> We experimented with electrotherapy after the unsuccessful tries with different stimuli. The test caused panic reactions, he was retreating and crying. I tried to calm him, promising that we will give him time to talk without any pressure. I believe he can do it. Regarding that different types of treatment increased his stress and hindered speaking (except for Glutarec which medication cannot be continued due to shortages) ... We try to involve him in written communication. He answers shortly, but when we are asking about his muteness, he gives no answer, puts the pencil down, and keeps his eyes forward. (OPNI, 0161–004053.335)

A few days later, changes in his medication (Actedron) affected his behaviour positively. The medical history reads: 'He is very vivid and motile, sometimes he is truly vicious [later corrected to aggressive], he hits other kids, plays violently but speaks no word' (OPNI, 0161–004053.335).

This short extract from his health report gives an insight into the state of Hungarian pharmacology. Glutarec (glutamic acid hydrochloride) was authorised in 1953 for use in the treatment of various degrees of oligophrenia, acquired degenerative brain lesions, schizophrenia, and the melancholic form of psychopathy. Upon his discharge, the boy was prescribed Andaxin, a Meprobamate-based drug. In a 1971 study, this drug is recommended in cases of conflict reaction, psychoneurotic or pre-electroshock fear (Siftár, 1971: 50, 62–3). Among the drugs prescribed to the boy was Actedron, an amphetamine derivative that was widely used before World War II to increase mental or physical performance (Ujváry, 2000). Although this chapter does not focus on changes in medication, it is worth mentioning that the growing effectiveness of drugs remarkably influenced the use of beds within Lipótmező. The shift from long to short-term hospitalisation and outpatient care changed the role of the healthcare staff and their way of exercising power (Foucault, 1999). Interestingly, the danger of a relapse and the emergence of a 'revolving door system' was very precisely recognised by clinicians in the cases of mutism and prevention was attempted. Lóránd pointed out: 'In cases where, despite our advice, the child was taken early, we did not succeed … Recovery is complete if there is no relapse in a foreign and unfavourable environment after leaving the hospital – but in most cases, it is necessary to get the help of an understanding parent and educator to achieve permanent asymptomatic relief' (Lóránd, 1961: 26).

Drugs and electric shocks did not help the boy in 1957. Three days later, on 11 July 1957, at the conference of doctors, a hypnotherapeutic plan was accepted and conducted by Blanka Lóránd herself. She summarised in her study: 'Regarding the total failure of previous therapeutical attempts, we turn to hypnotherapy, putting ourselves in the role of the mother and trying to talk to him' (Lóránd, 1961: 18).

The potential of hypnosis

At first reading, this kind of therapy may seem surprising, as it represents a shift from so-called active therapies (drugs, electroshock treatment) to psychotherapy. At the time active therapies were considered to be not only calming, but curing (Nyírő, 1962: 315). To which tradition can hypnotherapy in this case be linked – to a Pavlovian framework of stimulus–response patterns or to a legacy of depth psychology treatment approaches? Was the use of hypnotherapy in Lipótmező a sign of the renaissance of alternatives to Pavlovism?

The beginnings of Hungarian hypnosis research reach far back. Pál Ranschburg was the first researcher, who made hypnosis scientifically accepted in 1900 by separating it from animal magnetism. At the same time psychoanalyst Sándor Ferenczi (1873–1933) held more spiritualistic views and gave depth psychology hypnosis a place in everyday medical practice. Hypnosis had been spreading in Hungary since 1945. For ideological reasons, these approaches were labelled bourgeois and therefore suspicious in the 1950s. The recurrent narrative on hypnosis in socialist Hungary is that authors who promoted depth psychology hypnosis generally met with disbelieving or even hostile attitudes in the professional community. As a first assessment of this development from the early 1960s emphasises, scientific examination of the field had been intensified to meet this critique of its ideological roots: 'Hypnosis research and hypnosis therapy show a great boom after World War II. This renaissance of hypnosis is characterised by increased scientific demand and exact experiments, which slowly dispel any existing aversion, scepticism, and mystification in connection with this valuable method of psychotherapy and research' (Koronkai, 1964).

In any case, active alert hypnosis was still labelled as a mystical phenomenon in the mid-1970s (Gyimesi, 2018). It is worth noting that, while depth psychology hypnotherapy was being restricted ideologically in Hungary, the method lost popularity in the Western world as well. In the late 1950s, hypnotherapy did not belong to the most up-to-date or popular methods. Adult hypnosis attracted some attention in the treatment of war shock. The renaissance of child hypnosis did not start until the 1960s when major systematic research began. Wide use of the method took place only in the 1970s, accompanied by conferences, workshops and teaching sessions in self-hypnosis for children (Kohen and Olness, 2011).

However, suggestive hypnosis fulfilled the requirements of Pavlovian reflexology (Gyimesi, 2019) differently from depth psychology hypnosis, according to Freud. In this framework, fear and calmness were understood as neuro-physiologically opposing processes, and hypnosis could be used to weaken the link between stimulus and anxiety. Giving suggestions in hypnotic induction increased the occurrence of positive responses and made the patient react more strongly to the next suggestion. In other words, while electroshock therapy could be described as aversive conditioning, suggestive hypnosis involved the extinction and replacement of existing reflexes.

In communist countries, reflexology made the use of hypnosis possible. Although Pavlov underlined the importance of aversive therapies, his colleague Vladimir Bekhterev (1857–1927) explored suggestion and hypnosis as adjunct techniques (Davison, 2021). For Hungarian psychiatrists, traditionally the reference point had been Germany and, in the socialist era, the German Democratic Republic was set as positive role model for psychotherapy (Laine-Frigren, 2016). In 1959 and 1960, two highly recognised representatives of Hungarian clinical child psychology went abroad to study up-to-date practices of child psychiatry within the Eastern bloc. The reports on their visit to Leipzig (Hirsch, 1960) and to Leningrad (Liebermann, 1961) revealed that hypnotherapy and suggestion were widely used in other socialist countries, too. A year later, Lucy Liebermann discussed the presentation of Ernst Kretschmer in Vienna. He supported the combination of autogenic training, medication, hypnotherapy and psychotherapy to retune the whole personality (Liebermann, 1962). In 1962, neuroscientist Ferenc Völgyesi published *Az orvosi hipnózis* (Medical hypnosis). Völgyesi showed a certain talent in political self-promotion: he dedicated one chapter in his book to the hypnotherapeutic experiences of Engels with a 12-year-old boy (Völgyesi, 1962: 130). Mixing Pavlovian theories with political slogans could satisfy political trends (Gyimesi, 2018).

At Lipótmező, hypnotherapy had been used in several cases already a few years after the end of the war. However, it is not clear from the treatment histories in which exact ways the hypnotherapies were carried out. Examples from the adult ward include the treatment of alcoholism or obsessive-compulsive neuroses. For example, in 1952, a 16-year-old boy was hypnotised by Blanka Lóránd. Although he had been stuttering since he was four, it had become a serious problem only a year before his admission. His parents always asked him to speak slowly and this sometimes led to arguing and nagging.

The mother often cried in the presence of the patient, who would reply that it made things worse. When the boy was treated with hypnotherapy his condition improved in a week. The treatment history does not include any other methods (OPNI, 0161–007175 424).

This case appears rather atypical as hypnosis was generally only used after unsuccessful treatment attempts with drugs or electrotherapy. Lóránd described sixteen cases in her 1961 study on infantile mutism, but she used this method only once. The typical design for treatment was to start with medication, and if it failed, electrotherapy was used. If that did not work either, they tried hypnosis, like in this case.

The fact that Lóránd described the hypnotherapy performed on the adolescent boy of our case history in 1957 is a distinct feature. And it is very clear from the description that she did not only work with suggestion here, but also aimed at processing the trauma:

> In hypnophase, we will give him the instruction that he is at home with the parents (we call him the name used by his mother), and slowly we substitute us with the role of the mother (Your mother is sitting next to you, cling to her ... etc). We must remind him of the trauma and we will talk to him when he becomes alert. The first time he was uneasy, he started fidgeting. The second occasion was slightly more successful as he indicated with his eyes that he wants to recover and become like the other children. Although he was motivated for the treatment on the third occasion, he remained mute. The therapy that was of great expectations failed because of the mother's arrival. She told them that she will give birth soon and needed every help including the boy. The child was really happy to see his mother, he told her in tears that he was homesick even though everybody is so nice here except the kids who are making fun of his dumbness.

What is striking about the description is that in the attempted hypnosis, the therapist places herself in the role of the mother and works towards processing the trauma by with the help of the parental relationship with the child. This work with the therapeutic relationship is an indicator for the use of depth psychology therapy approaches. Thus, they were not rejected but integrated into the treatment. The case shows that psychiatrists had scope for eclectic practice beyond the political dogma in the case of hypnotherapy.

What is also remarkable is the doctors' acceptance of the boy's discharge in the middle of the therapy. This shows the level of parental agency. Therapies or observation stays in Lipótmező were interrupted only rarely until 1960. In these cases, the parents, generally described as 'worried', assuming overprotective attitudes, appeared a few days after their children's hospitalisation and, 'despite the counsel' or 'notice' of the doctors, took them home. The final report of the boy from 1957 registered no changes in his status and suggested a cure with the anxiolytic Andaxin to reduce his anxiety.

The therapeutic design in 1959–60

In November 1959, the boy returned to Lipótmező. In the two years after his interrupted therapy, he remained mute and became unable to continue his studies. He left school and started to work as an unskilled labourer in masonry. The following is written about the new admission in his medical history: 'There was still no complaint about his behaviour, he was loved by his colleagues, but he talked to no one except for his mother. He said that he desired to be healthy again.'

This time too, written communication was supported by the psychiatrists, and it turned out to be more effective. Some of his answers were preserved in his medical documentation:

[What would you like to be?] Miner to cut coal for the Motherland. I will finish elementary school.

Do you have a speech disorder? No.

Who mocks you? Lajos and Pászti, every evening. They hide under my bed and draw it. They are calling me deaf and dumb.

Do you agree to shock therapy? I dare, but only once.

Which nurse do you love the most? Nurse Kati.

The boy's medical file contains a detailed diary of his previous treatment in 1957 and a description of the treatment this time in 1959–60. One might expect the therapeutic process to be continued where it was interrupted, but it was not. The same order of therapeutic approaches was followed as during his first stay. This time too, an attempt was made to treat him with electroshock therapy, which was unsuccessful again. When the boy was taken to the central office 'he got slower with every step we were nearer to the room. He stopped dead in his tracks and started to protest furiously when he sees the machine. What are you afraid of? He gives written answers: the electro-shock.' In her study, Lóránd recalled the incident as follows: 'He came obediently to the doctor, but on seeing the Pantostat he turned pale, began to tremble, and then produced a stormy panic reaction, and tried to escape. When he was relieved, he seemed to be very ashamed of his cowardice. We are reintroducing hypnotherapy' (Lóránd, 1961: 18).

The next day the doctors decided to continue the treatment with hypnotherapy: 'He reacts well: he whispers his name in hypnosis and answers questions with a few words.'

On 6 January 1960, 'he gets bromide before the treatment, and he has to fixate for a long time before the hypnosis could start. He talks more, he even uses sentences, but he is still whispering.' For the following day, it is described that a posthypnotic suggestion took place in which he was instructed to answer the questions of a nurse. On 8 January, 'he explosively starts talking loudly, he says his name, suddenly he raises his hands, squeezes the fingers and the rest becomes easier. There is a boy in the department who stutters. We suggested him as a friend. They play board games and have a cigarette in the office of the special education teacher.' Nevertheless, his peer relationship was burdened with conflicts. In December, he wrote: 'Cili spit on me and Aunt Zsuzsa told me to slap her. I don't. Remember. Clearly. I want to go home at Christmas. My soap has been stolen.'

Suggestion helped him to talk with ever more nurses and doctors, but he hardly spoke to children except for his friend. His peers revealed that they thought 'he only pretends that he cannot speak. That is why we tickled him.' He beat a smaller kid for allegedly taking his cigarettes. At the same time, he showed a growing interest in girls.

His therapy stopped in the middle of January 1960 due to the illness of his doctor Lóránd. During these days he kept talking but only to 'the old acquaintances'. The therapeutic breakthrough happened on 18 January under hypnosis: 'We asked him to talk to us about his puppy being shot. We have asked him about this before but in the unconscious phase he could only say the name of the dog.'

According to the parents' narrative, 'when he was six, a dog by his side was shot and then he fainted. He was unconscious for only a few seconds, he turned pale but had no convulsions. After his awakening, he remained silent and only after half a year started to talk to his parents in a very low voice and only if there was no one else present.' The boy's handwritten version of the story was also preserved in the medical file: 'The dog was called Bodri. And this dog was very naughty. A border patrol came. I stood beside the dog. The soldier was drunk. He shot the dog and I got frightened.'

During hypnotherapy on 18 January 1960, the boy explained that he and the dog were the same age, and he liked the animal very much for being his perpetual playfellow. A drunken border guard shot the dog for barking at him. The first shot reached the dog's neck which made the animal flee to a barn. When it came out of the building, the guard shot it again. He had to watch while the dog died. He felt sorrow and the scene returned in his dreams. The medical file reads: 'He could not remember how he stopped speaking, but he remembers clearly that he was really scared because of strangers, and he could not formulate words ... He wants to study, finish school and become a carpenter.'

On the same day, the boy left the institute in 'cured' status. Throughout the description, it is clear that the 1959–60 treatment was aimed at coming to terms with the trauma, in addition to utilising suggestion. The fact that he was able to talk about the traumatising events was seen as crucial for his healing.

Two weeks later, the mother wrote a letter to the institute, addressing Blanka Lóránd:

Dear Department Chairman, please!

I inform the dear Department Chairman that the results of my son are very good. He speaks openly, I can send him to the shop. There is not a single error in his speech. He started the fourth class that he would finish this year and he would continue his studies at night school. He has had a part-time job since the first of February. His only trouble is his great anxiety. We ask him politely to hold back himself. He wants everything the way he likes. So, I humbly ask the dear Department Chairman to send us medicine that would help. To stop his anxiety. Please send us the recipe for the medicine you prescribed so we can order it from the local doctor. My dear Department Chair, we would like to thank you for your nice, conscientious knowledge and healing.

We will not keep him closed. The Népszabadság newspaper likes to promote this beautiful science. My son used to say that everybody was so nice to him as his mum and dad. We kiss your hands with love. My son also sends his greetings to everybody, to the dear Department Chairman, and to the kind nurses, too. Please, dear Department Chairman, answer us regarding medicine and everything. With love.

The letter not only registers the improvements, but also reveals that the cure was not as complete as the documentation suggested.

Conclusion

Some important biographical elements of the boy coincide with crucial years in the history of Hungarian psychiatry. His elective mutism emerged in 1950, one of the darkest years of Hungarian Stalinism, characterised by political arbitrariness, economic hardship and, in relation to psychiatry, by the doctrinal suppression of certain psychological and psychiatric trends. Although this is not, of course, a causal relationship, the boy's microhistory in some ways illustrates the macrohistory of Hungarian society. The boy's mutism and trauma were related to an encounter with a member of the armed forces. Such encounters were frequent for civilians between 1944 and 1960 during the deportations, the Stalinist terror, the crushing of the 1956 revolution and the collectivisation of agriculture. The silencing of the boy can also be paralleled in a figurative sense to the suppression of the voices of representatives of the 'bourgeois' traditions in science.

The present case study investigated practices in child psychiatry before the medical specialisation of this field came about in 1965. The study revealed that the effective functioning of the institution was hindered by financial obstacles, drug shortages and the low number of doctors. Once, the therapy had to be interrupted for a week when the doctor got sick. Effective operation depended on the individual's capacities and efforts.

The case shows a certain dichotomy: while diagnostic practices followed the tradition of the organic approach, the choice of therapeutic methods was eclectic (drugs, electroshock treatment, hypnosis). In the pathogenesis, the forced right-handedness of the child was considered more important to be taken into account than environmental aspects. The psycho-trauma in early childhood was mentioned, but his doctors paid little attention to social factors that aggravated the patient's condition, like moving, financial hardship of the family, death of relatives or the mother's institutional treatment. Iatrogenic effects were not discussed either: from today's perspective, the boy's encounters with electroshock therapy can be regarded as re-traumatisation.

As shown in the chapter, a certain eclecticism can be detected in the therapeutic design. The hypnotherapy carried out was a psychotherapeutic method and had a different quality from the electroshock therapy. Nevertheless, the contrast between the methods was limited by the fact that suggestive hypnosis was not considered taboo but conformed to a large extent to Pavlovian reflexology. In this respect, the therapies carried out on the boy (medication, electroshock treatment, hypnotherapy) were in line with Pavlovian doctrine. And although the boy reacted with fear to electroshock therapy, and hypnotherapy proved effective in the boy's case, it is striking that the same sequence of therapies – medication, electroshock, hypnotherapy – was maintained in both the 1957 and the 1960 treatments.

However, the detailed description of the hypnosis carried out clearly shows that Lóránd did not limit herself to positive reinforcement through suggestion, but also aimed at working through the trauma and at utilising the therapeutic relationship for the curative process. This openness to depth psychology approaches reveals the individual scope of the doctor in hypnotherapy and corresponds to the observation on the therapeutic practice at Lipótmező that the professionals here were open to anything that was deemed useful (Laine-Frigren, 2016).

In addition, the boy's treatment took place in a period characterised by changes regarding the ideological influence on scientific work. The early term in office of President János Kádár since 1956 saw Pavlovism increasingly lose its binding force and influence in research, while international trends gained in importance. This became visible, for example, in the increasing acceptance of psychoanalysis in theoretical writings.

Even though Lóránd presented the boy's case as a successful healing story in her 1961 study, her therapeutic work was not addressed in Hungarian hypnosis history. Based on her professional merits, colleagues insisted that she be awarded a doctorate after her retirement in 1967, but the request was rejected. Not least because of the lack of academic embeddedness, the therapeutic work taking place in Lipótmező became a forgotten chapter in the history of Hungarian hypnotherapies (Gyimesi, 2018).

Funding

This study was supported by the MTA BTK Lendület Ten Generations Research Group. Magyar Tudományos Akadémia Bölcsészettudományi Kutatóközpont is the Hungarian Academy of Sciences Research Centre for the Humanities. The Lendület programme, a part of the Academy, strives to form research teams in host institutions to explore emerging research topics.

Notes

1 The documentation of the National Institute of Neurology and Psychiatry (OPNI) is preserved in the Országos Kórházi Főigazgatóság (National Directorate General for Hospitals), Budapest. In further references to this collection, the abbreviation OPNI is used. In particular, the case dealt with in this chapter can be found under number 0161-004053.335. Citations in the following pages, when not differently specified, are taken from this file.
2 Also published in German (Lóránd, 1960).
3 The decline in scientific status and popularity of Freudian psychoanalysis was a worldwide post-war phenomenon (Micale, 2014), but their repression in the Eastern bloc brought psychoanalysis into the political arena.
4 Director István Hollós (1872–1957) promoted 'humanistic' psychiatry and believed in the effectiveness of open-door care (Szokolszky, 2016).
5 This is demonstrated by the example of Lenke Rugonfaly. She was the daughter of a high-ranking military officer and after acquiring her diploma in 1940 she worked as an ophthalmologist. However, in 1951 she can be found among the staff members of the Men's Department in Lipótmező (*Orvosi Hetilap*, 1951).
6 This optimism was based on three assumptions. First, it was assumed that Soviet science was superior to others in understanding and curing diseases. Second, mental diseases provoked by external factors (syphilis, alcohol) were expected to be covered by an effective prevention programme. Third, neuroses and anxiety were understood as results of the repressive conditions in capitalism. Therefore, the development of socialism would diminish these disorders.

References

Angyal, Lajos and Juba Adolf, 1943, 'Tapasztalatok az elektroshock-kezeléssel a budapesti elmeklinika anyagán' [Experiences with electroshock treatment at the Budapest Mental Health Clinic], *Orvosi Hetilap*, 87:27, 327–9.

Bakonyi, Péter, 1984, *Téboly, terápia, stigma* [Madness, therapy, stigma] (Budapest: Szépirodalmi Könyvkiadó).

Bottoni, Stefano, 2017, *Long Awaited West* (Bloomington, IN: Indiana University Press).

Brunecker, Gyöngyi, 1968, 'Adatok a gyermekpszichiátria fejlődéséhez' [Data on the development of child psychiatry], in Böszörményi Zoltán (ed.), *Az Országos Ideg- és Elmegyógyintézet 100 éve* (Budapest: n.p.), pp. 291–302.

Davison, Kate, 2021, 'Cold War Pavlov: Homosexual aversion therapy in the 1960s', *History of the Human Sciences*, 34:1, 89–119.

Doboş, Corina, 2015, 'Psychiatry and ideology: The emergence of "asthenic neurosis" in communist Romania', in Mat Savelli and Sarah Marks (eds), *Psychiatry in Communist Europe* (Basingstoke: Palgrave Macmillan), pp. 93–116.

Eysenck, H. J., 1954, *Uses and Abuses of Psychology* (Harmondsworth: Penguin Books).

Feinberg, Melissa, 2021, *Communism in Eastern Europe* (New York: Routledge).

Fekete, János, 1961, 'Intézetünk rövid története az Országos Tébolydától az Országos Ideg- és Elmegyógyintézetig' [A brief history of our institute from the National Lunatic Asylum to the National Institute of Neurology and Psychiatry], *Ideggyógyászati Szemle*, 14:2, 56–63.

Ferenczy, Ágnes, 2014, 'Nincs két egyforma autisztikus vagy autista' [No two autisms or autistic people are identical], *Esőember*, 18:1, 15–17.

Foucault, Michel, 1999, *Les anormaux: Cours au College de France (1974–1975)* (Paris: Hautes Etudes, Calliinard).

Frosh, Stephen, 2019, 'Psychoanalysis in troubled times: Conformism or resistance?', in Anna Borgos, Ferenc Erős and Júlia Gyimesi (eds), *Psychology and Politics: Intersections of Science and Ideology in the History of Psy-Sciences* (Budapest: Central European University Press), pp. 127–51.

Gegesi Kiss, Pál, 1955, 'A pavlovi szemlélet alkalmazása magyar gyermekgyógyászatban' [Applying the Pavlovian approach in Hungarian paediatrics], *Gyermekgyógyászat*, 6:3, 65–72.

Gyimesi, Júlia, 2018, 'Hypnotherapies in 20th-century Hungary: The extraordinary career of Ferenc Völgyesi', *History of the Human Sciences*, 31:4, 58–82.

Gyimesi, Júlia, 2019, 'Anomalies of demarcation in light of the nineteenth-century occult revival', in Anna Borgos, Ferenc Erős and Júlia Gyimesi (eds), *Psychology and Politics: Intersections of Science and Ideology in the History of Psy-Sciences* (Budapest: Central European University Press), pp. 23–37.

Herczeg, Ilona, 1993, 'A gyermekpszichiátriai osztály története' [The history of the child psychiatry department], in Kárpáti Miklós, Kuncz Elemér and Kundra Olga (eds), *Az Országos Pszichiátriai és Neurológiai Intézet 125 éves* (Budapest: Animula), pp. 51–5.

Hirsch, Margit, 1960, 'Beszámoló a Német Demokratikus Köztársaságban tett tanulmányútról' [Report on the visit to the German Democratic Republic], *Magyar Pszichológiai Szemle*, 17:2, 202–7.

Janos, Andrew C., 1996, 'What was communism: A retrospective in comparative analysis', *Communist and Post-Communist Studies*, 29:1, 1–24.

Kohen, Daniel P. and Karen Olness, 2011, *Hypnosis and Hypnotherapy with Children* (New York: Routledge).

Koronkai, Bertalan, 1964, 'Hypnosiskísérletek periódusos myoplegiás betegen' [Experimental hypnosis in periodic myoplegia], *Ideggyógyászati Szemle*, 17:5, 139–50.

Kovács, József Ö., 2014, 'The forced collectivization of agriculture in Hungary, 1948–1961', in Constantin Iordachi and Arnd Bauerkämper (eds), *The Collectivization of Agriculture in Communist Eastern Europe: Comparison and Entanglements* (Budapest: Central European University Press), pp. 211–42.

Kovai, Melinda, 2015, 'The history of the Hungarian Institute of Psychiatry and Neurology between 1948 and 1968', in Mat Savelli and Sarah Marks (eds), *Psychiatry in Communist Europe* (Basingstoke: Palgrave Macmillan), pp. 117–33.

Kovai, Melinda, 2019, 'The social roles and positions of the Hungarian psychologist intelligentsia between 1945 and the 1970s: A case study of Hungarian child psychology', in Anna Borgos, Ferenc Erős and Júlia Gyimesi (eds), *Psychology and Politics: Intersections of Science and Ideology in the History of Psy-Sciences* (Budapest: Central European University Press), pp. 185–205.

Laine-Frigren, Tuomas, 2016, *Searching for the Human Factor: Psychology, Power, and Ideology in Hungary during the Early Kádár Period* (Jyväskylä: University of Jyväskylä).

Lászlófi, Viola, 2019, 'Work as a cure for mental illnesses? Opportunism and seeking ways in psychology and psychiatry in the first decades of state socialism in Hungary', *Canadian Slavonic Papers / Revue Canadienne des Slavistes*, 61:2, 164–85.

Leuenberger, Christine, 2007, 'Cultures of categories: Psychological diagnoses as institutional and political projects before and after the transition from state socialism in 1989 in East Germany', *Osiris*, 22:1, 180–204. doi: 10.1086/521748.

Liebermann, Lucy, 1961, 'Beszámoló tanulmányutamról a Szovjetunóban' [Report on my study visit to the Soviet Union], *Magyar Pszichológiai Szemle*, 18:3, 347–51.

Liebermann, Lucy, 1962, 'Beszámoló a Wieni Pszichoterápiai Nemzetközi Kongresszusról (1961)' [Report on the International Psychotherapy Congress in Vienna, 1961], *Magyar Pszichológiai Szemle*, 19:2, 201–7.

Lóránd, B., 1960, 'Katamnese elektiv mutistischer Kinder', *Acta Paedopsychiatrica*, 27, 273–89.

Lóránd, Blanka, 1961, '*Az elektiv mutizmusos gyermekek katamnezise*', *Ideggyógyászati Szemle*, 14:1, 16–27.

Micale, Mark S., 2014, 'The ten most important changes in psychiatry since World War II', *History of Psychiatry*, 25:4, 485–91.

Nyírő, Gyula, 1962, *Psychiatria* [Psychiatry] (Budapest: Medicina Kiadó).

Orvosi Hetilap, 'A Pavlov Ideg-Elme Szakcsoport Vándorgyülése' [Congress of the Pavlov Section on Neurology and Psychiatry], 1951, *Orvosi Hetilap*, 92:32, 1083–4.

Ranschburg, Pál, 1943, 'Adatok az endogén kedélyi psychoneurósisok és sajátképpeni elmebántalmak aktív gyógykezelésének kérdéséhez' [Data on the active treatment of endogenous mood psychoneuroses and idiosyncratic mental disorders], *Orvosképzés*, 33:4, 109–46.

Shorter, Edward, 2013, 'The history of pediatric ECT', in Ghaziuddin Neera and Walter Garry (eds), *Electroconvulsive Therapy in Children and Adolescents* (Oxford: Oxford University Press), pp. 1–17.

Siftár, Imre (ed.), 1971, *Tájékoztató gyógyszerkészítmények rendelésére* [Information on ordering medicines] (Budapest: Medicina).

Szakács, Ferenc and Emőke Bagdy, 1993, 'Klinikai pszichológia az intézetben' [Clinical psychology in the institution], in Kárpáti Miklós, Kuncz Elemér and Kundra Olga (eds), *Az Országos Pszichiátriai és Neurológiai Intézet 125 éves* (Budapest: Animula), pp. 33–46.

Szokolszky, Ágnes, 2016, 'Hungarian psychology in context: Reclaiming the past', *Hungarian Studies*, 30:1, 17–56.

Ujváry, István, 2000, 'Az amfetamin-típusú drogok kultúrtörténete, kémiája, farmakológiája és toxikológiája' [Cultural history, chemistry, pharmacology and toxicology of amphetamine drugs], *Psychiatria Hungarica*, 15:6, 641–87.

Varga, Ervin, 1964, 'Megfigyeléseim az angol orvosi pszichológiáról' [My observations on the medical psychology in England], *Magyar Pszichológiai Szemle*, 21:1, 99–103.

Vekerdi, László, 1984, '"Permanens kritikai jelenlét hatotta át az egész klinikát
…" Interjú Tariska István professzorral Sántha Kálmánról' ['There was
a permanent critical presence throughout the clinic …' Interview with
Professor István Tariska about Kálmán Sántha], *Magyar Tudomány*,
29:7–8, 590–9.

Vetró, Ágnes, 1999, 'Child and adolescent psychiatry in Hungary', in H.
Remschmidt and H. van Engeland (eds), *Child and Adolescent Psychiatry
in Europe: Historical Development, Current Situation, Future Perspectives*
(Darmstadt: Steinkopff), pp. 151–64.

Völgyesi, Ferenc, 1962, *Az orvosi hipnózis* [Medical hypnosis] (Budapest:
Medicina Kiadó).

III

Reflections

8

Changing attitudes: psychoanalytic therapy of psychoses in 1950s clinical psychiatry

Marietta Meier

In 1951, Manfred Bleuler, the director of Burghölzli, the Psychiatric University Hospital of Zurich, published a widely acclaimed, comprehensive overview of 1940s schizophrenia research in one of the most renowned German-language psychiatric journals. This paper strongly influenced the development of German-speaking psychiatry (Schneider, 1954: 873).[1] The article concludes by stating that the physical treatment methods introduced ten to fifteen years ago did not meet expectations. Meanwhile, it was clear that therapies such as fever, sleep and shock cures had purely symptomatic effects and were unsatisfactory, as they only worked temporarily or not at all. The flood of research on physical treatment methods could, therefore, not hide the 'fact that hopes have shifted ... from physical treatment to psychotherapy'. For a long time, it was generally assumed that schizophrenic people could not be influenced by psychotherapy, but now this method had begun to be used to treat psychosis (Bleuler, 1951: 427–9).

The statement that hopes had shifted to psychotherapy in the treatment of psychoses may have surprised many readers of the research report. Four decades after the introduction of the concept of schizophrenia in psychiatry, the following view dominated: that schizophrenia was a biologically determined, inexorably progressing disease process, and that no conclusions about the disease could be drawn from the life history of the patients.[2] Bleuler, who, like his father Eugen, researched schizophrenia, had always advocated a 'psychotherapy of the everyday'. For psychoses, however, he had previously refused psychoanalytic treatment (Müller, 1961: 355). What had happened?

In the fall of 1949, Bleuler travelled to the USA for eight and a half months, where psychoanalysis had gained increasing influence since the end of World War II. In contrast to Europe, where analysts concentrated on the therapy of neurosis, some psychiatrists there had also begun to treat schizophrenic patients psychotherapeutically.[3] Various methods were applied. However, all approaches were based on the assumption that people with schizophrenia had been exposed to severe trauma in their early childhood. The therapy was intended to give the patients some of the love and care that their parents had denied them and thus heal them.[4]

Bleuler's experiences with analytical psychotherapy for psychoses during his research semester in the USA had not only had an impact on his overview of schizophrenia research. After returning to Switzerland in spring 1950, he submitted an application to the Rockefeller Foundation to establish a 'thorough modern postgraduate training in differentiated psychotherapy' at Burghölzli and investigate the interaction between endocrine and psychological disorders in the course of long-term psychotherapy.[5] Henceforth, Bleuler's research interests focused on psychotherapy. This had played an important role at Burghölzli in the beginning of the twentieth century, but then lost importance in the inpatient clinic (Müller, 1958: 456).[6]

When the application was approved, the hospital began to deal intensively with individual analytically oriented psychotherapy for schizophrenia in 1951. As Bleuler emphasised, the new method could not benefit many patients for the time being, but was primarily in the interest of research and teaching. The aim was to extend the initial encouraging experiences and to test them scientifically. Additionally, the new approach was incorporated into the training of psychiatrists and nursing staff.[7]

Bleuler, cautiously open to innovation, was likely the first European psychiatrist to try psychoanalytic therapy for psychoses in a state hospital after World War II. Analysing medical records, further internal clinic documents, correspondence and publications, this psychotherapeutic attempt is examined hereafter. By pursuing a cultural-historical praxeological approach, I ask how actors behave and give meaning to their behaviour. Therefore, what psychiatric practices – in other words, patterns of perception, interpretation and action[8] – can be identified by source analysis? Answering this question, I also explore the broader sociocultural context of these patterns, both in everyday clinical practice and at the level of psychiatric discourse. Furthermore, the consequences of engaging with these methods, as well as changes in psychiatric patterns, are examined.

The last goal is not intended to postulate simple causalities for change. First, it can be assumed that in a complex institution like psychiatry, different and sometimes contradictory patterns can be identified at the same time. This holds true all the more when the focus is on everyday clinical practices. Second, the trial, as the research was called, took place in a setting that was influenced by numerous uncontrollable factors and had to adapt to the conditions of everyday life in the institution. Third, it is important to investigate whether and to what extent the new therapy had an effect on these conditions. My interest, therefore, is concentrated on the interaction processes between the new method and the relations among various groups of actors, institutional routines, the clinical setting as well as further therapeutic approaches. As I will show, the trial did not so much contribute to answering the question under investigation – to what extent schizophrenic patients can be influenced by analytical psychotherapy – as it resulted in changes in everyday clinical practice as well as at the level of psychiatric discourse.

'Not a processing disease, but a disaster reaction': psychoanalytic therapy for schizophrenia

In the eyes of European psychiatrists who did not see the term psychotherapy in a negative light,[9] psychotherapy had long been practised in their clinics. They defined it as milieu and occupational therapy, which was called 'collective psychotherapy', as well as 'individual psychotherapy' (Müller, 1949: 20–1). The latter included all non-somatic treatment methods that a doctor granted directly to an individual patient. For psychotherapy in the sense of long-term talk therapy in an individual setting, resources were lacking. Furthermore, it was assumed that the method was suitable only for mild mental disorders.

Psychoanalytically oriented psychotherapy for psychoses was based on completely different premises. Here, a great deal of time and effort was invested in the therapy of an individual patient. Psychoanalytic psychotherapy, analytic psychotherapy or – as it was called later – dynamic psychotherapy (or psychotherapy)[10] did not necessarily mean a talking cure on the couch in the Freudian sense. However, the approach explained the patient's illness through their biography and aimed to heal the traumas they had suffered and thus their mental disorders. This could be done in different ways, such as through speaking, whereby the patients themselves were not required to answer, or through other actions.

For the attempts at Burghölzli, the work of John N. Rosen and Marguerite Sechehaye was decisive. Bleuler had become personally acquainted with Rosen and his direct analysis approach during his stay in the USA. Sechehaye was an internationally known psychologist and psychoanalyst from Geneva with her own practice, who had developed *réalisation symbolique*, a method based on the symbolic satisfaction – realisation – of basic needs that had been denied to the patient before. She had treated a young, severely schizophrenic girl with this method for ten years and had cured her (Meier, 2015: 264). Such breakthroughs, confirmed by independent experts and discussed in professional circles, challenged the view that schizophrenia ultimately led to a 'final defect state'. Furthermore, the insight that somatic therapies did not have a specific effect increased acceptance to see 'even in schizophrenia not a processing disease but a catastrophic reaction of a person in distress and brokenness'.[11]

Once the new method had been studied at Burghölzli and applied on a trial basis to a larger number of patients, the first longer-term therapies, which are analysed below, followed in 1952. Under Sechehaye's guidance, two doctors treated three selected severely schizophrenic patients[12] according to the method of *réalisation symbolique*.[13] Two of the patients were considered chronically ill and had already been in the clinic for quite a while. Burghölzli was a university hospital with a teaching and research mandate, but unlike university clinics in other countries, it treated more than just acute cases. The doctors saw their patients daily. The duration of each meeting differed, depending on the patient's condition, the situation in the ward and their own time availability. The psychotherapeutic attempts were supported by a male and a female nurse who were intensively involved with the individual patients – whether it was spending hours trying to feed them, getting them to draw, or taking them for a walk in the clinic park or even on an excursion.[14]

The two doctors closely exchanged information with the nursing staff about the three patients and discussed the therapeutic course with Sechehaye every fortnight.[15] In addition to the medical history, they kept a protocol on each patient, recording how they behaved during the therapy and what the nurses observed during the rest of the time. The documentation also contained the doctor's impressions and reflections, as well as short summaries of Sechehaye's feedback. According to the two doctors, they spent a total of 300, 500 and 600 hours on the three patients respectively during the therapies, which lasted between six and twelve months.[16] This meant an average of more than one and a half hours per day for each person. Compared to the time available for the other patients, this was an enormous effort. In the 1950s, one doctor at Burghölzli was responsible for an average of about thirty patients, one nurse for about three.[17]

Sechehaye, followed by two psychiatrists and psychoanalysts from nearby, introduced all the clinic's residents to psychotherapy. Volunteer doctors, with or without adequate salaries, offered to provide psychotherapy out of enthusiasm for the method. Lay people interested in psychology supported the efforts.[18] With donations, money was raised for these concerns.[19] At the end of 1952, a doctor was employed who treated several schizophrenic patients psychotherapeutically every day and supervised the therapies carried out by other staff members. In 1955, two posts for nurses engaged in psychotherapy were created. Apart from collaborating with Sechehaye, Bleuler continued to maintain contact with therapists in the USA. In the seminars and colloquia of the Zurich Institute for Medical Psychotherapy, founded in 1954, theoretical problems and individual cases were regularly lectured on and discussed (Müller, 1961: 355; Meerwein, 1965: 86–7).

Analytical psychotherapy met with great interest in clinical psychiatry outside Zurich and Switzerland. This is shown by the many enquiries Bleuler received. Patients or their relatives requested inpatient psychotherapeutic treatment at Burghölzli. Numerous foreign doctors and psychologists at the beginning of their careers came to Zurich for a traineeship to learn about the method.[20] The attempts were presented in publications and papers in various languages and received international attention. In 1956, a new volume of a renowned German textbook on psychiatry was published, which included a contribution on analytic psychotherapy in psychoses (Benedetti, 1956). In the same year the first international symposium on the psychotherapy of schizophrenia took place in the French-speaking part of Switzerland, with papers and discussions being published afterwards (Benedetti and Müller, 1957). More followed in various other European countries. In this way, analytical psychotherapy for psychoses began to be studied in many European places, even in regions where the method was hardly used or not used at all (Bister, 1976: 750; Kulenkampff, 1985: 133; Schott and Tölle, 2006: 399–400, 465–6, 471–2).[21]

'The rose' and 'the codex': making sense of pathological behaviour

15 January 1952. Today first attempt to get in contact with patient. Patient, …, had spontaneously sat up in bed at Christmas while listening to a musical performance of the song 'A boy saw a little rose growing'.[22] He smiled and sang along. In the following days, it was observed that the otherwise always mute catatonic could spontaneously start to rant and rail. Appropriate to the symbolic meaning of the rose, we brought him a small red rose and gave him a poem, 'To the Rose' by Hölderlin. At first, he pushed everything aside, turned away and threw the letter down in a negativistic manner, demanded to go back into the hall, even shouted that one should go outside. The reaction was rather aggressive; he tore the rose apart when we left him alone.[23]

These are the opening words of the documentation on the psychotherapeutic treatment of Carl Schmid, one of the three patients included in the trial of Sechehaye's method of *réalisation symbolique* over a year. The delivered part of the protocol refers to the first two months of the therapy and contains twenty-eight typewritten pages. The four and a half years before psychotherapy are documented in seventeen pages of medical history. In the following, Schmid's case is used as an example to describe and analyse the therapeutic attempts. Occasionally, additional sources are consulted: the files of the other two patients who were treated in the context of the trial, as well as other hospital files and publications.

Schmid was a 30-year-old patient in the 'unruly' ward diagnosed with 'chronic schizophrenia'. At Burghölzli, he had shown 'from the beginning the picture of a severe catatonic stupor with complete mutism' and quickly developed into 'one of the most difficult patients'. He was permanently bedridden, showed no reaction to his surroundings, resisted all treatment and had to be fed by tube. The various somatic cures attempted had hardly shown any effect and had been completely abandoned after a heart defect was found.[24]

Michel Foucault described the doctor as a decoder who filters out elements from the 'noise' that the patient sends according to a certain code and links them – again using a code – to stable units of meaning (Foucault, 1999). Foucault made this comparison to explain how doctors, so to speak, created diseases. However, it also works to describe how *réalisation symbolique* proceeded. Schmid's reaction to the song 'A boy saw a little rose growing' was probably not only the reason why he was chosen for the trial, but also led to the first symbolic object the therapy began with. In the following months, the attending doctor observed the patient, looked for clues of symbols in his behaviour and deciphered them. Then, with the help of symbolic objects, she tried to 'break the patient's rigidity', to show him that someone understood him and made an effort to satisfy his present and past needs. In this way, they hoped it would be possible for him to gradually leave his own world and thus his illness, which was the only place for him where he could still exist.[25]

While the nurse tried for hours to get some food into Schmid at the beginning of the therapy, the doctor mainly talked to him, even when he showed no reaction. 'I hold', she wrote on the fourth day, 'a monologue with the patient'. After a week, Schmid managed to elicit a few words. However, the search for symbols that would enable finding a common language with him remained difficult. When Schmid repeated the expression 'iron contestation' several times, the doctor noted that it seemed to be 'a specific symbol', but got nowhere this way. She began to show the patient pictures and realised that this was a chance to start a conversation with him. Therefore, Schmid was given drawing material, hoping that he would reveal more about himself through drawings and subsequent dialogues.[26]

With psychotherapy, not only did the patient's mutism disappear but also his food refusal. Schmid accepted being nourished after only a few days. After two weeks, he no longer had to be fed by tube, and one month later he ate on his own for the first time without having to be asked. A good two months after starting the therapy the severely underweight man had gained ten kilograms. This success was related to the fact that Schmid was now talking, which gave insight into his delusional system. The doctor and the nurse noticed that the patient believed he could not and should not eat because a 'codex' or 'earthman' lived in his mouth and went into a state of anxiety when he was forced to eat. Therefore, they repeatedly assured him 'that the mouth was empty of this codex'. The doctor also told Schmid that she knew his hallucinations were real and distressing for him. However, she and the nurse were supposed to protect him from them and to help him regain 'superiority' over the hostile forces.[27]

The patient's undesired behaviour was met with empathy. It was not simply interpreted as some symptom of illness, but explained with certain elements of his delusional system or psychoanalytical patterns of interpretation. For example, the doctor recorded in the treatment protocol that Schmid had thrown a book of poetry down the stairs. She returned it to him and explained that she knew for sure 'that he had not thrown the booklet away, that he was not responsible for it' [but the codex was]. The fact that Schmid initially spat when approached, she interpreted as his only possible defence. When he wet the bed several times, she instructed the nurses not to scold him at all and added, explaining, 'Madame Sechehaye thinks it is a sign of life, one should rather praise him for it, tell him we are glad he gives such a sign of life. Perhaps an awakening of repressed sexuality.'[28]

'I was afraid he might relapse': changing the psychiatric self

According to psychoanalytic therapy, the way in which a disorder manifested depended partially on the doctor. Therefore, the texts written in the context of such therapies were not only about the patient, but also about the therapists and their thoughts and feelings (see Meier, 2022). Once Schmid did not give a single answer for an entire hour, his doctor wrote the following day, 'I was afraid …

he might relapse. But since he continued to eat and work well and regularly, my fear calmed down.' At the same time, she stated that her goal was to show the patient that she could wait patiently until he spoke more of his own free will.[29]

Doctors who were engaged in the analytical psychotherapy of psychoses thus developed a different understanding of the mentally ill and their own work. Their psychiatric self changed: the intensive involvement with particular patients and the attempt to understand their illness on the basis of their individual life stories enabled them to perceive mentally ill people as personalities, to develop a closer relationship with them and to understand madness no longer just as something different and strange. They learned to pay attention to their own emotions, to critically reflect on their behaviour and to record such aspects. In texts, they spoke of themselves in the first person singular. The 'referent' appearing in the third person and the otherwise usual passive constructions rarely occurred. This applies to the therapy protocols and medical histories of the treated patients, as well as to published case histories of psychotherapies for psychoses. In contrast to other case studies from clinical psychiatry, such contributions usually focused on one case but discussed it in detail (see, for example, Schweich, 1953; Benedetti, 1955; Meier, 2022).

Nevertheless, it would be problematic to build up a dichotomy between the 'common' clinical psychiatry of the 1950s and the 'more humane', 'emancipative' psychoanalytic therapy of psychoses. First, in texts not written in a psychotherapeutic context, there were sometimes expressions such as 'tragic defective state',[30] in which the writing doctor let feelings shimmer through. Second, there were also limits in analytical therapy: patients who were found unsuitable for psychotherapy and not worth starting or continuing therapy because they did not meet certain conditions.[31] Thus, the approach was also characterised by clear expectations and power asymmetry. It was the doctors who explained the patients' illnesses and symptoms and knew what was good for them.

In Schmid's treatment protocol, for example, there are expressions such as 'defiance' or 'In the ward he [the patient] complies well' – formulations that were commonplace in clinical psychiatry at that time. Some entries show that the doctor reproached the patient if he spat or did not answer for a long time. She 'demanded' certain things from him and touched him even when he was visibly uncomfortable. Various statements suggest that she perceived and treated Schmid less as an adult than as a child. Thus, she once wrote, 'The patient was very sweet in the ward today.'[32] In publications, some authors also tended to heroise their great time and human commitment.[33]

Finally, the documents from Burghölzli prove that the same doctor could observe, describe, evaluate and interpret patients' statements and behaviour differently. Depending on whether one took on the role of departmental doctor or that of psychotherapist, different expectations had to be fulfilled and different knowledge produced. However, the sources on psychoanalytic therapy for psychoses show that new patterns of perception, interpretation and action were created and learned within the framework of this approach – even in state hospitals. Or, as a representative of dynamic psychotherapy for psychoses put it in 1958: 'Whereas in the past it was a matter of course to cultivate the driest objectivity and to frown upon the personal touch in case reporting, whereas ... countertransference problems were at most alluded to in publications but not called by name, today we are more careless and freer in this respect' (Müller, 1958: 461).

'An extremely pleasing improvement – but by no means a cure': the aftermath

The psychotherapeutic attempt with the three patients was completed at the end of 1952. One of the treated patients was discharged on 23 December in a 'very good condition' and started a job in January. Two weeks before, his doctor travelled with him to the future place of work and noted the following day, 'You can really say that there was nothing left to see and sense ... of a schizophrenic defect, unless one is particularly trained.' In the last entry made in the medical history, he added in brackets the request to be contacted if the patient was to return to Burghölzli, even if he no longer worked there.[34] The woman chosen for the trial was also subjected to insulin cures, sleep therapies and some electric shocks during psychotherapy. Despite all these efforts, the patient, as it says in a report, 'sank more and more into the psychotic defect'. The 'special psychotherapeutic care' was therefore stopped at the end of November 1952 'because it was too unsuccessful and too exhausting'.[35]

Carl Schmid suffered a relapse in summer 1952. He worked in the garden without supervision in July and punched a woman 'in the face with his fist on the orders of the "codex"'. In August, he attacked the nurse who was taking care of him in the course of psychotherapy on an outing and again explained this aggression with the 'codex'. However, his condition improved anew; the psychotherapy continued for a few more months, and at Christmas he gave a musical performance with his therapist. Although he relapsed a bit after the end of the intensive treatment, he continued to feel much better than before. Schmid ate on his own, spoke of his own free will and pursued activities.[36] 'An extremely pleasing improvement – but by no means a cure' was Bleuler's conclusion, and there were no doubts that the result was due to psychotherapy.[37] Thus, by considering the disappearance or alleviation of symptoms as success, a pragmatic rationale of behaviour change becomes evident even in a psychoanalytically oriented clinical context.

According to Marguerite Sechehaye, the trial proved that psychotherapy, such as *réalisation symbolique*, could also be implemented in a large state hospital if a doctor could only concentrate on this task, count on the psychological understanding of the nursing staff and 'sacrifice' himself to the patients. The fact that these conditions were difficult to fulfil was related to a fundamental problem: the financial resources. Indeed, Burghölzli lacked the funds to continue with intensive psychotherapies. When Schmid's mother asked Bleuler if it was not possible that at least the nurse would continue to take care of her son, Bleuler replied that the resources were 'simply out of reach'. Moreover, they would have to be distributed 'more or less equally'. 'I would like to give each individual patient, as was the case with your son for a long time, a large part of the working time of a doctor and a nurse alone – but you must realise yourself that this is completely impossible.'[38]

In addition to the question of resources, ethical questions arose in a state clinic: was it permissible – outside of a trial – to invest so much in the therapy of a few patients when success was uncertain, and the large majority of patients did not benefit from extensive treatment? Apart from the three intensive treatments, shorter psychotherapies were also conducted at Burghölzli in 1952. There were several improvements and even discharges.[39] According to Bleuler, further experience confirmed the impression 'that there were no schematic theories and no individual techniques that were decisive in psychotherapy'. Instead, it was more a matter of 'the personality of the psychotherapist and the harmony of the same with the personality of the sick person'.[40] Unless it was assumed that the theoretical framework was crucial, there was no need to concentrate only on individual, analytically oriented, long-term psychotherapies. Under the given circumstances, it was therefore obvious to focus more on time- and cost-saving methods in the future.

One solution adopted at Burghölzli was to increasingly consider patients who had not been ill for long and had only recently been hospitalised. According to a catamnestic overview from 1961, of the 94 schizophrenic patients who received psychotherapeutic treatment in an individual setting between 1950 and 1958, more than half had been hospitalised for a maximum of one month before starting therapy. About two-thirds of the patients treated left the clinic afterwards, whereby a good half of them continued psychotherapy on an outpatient basis for some time after discharge.[41] The duration of therapies decreased: 55 of the 94 patients were treated for between 10 and 100 hours, 28 for between 100 and 300 hours and 11 for over 300 hours. In addition to doctors, psychologists conducted therapies as well. Most of the treatments no longer applied a specific method but followed an eclectic approach (Müller, 1961).

The other solution aimed to treat several patients together. The practice of group psychotherapy spread throughout Europe after World War II (Henckes, 2011: 174–5). At Burghölzli, the method was introduced in 1953 and expanded in the following years. The groups were composed of 'suitable patients' with different diagnoses and were led by doctors, psychologists or nurses.[42] Group and individual therapy were usually combined with somatic cures, after the introduction of psychotropic drugs increasingly with medication. As in many other places, the opinion was held that somatic treatment could facilitate psychotherapy.[43] According to the recollections of former doctors, however, even in the 1960s, psychotherapy in the inpatient clinic remained a marginal phenomenon, despite efforts to find pragmatic solutions. In view of the low headcount, it was impossible to apply the method across the board. Around 1970, there was finally a shift to short-term psychotherapy in the sense of crisis intervention (Jenzer *et al.*, 2017: 140–2).

Therefore, what remained of psychoanalytic therapy for psychoses? Contemporary physicians emphasised mainly one point: to realise that they could also find access to seriously ill patients who had previously been assumed to be 'no longer human', and that in the course of psychotherapy, every symptom could change or even disappear. According to Bleuler, the relationship with patients and their individual fates had moved to the foreground: 'Diagnosing diseases has become subordinate to delving into personal tragedies.' He also pointed out that the procedures had 'greatly enlivened the therapeutic attitude of the clinic's doctors and nurses as a whole', and in this way benefited not only specific patients but all of them.[44]

Furthermore, from studying medical files, clinical records and professional articles, it is apparent that doctors and nurses who engaged with psychotherapy began to critically reflect on themselves, their work and the social role of psychiatry (cf. Müller, 1960; Henckes, 2011: 174). A doctor in 1956 wrote that psychiatrists often mixed social and emotional order and valued social order too highly (Ernst, 1956: 355, 365–6). Individual and common good, therefore, did not have to coincide. Doctors adopting such thoughts no longer saw themselves as unconditional guardians and defenders of the social order, but felt committed to their patients first. The focus tended to shift from abstract clinical pictures to the sick individual, from the goal of fitting patients into society and the clinical order to efforts to consider their individual needs (see, for example, Bally, 1956: 442).

Finally, the attempt with analytically oriented psychotherapy of psychoses not only brought new actors into play, but also contributed to a first differentiation of the medical clinic staff and a softening of their roles. As clinic director, Bleuler was crucial to the project because he initiated and supported it. On a practical level, however, he subsequently left the field to younger colleagues. With Marguerite Sechehaye, he engaged a woman who – as a female expert and freely practising psychologist and psychoanalyst – was, in two respects, a novelty at Burghölzli. Sechehaye was followed by other psychologists, and a new professional group entered the psychiatric hospital. In the context of intensive psychotherapies, nurses worked closely with the attending physician, took on new therapeutic tasks and later led group psychotherapies.

Analytic psychotherapy thus resulted in a fundamental, largely unintended change in psychiatric patterns of perception, interpretation and action. This change was driven by many other factors that influenced each other: the introduction of psychotropic drugs and reform efforts within psychiatry, for example, as well as sociocultural changes, such as the emergence of a new subject order that gave more weight to individuality than social adjustment (Meier, 2015: 310–5).

A final look at Carl Schmid and the second male patient included in the therapeutic attempt highlights the point that this thesis does not conceptualise change as a simple story of success or progress. Unlike his fellow patient who could leave the hospital after the trial and apparently never returned to Burghölzli, Schmid's life took a different path. When the research was completed at the end of 1952, his therapy was not continued. The worst symptoms had disappeared; the doctor and the nurse had to assume other tasks, and resources for longer-lasting intensive care were lacking. From 1953, the patient received neuroleptics. According to an entry in the medical history, his former doctor resumed psychotherapy at the beginning of 1954. Two years later, psychotherapeutic efforts by a nurse are noted. However, because any further information is missing, it can be assumed that their attempts did not last long. In 1967, Schmid was asked if he wanted to participate in group psychotherapy, but declined. The year before, he had taken up a job in the clinic library, and later he even worked outside the hospital.

Nevertheless, there were repeated phases in which Schmid refused medication, became abusive and wrote confused letters. He was obviously much better than at the beginning of the 1950s, but his condition remained too poor for discharge. Therefore, Carl Schmid remained at Burghölzli until he died in 1993 at the age of seventy-five. He had spent forty-six years in the hospital, more than half of his life. At the end, his patient record comprised four files, and the medical history had grown to 110 pages.[45] His dossier shows that in clinical psychiatry different patterns of perception, interpretation and action could run parallel, complement or even compete with each other at the same time. Apart from certain changes many practices remained static, and by no means all shifts went in the same direction.

Notes

1 For German-speaking psychiatry, the almost seventy-page article was important for several reasons: first, it was written by an internationally recognised expert in the field of schizophrenia research; second, English was not yet the international language of science, so overviews in the mother tongue were central for gaining an orientation on the state of research; third, in post-war Germany and Austria, it was difficult to gain access to publications from abroad, which is why foreign literature was received through reviews and research overviews (Meier, 2015: 85, 90–1).

2 On the transformation of the concept of schizophrenia from 1945 until the 1980s see Schmitt, 2018.

3 The first attempts to understand schizophrenic symptomatology psycho-analytically and to present it in case studies took place before World War I. In this context, Burghölzli played a central role because it was the first, and for a long time the only, European state psychiatric hospital interested in Freud's theory. After the initial enthusiasm and the departure of Carl Gustav Jung, Alphonse Mäder and Karl Abraham, however, there were no more publications on the psychoanalytical treatment of schizophrenia from Zurich. Until about 1940, the decisive factor for this subject were freely practising therapists and private sanatoria (see for example Müller, 1958; Stone, 1999: 587).

4 On the history of psychoanalytic therapy of psychoses see Hale, 1995; Vincent, 1996; Alanen *et al.*, 2009.

5 State Archives of Zurich (hereafter StAZH), Zurich, Z 99.247, Finanzierung wissenschaftlicher Arbeiten, Request by Manfred Bleuler to Rockefeller Foundation, 20 June 1950.

6 On the connection between Eugen and Manfred Bleuler's schizophrenia theory and the role of psychotherapy in psychoses at Burghölzli, see Benedetti, 1995.

7 StAZH, Z 99.253, Finanzierung wissenschaftlicher Arbeiten, Application by Manfred Bleuler to the State School Administration of Zurich, 13 June 1951.

8 Typical, widely used forms of perceiving, interpreting and acting in clinical psychiatry.

9 Clinical psychiatry in Europe seems to have been far more sceptical, not to say negative, about psychotherapy after World War II than psychiatry in the USA. That was one of the reasons why psychotherapy was introduced later in European state psychiatric institutions. However, there is not much research on this question, especially not for all European

countries. For publications on the history of post-war psychotherapy dealing with individual European countries, see for example Hutsche- maekers and Oosterhuis, 2004; Neve, 2004; Roelcke, 2004; Alanen, 2009; Fussinger, 2009; Fussinger and Ohayon, 2010; Marks, 2018; as well as the contributions of Gábor Csikós, Gundula Gahlen, Henriette Voelker, Despo Kritsotaki and Katariina Parhi in Chapters 1, 3, 5, 7 and 10, which provide further literature references.

10 See, for example, Bister, 1976: 746–7. During the 1950s, psychoanalyti- cally trained psychiatrists increasingly sought to speak of psychotherapy rather than psychoanalysis in a medical context (Fussinger, 2009: 184).

11 State Health Services of Zurich (hereafter SHSZH), 12.06.2, Heilanstalt Burghölzli, Tätigkeitsberichte von Direktor und Verwalter, Lecture by Manfred Bleuler to the Society of Physicians of Zurich, 24 January 1957, 11.

12 Manfred Bleuler himself neither did a teaching analysis nor did he conduct any psychotherapies. As far as I know, during his time as clinic director, he didn't have his own patients either.

13 StAZH, Z 99.262, Bleuler to the Board of the Jubilee Donation for the University of Zurich, 30 January 1953.

14 StAZH, Z 100.41821; Z100.45455; Z 100.46222.

15 To the general part of these meetings, which lasted for a year, all doctors and French-speaking, interested nurses at Burghölzli, the polyclinic and the child psychiatric service were invited. StAZH, Z 99.257, Wis- senschaftliches, Dissertationen, Bleuler to the doctors of the polyclinic and the child psychiatric service, 30 October 1951; Bleuler to the head nurses at Burghölzli, 30 October 1951.

16 StAZH, Z 999.261, Finanzierung wissenschaftlicher Arbeiten, Reports of the two attending doctors, n.d. and 10 December 1952.

17 StAZH, DS 104.1.9, Annual reports 1950–59.

18 The lay people who offered their support were apparently from Zurich and the surrounds. In the files of one patient who received psychotherapy, for example, there is a report from a teacher who wrote about a walk with the patient. StAZH, Z 100.45455, Report of the volunteer, July 1951.

19 StAZH, DS 104.1.9, Annual reports 1950–59.

20 StAZH, Z 99.252–273, Directorial correspondence 1951–54; DS 104.1.9, Annual reports 1950–59. Unfortunately, the names of these doctors and psychologists are not listed in the annual reports. One of the doctors was Martti Siirala, and one of the psychologists was Erena Adelson.

21 The contributions appeared not only in psychoanalytic, but also in psychiatric and medical journals. A search in PubMed revealed articles on the topic of psychotherapy or psychoanalysis of schizophrenia from

the following European countries: for the years 1950–59 Austria, Belgium, Czechoslovakia, Federal Republic of Germany, France, German Democratic Republic, Great Britain, Holland, Italy, Norway, Portugal, Switzerland, Spain, USSR; for the years 1960–69 Denmark, Federal Republic of Germany, Finland, France, Great Britain, Italy, Portugal, Spain, Sweden, Switzerland, USSR, Yugoslavia. See for example Gabe and Grotjahn, 1952: 653; Gál, 1951; Schweich, 1953; Bleuler, 1954: 841; Searles, 1956; Stierlin, 1957.

22 A folksong based on the poem 'Little Rose upon the Heath' by Johann Wolfgang von Goethe.

23 StAZH, Z 100.41821, Part 2, Protocol on psychotherapeutic treatment, 1, 15 January 1952.

24 StAZH, Z 100.41821.

25 StAZH, Z 100.41821, Part 2, Protocol on psychotherapeutic treatment, 2, 19 January 1952.

26 *Ibid.*, 2 and 4, 18 and 19 January 1952.

27 *Ibid.*, 4–7, 19–27 January 1952, 19, 28 February 1952.

28 *Ibid.*, 9, 31 January and 1 February 1952, 20–1, 4 March 1952, 28, 17 March 1952. As already mentioned, only part of the psychotherapy protocol has survived. There is no statement in the existing files that attempts to make overarching sense of the therapeutic dynamics in Carl Schmid's case.

29 *Ibid.*, 22, 8 March 1952.

30 StAZH, Z 100.16072, Part 2, Protocol on psychotherapeutic treatment, 42, 3 April 1952.

31 See for example StAZH, Z 100.43763, 20, 14 November 1951; Z 100.44885, 17–18, 30 September, 14 October and 4 December 1950; Z 100.45506, 36, 4 and 26 November 1953. Cf. Henriette Voelker's contribution in Chapter 10.

32 StAZH, Z 100.441821, Part 2, Protocol on psychotherapeutic treatment, 5, 23 January 1952, 6, 24 January 1952, 9, 27 January 1952, 17 February 1952, 12, 17 February 1952, 14, 18 February 1958, 16, 22 February 1952, 18, 29 February 1952.

33 A representative of the approach also mentioned the danger of self-heroisation: Müller, 1958: 461.

34 StAZH, Z 100.46222, 19, 17 and 23 December 1952.

35 StAZH, Z 99.261, Finanzierung wissenschaftlicher Arbeiten, Report of the attending doctor, 10 December 1952.

36 StAZH, Z 100.41821, Part 1, 20–4.

37 StAZH, Z 99.262, Bleuler to the Board of the Jubilee Donation for the University of Zurich, 30 January 1953.

38 StAZH, Z 100.41821, Bleuler to the mother of the patient, 5 May 1953.

39 StAZH, Z 99.262, Bleuler to the Board of the Jubilee Donation for the University of Zurich, 30 January 1953.

40 StAZH, 12.06.2, Heilanstalt Burghölzli, Tätigkeitsberichte von Direktor und Verwalter, Lecture by Manfred Bleuler to the Society of Physicians of Zurich, 24 January 1957, 11.

41 According to Müller, the fact that many therapies were discontinued after discharge can be attributed to various reasons: the therapists changed jobs or did not find the time to continue treating patients in addition to their work at Burghölzli. Alternatively, the patients did not want to continue the therapy or lived too far away to come to the clinic for therapy (Müller, 1961: 358). As far as I know, few schizophrenic patients were treated in private practices.

42 For a published report on a psychotherapy group at Burghölzli, see Adelson, 1953. For two later examples of clinical group psychotherapy in Europe, see Chapters 1 and 10 in this volume. The group psychotherapy in the Heidelberg Psychiatric University Clinic in the 1960s and 1970s was aimed at hospitalised patients who had entered the clinic specifically for this purpose (see Chapter 3). In contrast, the Open Psychotherapeutic Centre of Athens in the 1980s provided group psychotherapy for people who did not live in the clinic. For outpatient care see Chapter 5 on the treatment of young drug users in Finland, 1969–75.

43 According to the catamnestic overview of 1961, most of the ninety-four patients included in the study received psychotropic drugs before, during or after psychotherapy. Müller, 1961: 357. See also Adelson, 1953; StAZH, DS 104.1.9, Annual report 1959, 2.

44 StAZH, Z 99.261, Wissenschaftliches, Dissertationen, Bleuler to Sechehaye, 10 December 1952; Z 99.262, Bleuler to the Board of the Jubilee Donation for the University of Zurich, 30 January 1953; StAZH, 12.06.2, Heilanstalt Burghölzli, Tätigkeitsberichte von Direktor und Verwalter, Lecture by Manfred Bleuler to the Society of Physicians of Zurich, 24 January 1957, 3 and 14. Cf. Steck, 1957: 9.

45 StAZH, Z100.41821.

References

Adelson, Erena, 1953, 'Die psychotherapeutische Gruppe in der Heilanstalt: Praktische Erfahrungen und theoretische Erwägungen', *Psyche*, 7:7, 463–80.

Alanen, Yrjö O., Manuel González de Chávez, Ann-Louise S. Silver and Brian Martindale (eds), 2009, *Psychotherapeutic Approaches to Schizophrenic Psychoses: Past, Present and Future* (London: Routledge).

Bally, Gustav, 1956, 'Gedanken zur psychoanalytisch orientierten Begegnung mit Geisteskranken', *Psyche*, 10:7, 437–47.

Benedetti, Gaetano, 1955, 'Psychotherapie eines Schizophrenen', *Psyche*, 9:1, 23–41.

Benedetti, Gaetano, 1956, 'Analytische Psychotherapie der Psychosen', in Hans Hoff (ed.), *Lehrbuch der Psychiatrie: Verhütung, Prognostik und Behandlung der geistigen und seelischen Erkrankungen*, vol. 3 (Basel: Schwabe), pp. 787–806.

Benedetti, Gaetano, 1995, 'Die Bleulersche Tradition der Schizophrenielehre und das Burghölzli als Stätte der Psychotherapie bei Schizophrenen', *Schweizer Archiv für Neurologie und Psychiatrie*, 146:5, 195–9.

Benedetti, Gaetano and Christian Müller (eds), 1957, *Internationales Symposium über die Psychotherapie der Schizophrenie, Lausanne, Oktober 1956 / Symposium international sur la psychothérapie de la schizophrénie, Lausanne, Octobre 1956* (Basel: Karger).

Bister, Wolfgang, 1976, 'Über das neue Verständnis für die schizophrenen Psychosen', in Dieter Eicke (ed.), *Die Psychologie des 20. Jahrhunderts: Freud und die Folgen*, vol. 2 (Zurich: Kindler), pp. 738–59.

Bleuler, Manfred, 1951, 'Forschungen und Begriffswandlungen in der Schizophrenielehre 1941–1950', *Fortschritte der Neurologie und Psychiatrie*, 19, 385–452.

Bleuler, Manfred, 1954, 'Zur Psychotherapie der Schizophrenie', *Deutsche Medizinische Wochenschrift*, 79, 841–2.

Ernst, Klaus, 1956, '"Geordnete Familienverhältnisse" späterer Schizophrener im Lichte einer Nachuntersuchung', *Archiv für Psychiatrie und Zeitschrift Neurologie*, 194, 355–67.

Foucault, Michel, 1999, 'Botschaft oder Rauschen?', in Michel Foucault and Jan Engelman (eds), *Botschaften der Macht: Der Foucault-Reader, Diskurs und Medien* (Stuttgart: Deutsche Verlags-Anstalt), pp. 140–4.

Fussinger, Catherine, 2009, 'Psychiatres et psychanalystes dans les années 1950: Tentations, tentatives et compromis: Le cas suisse', in Jacques Arveiller (ed.), *Psychiatries dans l'histoire: Actes du 6e Congrès de l'Association européenne pour l'histoire de la psychiatrie* (Caen: Presses universitaires), pp. 171–88.

Fussinger, Catherine and Annick Ohayon, 2010, 'Psychotherapy in Switzerland and France in the 1950s: Similar controversy, different solutions', in Waltraud Ernst and Thomas Müller (eds), *Transnational Psychiatries: Social and Cultural Histories of Psychiatry in Comparative Perspective, c.1800–2000* (Newcastle: Cambridge Scholars Publishing), pp. 272–95.

Gabe, Sigmund and Martin Grotjahn, 1952, 'Neuere Fortschritte in der analytischen Psychotherapie der Psychosen', *Psyche*, 5:11, 653–61.

Gál, Paul, 1951, 'Zur Psychotherapie der Schizophrenie', *Monatsschrift für Psychiatrie und Neurologie*, 121:1, 1–8.

Hale, Nathan G. Jr, 1995, *The Rise and Crisis of Psychoanalysis in the United States: Freud and the Americans 1917–1985* (New York: Oxford University Press).

Henckes, Nicolas, 2011, 'Reforming psychiatric institutions in the mid-twentieth century: A framework for analysis', *History of Psychiatry*, 22:2, 164–81.

Hutschemaekers, Giel J. M. and Harry Oosterhuis, 2004, 'Psychotherapy in the Netherlands after the Second World War', *Medical History*, 48:4, 429–48.

Jenzer, Sabine, Willi Keller and Thomas Meier, 2017, *Eingeschlossen: Alltag und Aufbruch in der psychiatrischen Klinik Burghölzli zur Zeit der Brandkatastrophe von 1971* (Zurich: Chronos).

Kulenkampff, Caspar, 1985, 'Erkenntnisinteresse und Pragmatismus: Erinnerungen an die Zeit von 1945 bis 1970', in Klaus Dörner (ed.), *Fortschritte der Psychiatrie im Umgang mit Menschen: Wert und Verwertung des Menschen im 20. Jahrhundert* (Rehburg-Loccum: Psychiatrie Verlag), pp. 127–38.

Marks, Sarah (ed.), 2018, 'Psychotherapy in Europe', *History of the Human Sciences*, 31:4, 3–12.

Meerwein, Fritz, 1965, *Psychiatrie und Psychoanalyse in der psychiatrischen Klinik* (Basel: Karger).

Meier, Marietta, 2015, *Spannungsherde: Psychochirurgie nach dem Zweiten Weltkrieg* (Göttingen: Wallstein).

Meier, Marietta, 2022, 'Third person: Narrating dis-ease and knowledge in psychiatric case histories', in Rob Boddice and Bettina Hitzer (eds), *Feeling Dis-Ease in Modern History: Experiencing Medicine and Illness* (London: Bloomsbury), pp. 103–20.

Müller, Christian, 1958, 'Die Pioniere der psychoanalytischen Behandlung Schizophrener', *Der Nervenarzt*, 29, 456–62.

Müller, Christian, 1960, 'Die psychiatrische Klinik und die Psychotherapie der Schizophrenen', in Gaetano Benedetti and Christian Müller (eds), *2. Internationales Symposium über die Psychotherapie der Schizophrenie, Zürich 1959 / 2e Symposium international sur la psychothérapie de la schizophrénie, Zurich 1959* (Basel: Karger), pp. 291–6.

Müller, Christian, 1961, 'Die Psychotherapie Schizophrener an der Zürcher Klinik: Versuch einer vorläufigen katamnestischen Übersicht', *Der Nervenarzt*, 32, 354–68.

Müller, Max, 1949, *Prognose und Therapie der Geisteskrankheiten*, rev. edn (Stuttgart: Georg Thieme Verlag).

Neve, Michael, 2004, 'A commentary on the history of social psychiatry and psychotherapy in twentieth-century Germany, Holland and Great Britain', *Medical History*, 48, 407–12.

Roelcke, Volker, 2004, 'Psychotherapy between medicine, psychoanalysis, and politics: Concepts, practices, and institutions in Germany, *c*.1945–1992', *Medical History*, 48:4, 473–92.

Schmitt, Sandra, 2018, *Das Ringen um das Selbst: Schizophrenie in Wissenschaft, Gesellschaft und Kultur nach 1945* (Munich: De Gruyter Oldenbourg).

Schneider, Kurt, 1954, 'Zur Frage der Psychotherapie endogener Psychosen', *Deutsche Medizinische Wochenschrift*, 79, 873–5.

Schott, Heinz and Rainer Tölle, 2006, *Geschichte der Psychiatrie: Krankheitslehre, Irrwege, Behandlungsformen* (Munich: C. H. Beck).

Schweich, M., 1953, 'La psychothérapie des schizophrènes. A propos d'un cas clinique aperçu général du problème', *L'Encéphale*, 42, 63–87.

Searles, Harold F., 1956, 'Verlaufsformen der Abhängigkeit in der Psychotherapie von Schizophrenen', *Psyche*, 10:7, 448–81.

State Health Services of Zurich, 1957, 'Tätigkeitsberichte von Direktor und Verwalter, Entwicklungsrichtungen in der Psychiatrie von heute', lecture by Manfred Bleuler to the Society of Physicians of Zurich, Heilanstalt Burghölzli, 24 January.

Steck, Hans, 1957, 'Allocution', in Gaetano Benedetti and Christian Müller (eds), *Internationales Symposium über die Psychotherapie der Schizophrenie, Lausanne, Oktober 1956* (Basel: Karger), pp. 7–9.

Stierlin, Helm, 1957, 'Die Schizophreniebehandlung in der Klinik: Anmerkungen zur psychotherapeutischen Technik', *Psyche*, 11:7, 459–71.

Stone, Michael H., 1999, 'The history of the psychoanalytic treatment of schizophrenia', *Journal of the American Academy of Psychoanalysis*, 27:4, 583–601.

Vincent, Thierry, 1996, *'Pendant que Rome brûle': La Clinique psychanalytique de la psychose de Sullivan à Lacan* (Strasbourg: Editions Arcanes).

9

In the wake of Goffman? Doing social sciences at the site of psychiatry in Austria

Monika Ankele

In April 1974, two postgraduate students of the Institute for Advanced Studies (IHS) and a doctoral student of the University of Vienna had their first working day at the psychiatric hospital Baumgartner Höhe in Vienna (PKH). They had applied as ward assistants in order to conduct empirical research on the quality of inpatient psychiatric care and the actions of psychiatric nurses that mediated it, using the method of covert participant observation. Under their white work coats, which identified them as part of the nursing staff, they carried writing pads and pens, the tools of the field researcher. The notes they recorded in unobserved moments provided the source material for a study that was led by Austrian sociologist Jürgen M. Pelikan. He initiated a comprehensive project on the problems of nursing staff in Austria commissioned by the Ministry of Health and Environmental Protection, which included an analysis of patient care and staff work in hospital departments (without further specification). The selection of a psychiatric hospital for this study was inspired by the students' reading of the book *Asylums* by the American sociologist Erving Goffman. For the covert participant observation at the PKH, Pelikan had acquired the consent of its medical director, Wilhelm Solms-Rödelheim, as well as of the head of the works council.

Four years later, in 1978, the study was complete: the data from the covert participant observation were complemented by a question-naire study with the nurses of the hospital and an analysis of the structural conditions under which the staff had to act. One of the aforementioned ward assistants, Austrian sociologist Rudolf Forster, and the project leader Pelikan, presented the results firstly to the Viennese City Councillor for Health and Social Affairs, the physician and social democrat Alois Stacher, and the newly appointed medical director of the PKH, Eberhard Gabriel. As Forster explained, the researchers declared their intention to make the results of their study available to the public to make it clear that the situation in the hospital was unbearable and fundamental reform was urgently needed. To alleviate the tensions which inevitably lay in the air, the sociologists had suggested inviting the internationally acknowledged social psychiatrist Hans Strotzka, a promotor of cooperation between medicine and sociology in Austria. At the end of the meeting, Stacher agreed to give a joint press conference with the researchers and to announce a profound reform of psychiatric services in Vienna.[1]

The sociological study by Forster and Pelikan (1978) will be the focus of this chapter, which offers a multilayered contextualisation on the interdependence of sociology, psychiatry, the public and politics in Austria in the 1970s. Following the topic of the volume, 'doing psychiatry' is explored here in the sense of doing social sciences at the site of psychiatry. From the late 1950s, social scientists began to enter the psychiatric hospital, using it as a field of research. In this respect, the approach by Forster and Pelikan was not unique, but it was unique for Austria (at least at the time when the study started) and considered to be an important component for psychiatric reform. In this chapter, the sociological research practices being examined will be conceived of as reflective practices that were intended to have an impact on the institution by getting the responsible authorities, politicians, doctors and staff to take action and improve the patients' living conditions inside and outside the institution. The sociologist became a consulting expert who, through the position of the outsider, gained different insights into the closed world of the hospital and, based on these insights, offered policymakers proposals for change. What Christina Malathouni states in her contribution to this volume on the role of the architect in the context of psychiatric reform in post-war England applies to the social scientist in the case of my chapter: 'S/he joined the larger pool of reform actors.'[2] There were at least three aspects that contributed to this, which I will elaborate on in the following: firstly, the general boom in the social sciences after World War II, a boom that reached Austria rather late and on a small scale, and their interest in the psychiatric hospital as a subject of research; secondly, the response and support that the social sciences received from the 'modernisation agenda' of social democratic politics in Austria (Rehor, 2019); and thirdly, the crisis that institutional psychiatry and inpatient care faced in these years, which led to a willingness of reform-oriented psychiatrists to open their institutions up to experts from outside to let them analyse their workplace and the daily activities at site, although this willingness was rather rare among the directors of Austrian psychiatric hospitals at the time the study took place.

In my chapter I refer to contemporary publications and printed sources. I also had conversations with the psychiatrist Eberhard Gabriel, who was the hospital's medical director from 1978 to 2004, and the sociologist Rudolf Forster, who together with Jürgen M. Pelikan initiated, conducted and wrote up the study in focus here. Administrative and medical files from the PKH Baumgartner Höhe (today Clinic Penzing) from the period in question were not accessible, as they are being transferred to the Vienna City and Provincial Archives at the current time (September 2021). Since there was no evaluation of the proposed reforms and their implementation at the PKH after the publication of the study, their effects on the institution, which must be located in a larger context of the reorganisation and restructuring measures of psychiatric care in Vienna, can only be made visible to a very limited extent.

The presentation of the study

When, on 19 June 1978, the study by Pelikan and Forster was presented at a joint press conference by the Austrian Minister of Health Ingrid Leodolter[3] the physician and social democrat Alois Stacher and the two sociologists, its findings of serious shortcomings in patient care at the PKH Baumgartner Höhe came as little surprise.[4] From the mid-1970s onwards, the number of reports critical of psychiatry had increased in Austrian newspapers and magazines, and public television had also turned its attention to the topic (Irschik, 2017). Undercover stories by journalists (Fritsch and Mayer, 1978) and researchers (Weiss, 1976)[5] as well as reports by people with psychiatric experience (Eva P., 1977; Meissner, 1976) were published and particularly targeted the nurses for their handling of the patients. Groups such as the Society for Democratic Psychiatry Vienna and the Scientology-supported Austrian Society for the Protection against Violations of Human Rights by Psychiatry were founded, the Italian reform psychiatrist Franco Basaglia attended a discussion event in Vienna, and leaflets were written and distributed to patients' relatives at the gates of Baumgartner Höhe (Gesellschaft für Demokratische Psychiatrie Wien, 1979: 9–11). The publication of the final report on the situation of psychiatry in the Federal Republic of Germany (1975) revealing the deplorable conditions in the psychiatric hospitals there had also received professional response in Austria (Rehor, 2019: 322). Overall, there was already enormous public pressure in the run-up to the presentation of the study that, firstly, provided insights into one closed institution and, secondly, confirmed that negative ideas prevailed about psychiatry and the treatment of the sick in Austrian society. By using the methods of empirical research to collect and analyse the data of one psychiatric hospital, the study provided a scientific foundation for public criticism. But unlike the majority of reports published in Austria so far, it did not focus on criticism of the nurses, but instead defused it by highlighting the structural determinants that impacted the work of staff as well as the living conditions of patients in the hospital – i.e. the shortage of qualified staff, the obsolete state of the premises, the meagre endowment of the wards – all traceable to decades of serious underfunding and political neglect. After the press conference, public reactions were not lacking and newspapers reported extensively on the shocking findings of the study: 'The Prison Inmates Are Better Off'[6] (*Kronen Zeitung*, 1978), 'Vienna: Scandalous Conditions at Psychiatric Hospital' (*Neues Volksblatt*, 1978), 'Psychiatric Hospital Vienna: Human Dignity – Perhaps in Five Years' (*Volksstimme*, 1978) were some of the headlines of the Austrian daily newspapers. Even the image of the 'snake pit' – borrowed from the title of a novel critical of psychiatry by Mary Jane Ward (1946) and the film based on it, which was released two years afterwards – was used to describe the conditions in the hospital (Schwarz, 1978). The *Kronen Zeitung* (1978), the most widely read daily newspaper, listed in its article on the press conference several observations that the sociologists had made during their research at the hospital, which clearly demonstrated that basic human needs were disregarded and neglected. The report mentioned that clothes were randomly handed out and often did not fit, special requests outside of routine meals were hardly ever fulfilled, there were still tin bowls in use in which food was often served cold, the sanitary facilities were a disaster, too many patients were housed in one room and furnishings like bedside cabinets were lacking. The report also pointed to a lack of trained staff and noted that there was just one doctor for every ninety patients. The article also referred to the extensive medication and lack of psychotherapeutic treatment.

At the press conference, to defuse the expected public criticism, Stacher pointed to improvements that had already been initiated, such as the extension of visiting hours, the improvement of training opportunities for staff, the amendment of the house rules, the abandonment of gender segregation and the change to private clothing. Pelikan and Forster presented their ideas for a reform programme and Stacher publicly promised its implementation.[7] The introduction of the new medical director, Eberhard Gabriel, was intended to embody this new beginning. In the context of a public already sensitised to abuses in psychiatric hospitals, the study provided politicians with a starting point to tackle the reform of psychiatric care. On 2 April 1979, a target plan (Presse- und Informationsdienst der Stadt Wien, 1979) for psychiatric and psychosocial care in Vienna was unanimously adopted by the city council, building on the study (Gabriel, 2007: 118; Presse- und Informationsdienst der Stadt Wien, 1979: 5) as well as on further enquiries that had been carried out since 1977.[8] Psychiatric reform in Vienna was the first comprehensive reform project in Austria, and remained the only one for quite a while.

The place of the study: the psychiatric hospital Baumgartner Höhe

The subject of research was the psychiatric hospital Baumgartner Höhe, which opened in 1907 as the Lower Austrian Provincial Sanatorium and Nursing Homes for the Mentally and Nervously Ill 'Am Steinhof'.[9] Located on a hill in the west of the city, the Art Nouveau-style complex with 34 hospital pavilions was intended to accommodate 2,200 patients. The area of 970,000 square metres was divided into a nursing home for the incurable, a sanatorium for the curable and a sanatorium for the paying sick (*Der Bautechniker*, 1907: 465). Following the concept of the colonial asylum, gardens, agricultural land and workshops provided opportunities to occupy the patients and, in keeping with the modern approaches of the time, to offer an apparently freer kind of treatment. In the years of the First Republic (1918–38), the Great Depression, financial cuts and a dramatic increase in admissions left their mark on daily life in the hospital. After World War II and National Socialist crimes and murders (Czech *et al.*, 2018), nothing was left of the glamour and spirit of optimism that had surrounded the institution when it was founded. Its consistent underfunding had a deep impact on the material and personnel resources (Schäfer, 2016). This did not improve even when, in 1956, the Hospital Act put psychiatric hospitals on an equal footing with general hospitals (Forster, 1997a). In the outdated and largely unrenovated buildings, newer (psycho)therapeutic approaches had little or no place, psychotropic drugs were widely used and biological concepts of illness were dominant in the doctors' attitude towards patients. Even the establishment of a rehabilitation centre in 1962, which worked closely with the Social Welfare Office and the Labour Office of the City of Vienna and was supposed to support the patients' return to work (Gabriel, 2007: 109), benefitted only a small proportion of the patients.

When the research group of the IHS started its study in 1974, the Baumgartner Höhe was still the largest psychiatric hospital in Austria. It cared for more than 2,600 patients, most of whom had been compulsorily admitted. Among men, 'alcoholism' (40 per cent) was the most frequent admission diagnosis; among women, it was 'mental disorders of advanced age' (32 per cent).[10] The hospital also cared for 200 to 300 permanently hospitalised mentally disabled patients. Those patients who were discharged relatively quickly after their admission were contrasted with the group of patients who had already spent several years – some more than ten years – in the hospital. For trained nurses, the Baumgartner Höhe was an unpopular place to work, and the resignation rate was high. This was the situation on site when Forster and his two colleagues entered the hospital in their role as ward assistants.

Smuggling oneself in: the sociologist as participant observer

In the 1960s and 1970s, for social science studies that chose psychiatry as their object of investigation (covert) participant observation and interaction analysis were often the chosen methods (Reimann, 1973: 247). As Forster reported, he read Goffman's (1973) book *Asylums* when he was a scholar at the IHS. Inspired by his approach and method, Forster, in the context of a large research project on the nursing staff (Forster *et al.*, 1975), saw the opportunity had come 'to experience the functioning of a presumably "total institution" from the inside, i.e. "up close" and yet protected by the role of the semi-outsider' (Forster, 1997a: 11). Without having worked scientifically on psychiatry before, the idea arose to smuggle oneself into the PKH to carry out covert participant observation in the wards. After consulting the medical director and the works council, Rudolf Forster, Dimiter M. Hoffmann and Monika Hoffmann-Paast applied as ward assistants (Stationsgehilfen) in the hospital (Forster, 1997a: 11–18). It was not unusual at that time for someone who had a different education or had never worked in the medical field before to get a job as a ward assistant at the PKH, as staff were rare and in demand. The only requirement was that he or she completed a nursing course within two years. As ward assistants, they had to support the graduate nursing staff in their activities such as making beds and serving meals. In April 1974, the three researchers started to work in different wards with the aim of 'getting to know and systematically documenting the living conditions of the patients and the working conditions of the staff for a few months' (Forster, 1997a: 11). As Forster recounted in conversation, he carried a small pocket diary and a pen with him during the work to make notes in unobserved moments – usually in the toilet.[11] After three and a half months, they finished their work at the PKH.

The study by Forster and Pelikan was not to be the only sociological study based on participant observation at the Baumgartner Höhe. Years later, from April 1980 to May 1981, the sociologist Karl Schwediauer investigated the 'social situation of mentally ill persons' there, with a corresponding approach, as part of his diploma thesis. Schwediauer was working in one of the two communication centres at the PKH when he decided to apply for a job as a ward assistant

to conduct covert participant observation in a men's ward (Schwediauer, 1984: 10–11). He later returned to his position at the communication centre where he had intensive conversations with patients.
He described his work as an extension of the study by Forster and
Pelikan, while the study of Goffman also provided him with important
ideas (Schwediauer, 1981: ii; 1984: 10).[12] In contrast to Forster and
Pelikan, who chose a so-called needs approach to systematically
analyse the patient's situation in the hospital,[13] Schwediauer's interest
lay in recording life in the institution from the perspective of the
patients, whom he therefore interviewed. The covert participant
approach that sociologists chose as a method of research was also
used by journalists at that time (and not only then) to gain insights
into the closed life of a psychiatric hospital. In 1978, the Baumgartner
Höhe became the subject of an undercover report by photographer
and journalist Gerhard Mayer titled 'Cultivated Insanity', which
was published in the news magazine *profil* (Mayer, 1978).[14] Mayer,
like Forster and his colleagues, was also hired as a ward assistant
and reported on the dehumanising conditions in the hospital. Neither
the journalists nor the sociologists reflected on the ethical aspects
of their research method.

Excursus: the patient's perspective

Even though the inclusion of the patient's perspective was expressed
as a concern in the study by Forster and Pelikan, to counteract the
'concentration of knowledge among professionals' (Forster and
Pelikan, 1978: 6–7), patients were not interviewed. In the final
report, the researchers reasoned as follows: '[C]ommunication
problems due to drug-induced attenuation of the patients as well
as due to illness and hospitalism; validity problems due to the
dependent position of the patients; irritation of the staff' (Forster
and Pelikan, 1978: 11). The researchers thus followed the zeitgeist
of those years, which gave only limited credibility to patients' narratives. When asked why the study claimed to take a patient perspective, but did not ask patients about their needs, Forster explained
that patients were 'delegitimised' at that time. People with a mental
illness were still stigmatised, their statements untrustworthy. Therefore,
demands for reform of the psychiatric hospital and psychiatric care

could not be based on their voices. Even though the sociologists thus moved within the existing paradigm of psychiatry, the reality of the patients' life in the PKH, the scarcity and deprivation they experienced, nevertheless gained visibility within the framework of the study. A needs approach was chosen for 'the conceptualisation of the psychosocial situation of the patient' (Forster and Pelikan, 1978: 7), which placed the focus of the researchers on the care of the patients and on the satisfaction of their needs. To this end, they conducted a questionnaire survey with the nurses in the second part of their study. In this way, they were able to link nursing practice with patient care.

The influence of social science research on political action in Austria in the 1970s

The study by Forster and Pelikan was conducted at the IHS, which was founded in 1963 with funds from the Ford Foundation as a postgraduate, non-university training centre for the empirical social sciences. Its founding coincided with the boom phase that sociology experienced in Western Germany in the years following World War II, when it was assigned central educational tasks in the context of re-education and was seen by both academics and politicians as playing an enlightening role (Neun, 2018: 505).[15] In Austria in the 1970s, the IHS formed 'the nucleus of sociology and social research that was halfway in keeping with the times' (Fleck, 2018: 328). It promoted international exchange and became the 'sole producer of young sociologists' during this period (Fleck, 2016: 1). Pelikan was head of the Department of Sociology at the IHS from 1972 to 1978. Forster came there in 1972 as a postgraduate student after studying psychology.[16] Both Pelikan and Forster later received professorships in sociology at the University of Vienna and, in 2017, they were awarded the Great and Golden Decoration of Honour for Services to the Republic of Austria for their academic work.

As Christian Fleck – himself an Austrian sociologist and contemporary witness – put it in his historical portrayal of the IHS, in the years of the student movement the 'exponents of the rebellion' were 'almost all taken in as scholars' through the intervention of the Social Democratic Federal Chancellor Bruno Kreisky, who was a member of the executive committee of the IHS (Fleck, 2016: 5). Fleck described it as Kreisky's calculation to place the 'revolucers' in the IHS, where they 'would [do] less harm than if they were left to roam free' (Fleck, 2016: 5). Irrespective of how Fleck's description is to be evaluated, it at least allows for a political classification of the institute, its proponents and its atmosphere. Particularly in the 1970s, the institute increasingly succeeded in acquiring third-party funding projects and in receiving research assignments from the government (Fleck, 2016: 7). These included, from the field of medical sociology,[17] a study on the 'Investigation of the Problems of Austria's Nursing Staff' (Forster *et al.*, 1975), already mentioned in the introduction, of which the study in question was a part (Pelikan and Leitner, 1974; Forster *et al.*, 1975). The general research at the IHS, which among other topics included a widely received system analysis of healthcare in Austria led by German political scientist Frieder Naschold (1975), delivered important diagnoses which could be used to argue for or justify political decisions, or as a basis for them.

Regarding the funding of social science research projects by politics, Fleck noted that 'in the 1970s, the socialist government … was generous with the [freehand] allocation of research assignments' (Fleck, 2018: 1003), and he explained with regard to the impact of the social sciences on politics: 'The government, subscribed to reforms, expected help from social science research in identifying the need for reform as well as in orchestrating the call for change in a publicity-effective way' (Fleck, 2018: 1003). In this context, the methods and findings of empirical social science research in particular were seen as holding special potential for the analysis and solving of current societal problems. The Austrian Research Conception, published in 1972 by the Federal Ministry of Science and Research (BMWF), stated that 'system analyses in all their variants, empirical social research in general … are important instruments for the examination and control of the socio-economic reproduction and life process and … can be made serviceable for … the improvement of the quality of life' (BMWF, 1972: 29, quoted in Knorr *et al.*, 1975: IV/II/66).[18] In these years, the social sciences and politics became more closely connected, sometimes even forming alliances and providing important resources for both sides. As Forster explained, in many cases it was the researchers who submitted proposals for projects to politicians. Thereby, the objectives were not always clearly specified, which opened up scope for the researchers.

In these years, the institution of sociology gained high recognition (Clemens, 2001; Neun, 2018). The discipline experienced an expansion, both at universities and through the funding of non-university institutions that – like the IHS – gave new impetus to research and politics. Sociology was presented as a medium of social criticism and, at the same time, as an application-oriented science that provided instructions and tools for sociopolitical change (Knorr *et al.*, 1974; Knorr *et al.*, 1975).[19] This gave the field the status of a leading discipline and made it attractive, especially for the left-wing student movement, as it not only analysed social structures and their underlying mechanisms with the detached gaze of a scientist, but took a stand. Sociology stood for combining research and action, analysis and activism. In the context of the reform discussion, sociology took on the role of a 'planning science' – also in the field of psychiatry – that scientifically justified, guided and secured the implementation of reforms (Giesen, 1982: 135, quoted in Clemens, 2001).[20] This was also intended to be the case in Vienna with the study by Forster and Pelikan.

The psychiatric hospital as an object of study for the social sciences

Looking back to the 1960s, Ernst von Kardorff stated that there was a 'break-in of sociology into psychiatry' (von Kardorff, 1985: 240; see also Forster, 1997a: 70–1) when social science critiques of psychiatry, its institutions, its treatment concepts and its illness paradigm started in the USA. Von Kardorff himself is a psychologist and sociologist who was a researcher in Germany in the 1970s and 1980s.[21] Formative for the sociological research (and criticism) of psychiatry in these years was the study *Asylums: On the Social Situation of Mental Patients and Other Inmates* by the sociologist Erving Goffman (1922–82), which was published in 1961. His book is based on ethnographic fieldwork he conducted at St Elizabeths Hospital in Washington, DC from 1955 to 1956, when he was a visiting scientist at the Laboratory of Socio-Environmental Studies of the National Institute of Mental Health (NIMH) (Hettlage and

Lenz, 1991: 11).[22] Using the method of participant observation, Goffman studied the practices and interactions of the 'inmates' of the hospital. St Elizabeths cared for over 7,000 patients, and Goffman conceived of it as a 'total institution' that regulated the work time, leisure time and life time of its inmates. For Goffman, the psychiatric hospital was perfect for investigating a social microcosm. There he could observe and analyse how the individual was shaped by social reality – this meant, in the case of psychiatry, the institutionally determined framework and the effects these structures had on the various actors – and how the inmates in turn reacted to this 'reality' by forming specific modes of behaviour. His sociological perspective showed that certain behaviours and actions could be explained as reactions to the conditions of the institution and its regulations – and not only as the expression of a certain disease pattern, as the medical view would suggest.

In the 1950s and 1960s, other researchers, mainly from English-speaking countries, also impressively demonstrated the damaging effects and destructive potential of large psychiatric hospitals for patients (Scull, 1980: 115–43) – those very places that had been conceived of in the early nineteenth century as a remedy to alleviate the suffering of the sick. Findings like those in Russel Barton's study *Institutional Neurosis* (1959) or in George William Brown and John Kenneth Wing's study *Institutionalism and Schizophrenia* (1970) were intended to supplement existing models of illness with social factors and bring to light the pathogenic influences of the psychiatric hospitals on their inmates.[23] In 1974, German psychiatrist Asmus Finzen edited a book titled *Hospitalisation Damage in Psychiatric Hospitals*. His volume contained a German translation of Barton's booklet and of Brown and Wing's study. This shows that corresponding approaches gained prominence in scientific communities in German-speaking countries.

Goffman's book, which was first published in German in 1972, translated by Nils Lindquist, gave the impulse for scientific studies to make the psychiatric hospital and its inmates the subject of research. As already mentioned, Goffman's book also inspired the project of Forster and Pelikan. As von Kardorff noted, with Goffman's analyses 'the social situation of the patients in the system of the institution became for the first time scientifically justifiable for discourse' (von Kardorff, 1991: 337). And he added: 'Here we see the historically rather rare case of a successful scientification of pre-scientific, moral indignation about the conditions in psychiatry in the medium of sociological criticism' (von Kardorff, 1991: 337). This put the growing public critique of the institution on another level.

In contrast to Goffman, whose study still maintained a sociological distance to the field of practice he was researching, Forster and Pelikan's study was directed at changing psychiatric practices and improving the living conditions of the patients inside and outside the hospital. In their role as 'undercover observers', the sociologists gained access to an institution that had hitherto been closed not only to the public, but also to researchers who did not come from the field of psychiatry. When it started in 1974, it was the first such study in an Austrian psychiatric hospital.[24] This required, as Forster and Pelikan, also for strategic reasons, repeatedly emphasised, 'an unusual degree of openness and willingness on the part of all those involved to self-critically question everyday routine actions and entrenched organisational structures' (Forster and Pelikan, 1978: ii).[25] That those working in and responsible for psychiatry opened themselves up to this perspective was explained by von Kardorff by the fact that 'a certain type of sociological analysis, which chose psychiatric practice as its object for illustrating sociological theoretical problems and questions, [encountered] a phase of disorientation and new beginnings within psychiatry itself' (von Kardorff, 1985: 240). For von Kardorff, it was also the crisis of the psychiatric institution that created 'a readiness to receive sociological ways of thinking and research results' (von Kardorff, 1985: 240) at this time. This is a conclusion that Eberhard Gabriel, who became the medical director of the PKH Baumgartner Höhe in 1978, also confirmed. The deplorable state of the psychiatric hospital must have been obvious to the people in charge there,[26] and studies like the one by Goffman could contribute not only in terms of raising awareness, but also in terms of providing evidence of the harmful effects of these places on the patients. As Gabriel explained, the sociologists' study was essential to get political attention and funds to restructure psychiatric care at the PKH, even though the serious shortcomings the study revealed were widely known beforehand. From this perspective, one can only conditionally agree with the following statement by the medical student Rolf Dieter Hemprich and the psychiatrist Karl Peter Kisker, who themselves had conducted covert participant observation in a closed men's ward in the Psychiatric University Clinic in Heidelberg in 1965:[27] 'If psychiatrists now know that their institutions are mostly conglomerates of pathogenic subcultures, it is because some among them have been fair enough to let their work environment temporarily become a sociological observatory' (Hemprich and Kisker, 1968: 433). Psychiatrists didn't only know it from then on, as a look into history shows,[28] but at the time in question, sociological investigation of the institutions made it easier to get political attention, especially at a time when sociology was ranked highly. Following the press conference in June 1978 where Forster and Pelikan presented the findings of their study, the journalist Sebastian Leitner polemicised in his column against Austrian bureaucratism, which only prompted politicians to act when shortcomings were scientifically prepared and presented in paper form: 'It is a time-honoured Austrian peculiarity that a scandal, an eyesore like this one, only becomes clearly visible when it takes on [on order] the official form of paper in file covers or at least that of scientific documentation' (Leitner, 1978). Leitner called the study 'a horrifying confession of failure and inhumanity' (Leitner, 1978). He didn't absolve the psychiatrists of responsibility, but supported the politicians who had the courage to publicly admit to the abuses that the study revealed and promised reforms.

Reflecting practices?

As Jürgen M. Pelikan stated at an interdisciplinary symposium at the PKH in 1982, views of reality in the social sciences and in medicine are complementary, whereby 'the social scientific paradigm ... also [captures] only one partial aspect of reality, but one that is quite essential for patients. In the context of professional practice, this aspect ... tends to be suppressed and repressed – after all, it means constantly questioning the appropriateness and meaningfulness of one's own professional practice' (Pelikan, 1983: 18). Just as reflection is an inherent tool of sociology, it can also stimulate reflection in those studied and interviewed. In contrast to the method of covert participant observation, the method of interviewing nursing staff (as it was applied in the second part of the study by Forster and Pelikan) about their daily routines, their interactions with the patients, their attitudes towards certain treatment methods, their opinion about certain patient needs, and so on, holds the possibility of initiating a process or maybe just a moment of critical reflection on one's own professional practice.

Although the sociological approach was significant for the preparation of the reform plan in Vienna, the influence of sociologists in the restructuring of psychiatric care or the reorganisation of the PKH was waning. This was already critically noted by Pelikan at the aforementioned eighth Steinhof Symposium initiated by Eberhard Gabriel in 1982 (Pelikan, 1983). The subject of the interdisciplinary symposium – which was itself a manifestation of reflecting on one's own professional practice and exchanging perspectives across disciplinary and professional boundaries – was 'patients in psychiatric hospitals'. This topic was outlined and discussed from the angle of the social sciences, psychiatry, health and social policy, and the institution (Presse- und Informationsdienst der Stadt Wien, 1983). In his presentation, Pelikan pointed out that there was no social-scientific evaluation of the reform steps at the PKH and clearly expressed his dissatisfaction about this (Pelikan, 1983). According to my conversation with Eberhard Gabriel, there was no money to implement an accompanying evaluation. According to my conversation with Rudolf Forster, there was no political interest in it anymore. Wherever the reasons may have been, the interest in sociological issues was pursued more intensively at the PKH than before: the booklet on the symposium also includes different reports by working groups (Arbeitsgruppen) that were established in the run-up to or during the symposium and focused on its topic. They consisted of multiprofessional teams (psychologists, social workers, physicians, nurses and head nurses, ward assistants, etc.), which obviously lacked sociologists. The groups, which had different institutional backgrounds, dealt with subjects like 'violence and psychiatry', 'How therapeutic is the therapeutic milieu?', 'How do patients, nurses, and doctors experience the problem of medication in the psychiatric hospital?' and 'Patients' wishes – limits and fulfilment' (Presse- und Informationsdienst der Stadt Wien, 1983). Referring to the last subject mentioned, the head of the nursing service and a psychologist from the PKH reported on a survey they had conducted there in October 1982, when the nurses handed out a questionnaire to all 1,682 patients. Three hundred and thirty patients filled in the questionnaires themselves, while 553 patients were assisted by nurses (Biebel and Bartuska, 1983: 96). The questionnaire consisted of ten questions on patients' wishes regarding food, drink, sleep, clothing, work, entertainment, liberties, care, security and help. It seemed to both connect to the study by Forster and Pelikan and fill a gap by engaging patients, which became a more and more common practice in these years when doing research on psychiatric hospitals.[29]

Without going into the details of these studies by the aforementioned working groups, they are nevertheless proof that a shift had taken place at the PKH. The hospital was now taking independent action to develop a reflective and analytical view of the conditions on site. These initiatives can be described as an adaptation of the sociological-reflexive approaches as undertaken by Forster and Pelikan in their study. In this case, however, the non-psychiatric experts did not come from the outside anymore but from within, they were now part of the institution, and were not only participating observers, but participants themselves.

Conclusion

At the beginning of this chapter, I outlined three points that I consider contributed to sociologists joining the larger pool of reform actors and which I will specify in this conclusion in regard to the situation in Vienna. Even though the boom in the social sciences reached Austria rather late, the 1970s nevertheless marked a stronger institutional anchoring of the discipline both within and outside the university. As an application-oriented science, sociological research in these years was directed at providing a basis for political decisions. The leading party in Austria (as well as in Vienna), the social democrats, was open to such approaches, as the sociologists' project met with the politicians' intentions for sociopolitical transformation. One particular subject that both researchers and the public increasingly turned to critically in the 1970s was the psychiatric hospital and its grievances. The study by Pelikan and Forster was inspired by Goffman's *Asylums*, but went beyond it. Unlike Goffman, the Austrian sociologists sought to impact the social reality of the patients at the Baumgartner Höhe, which they succeeded in doing because of the social and political conditions at the time when the study was presented. The willingness of Austrian psychiatrists to open up their institutions to experts from outside must not be overestimated, as Forster cautions. Even if the motives are left open, the example of the Baumgartner Höhe seems to have been an exception in this regard. The presentation of the study's results went hand in hand with the appointment of Eberhard Gabriel as the new medical director, who committed to implementing reforms that were partly based on the recommendations by Forster and Pelikan. The example of psychiatric reform in Vienna shows that the social sciences were able to exert influence, but to an extent that did not initially leave the existing paradigm of institutional patient care. Compared to other European countries (e.g. Italy), the closure of the large institutions was not the first, but the very last step of their reform proposals for Vienna. The first reform step focused on reshaping and adapting the institutions to contemporary standards. The institutions were lagging behind enormously in comparison to general hospitals and had to catch up. In the case discussed in this chapter, sociology seemed to take on a bridging function between the critical public, political decision-makers and reform-minded psychiatrists, condensing in it many intentions and hopes.

Acknowledgements

I thank Eberhard Gabriel, medical director at the Baumgartner Höhe Psychiatric Hospital from 1978 to 2004, and Rudolf Forster, sociologist and co-initiator of the study examined here, for standing by for discussions, providing me with literature and critically reviewing the chapter.

Notes

1 I thank Rudolf Forster for these remarks on the background of the press conference.
2 See the contribution by Malathouni in Chapter 4.
3 Leodolter, physician and politician of the Social Democratic Party of Austria (SPÖ), was the first minister of the Ministry of Health and Environmental Protection newly created under Federal Chancellor Bruno

Kreisky (SPÖ) in 1972. Under the minority government Kreisky led, the reform of the health system was declared to be a central task (Rehor, 2019).

4 Two days earlier, also in presence of Leodolter and Stacher, it had been presented to the staff of the PKH to prepare them for the public reactions the politicians expected.

5 For his thesis, psychologist Hans Weiss smuggled himself into the Valduna psychiatric hospital in the Austrian province of Vorarlberg as a ward assistant and published excerpts from his 'Nursing Diary' in the Austrian weekly magazine *profil* (1976). His research led to the resignation of the head of the hospital.

6 All newspaper articles concerning the press conference are collected in the 'Sozialwissenschaftliche Dokumentation der Arbeiterkammer Wien' and were read by the author: AK Bibliothek Wien [Vienna Chamber of Labour Library], Vienna, Sozialwissenschaftliche Dokumentation [Social science documentation].

7 Forster and Pelikan recommended starting the reform with the humanisation and modernisation of therapy and rehabilitation and ending it with the implementation of sectorised mental health care – a project that started in Vienna in the 1980s and will be completed in 2025 – and the establishment of day clinics and outpatient clinics. The Arbeiterzeitung noted that Stacher was sceptical about opening projects like Basaglia's model in Trieste. For Basaglia's reform projects, see Chapter 2 in this volume.

8 They focused on the image of the mentally ill in the media, the problems in gerontological psychiatric care in Vienna, neuropsychiatric care for children and adolescents and psychiatric patient care in Vienna (Presse- und Informationsdienst der Stadt Wien, 1979).

9 For the history of the institution, see Czech *et al.* (2018); Ledebur (2015); Gabriel (2007).

10 For the data, see Presse- und Informationsdienst der Stadt Wien (1979).

11 The pocket diary is no longer preserved.

12 When Schwediauer finished his diploma, a study by the sociologists Christa and Thomas Fengler entitled *Everyday Life in an Institution* (1980) was published in Germany. Asmus Finzen called their study 'the German Goffman' (Dörner, 1980: 5), while obviously not noticing – or even ignoring, as Forster suggested – the study by Forster and Pelikan.

13 With their approach they referred to the work of American psychologist Abraham Harold Maslow (Forster and Pelikan, 1980).

14 Mayer was honoured with the 'Dr. Karl Renner Journalism Award' for his story in 1979, see Wikipedia, *Dr.-Karl-Renner-Publizistikpreis*, https://de.wikipedia.org/wiki/Dr.-Karl-Renner-Publizistikpreis (accessed 1 November 2021).

15 In 1966, the social sciences and economics fields of study were established at the Faculty of Law of the University of Vienna and, in 1975, a separate Faculty of Social and Economic Sciences was founded (Fleck, 2018: 329).

16 In 1979, Pelikan founded the Ludwig Boltzmann Institute for the Sociology of Medicine and Health together with Hans Strotzka. Forster moved to this institute in 1981, where he worked on legal reforms of guardianship and involuntary hospitalisation together with Pelikan, a project in which sociological research had an even bigger impact on legal regulations and practice, as Forster explained. *Hohe Auszeichnungen der Republik Österreich für Jürgen Pelikan und Rudolf Forster*, www.soz.univie.ac.at/ueber-uns/archiv-meldungen/auszeichnungen/pelikan-und-forster-2017/ (accessed 24 September 2021).

17 In 1970, the subject 'medical sociology' was included in the *Approbationsordnung* (licensing regulations) for doctors in the Federal Republic of Germany and professorships for medical sociology were established at the medical faculties. The health report of the Federal Ministry for Youth, Family and Health of 1971 singled out 'medical sociology' as particularly worthy of support (Lepsius, 1973: 955). As Forster pointed out, Austria's medical elite successfully resisted the incorporation of medical sociology into medical education.

18 See the reference in Knorr *et al.* (1975) to the SPÖ economic programme of 1968, which stated the necessity of expanding social research and incorporating it into planning (Knorr *et al.*, 1975: IV/II/66–7).

19 In their project report completed at the IHS in 1974, Knorr *et al.* worked out the research foci of projects in the social sciences between 1969 and 1973. They stated that among the 723 projects they evaluated (which were funded by the Fund for the Promotion of Scientific Research and had in common that they concerned central aspects of social life) economics-related research dominated (35 per cent). Of the evaluated projects, 2.7 per cent could be assigned to the health sector. Of these, six out of the total of twenty projects were carried out by physicians with a focus on social psychiatry and medical sociology (cf. Katschnig et al., 1975 a, b). Three out of the twenty projects were research commissioned in 1973 and were 'connected with the new establishment of the Department of Social Psychiatry and Documentation at the Psychiatric University Hospital' (Knorr *et al.*, 1974).

20 For a critical examination of this application orientation of sociology see Heinrich and Müller (1980), Forster and Pelikan (1990).

21 He was a researcher in the project 'Modernisation of Psychiatric Care', funded by the German Research Foundation at the University of Munich from 1979 to 1982.

22 Environmental psychology as a new discipline also started in the context of research funding by the NIMH, which addressed the question of how the layout of psychiatric wards and their material environment influenced patients' behaviour (Ittelson *et al.*, 1977: 12). For the reception of this approach in Germany see the thesis by Schwarz (1980) entitled *Environmental Psychological Studies on the Influence of the Spatial Environment on the Behaviour of Inpatient Psychiatric Patients*. His supervisor was psychiatrist Hans Hippius, who was a member of the expert commission of the German Federal Parliament, which produced the report *The Situation of Psychiatry in the Federal Republic of Germany* (1975).

23 See, for example, the report *Psychiatric Services and Architecture* (Baker *et al.*, 1959), commissioned by the World Health Organization, in which Alex Anthony Baker, Paul Sivadon and R. Llewelyn Davies presented recommendations for the construction of future psychiatric hospitals and pleaded for architecture to be considered as a social factor influencing patients. On architectural practices, see the contribution of Malathouni in Chapter 4.

24 The study by Weiss was published in 1976. See also the impact of Frank Fischer's book *Irrenhäuser* (1969) on German discussions of psychiatric hospitals in the contribution by Gahlen in Chapter 3.

25 In the case of the study by Forster and Pelikan, only the medical director and the PKH works council knew about the covert participant observation. Later, when the nurses were interviewed as part of the study, they were informed of the ongoing research, but not about the previous covert participant observation.

26 Already in the early 1970s, psychiatrists founded the Reform Working Group Steinhof, as psychiatrist Georg Psota remarked in a lecture on 29 October 2021 at the Austrian Academy of Science. Forster took a critical view here: if psychiatrists were aware of the abuses in the hospitals, they were more likely to prevent them from being made public. He points out that, in 1975, the hospital directors blocked the publication of patient populations differentiated by institution as well as the publication of the high percentage of involuntary admissions (Forster, 1997b: 258–9).

27 Hemprich was smuggled into the ward in the role of a nurse. For Kisker and the Psychiatric University Clinic in Heidelberg, see Chapter 3.

28 Andrew Scull (Scull, 1980: 128) draws attention to this in his book on decarceration: 'With all due respect to sociologists who believe that our knowledge of society is built upon the advances of their particular discipline, it must be said that the recognition of the pernicious influence of these circumstances was highly developed early in the history of the asylum.'

29 In cooperation with physicians, sociologists and psychologists, methods
    for questioning long-term psychiatric patients about their needs and
    wishes were developed in the study by Mühlich *et al.* (1982), which
    was conducted in North Rhine-Westphalia.

References

Baker, Alex Anthony, R. Llewelyn Davies and Paul Sivadon, 1959, *Psychiatric Services and Architecture* (Geneva: World Health Organization).

Barton, Russell, 1959, *Institutional Neurosis* (Bristol: Wright).

'Baunachrichten', 1907, *Der Bautechniker*, 27:24, 465.

Biebel, H. and Heiner Bartuska, 1983, 'Patientenwünsche – Grenzen und Erfüllbarkeit', in Presse- und Informationsdienst der Stadt Wien (ed.), *Patienten im Psychiatrischen Krankenhaus: Verhandlungen des 8. Steinhof-Symposions* (Vienna: Vorwärts), pp. 96–8.

Brown, George William and John Kenneth Wing, 1970, *Institutionalism and Schizophrenia: A Comparative Study of Three Mental Hospitals 1960–1968* (Cambridge: Cambridge University Press).

Clemens, Wolfgang, 2001, 'Soziologie in der gesellschaftlichen Praxis: Zur Anwendung soziologischen Wissens und Qualifizierung von Sozialwissenschaftlern', *Sozialwissenschaften und Berufspraxis*, 24:3, 213–34.

Czech, Herwig, Wolfgang Neugebauer and Peter Schwarz, 2018, *The War Against the 'Inferior': On the History of Nazi Medicine in Vienna: Catalogue to the Exhibition of the Steinhof Memorial* (Vienna: Documentation Centre of Austrian Resistance).

Fengler, Thomas and Christa Fengler, 1980, *Alltag in der Anstalt: Wenn Sozialpsychiatrie praktisch wird* (Rehburg-Loccum: Psychiatrie Verlag).

Finzen, Asmus (ed.), 1974, *Hospitalisierungsschäden in psychiatrischen Krankenhäusern: Ursachen, Behandlung, Prävention* (Munich: R. Piper).

Fleck, Christian, 2016, *Soziologie in Österreich nach 1945* (working paper), pp. 1–27, www.researchgate.net/publication/304623812 (accessed 27 January 2022).

Fleck, Christian, 2018, 'Geschichte des Instituts für Höhere Studien in Wien', in Stephan Moebius and Andrea Ploder (eds), *Handbuch Geschichte der deutschsprachigen Soziologie: Geschichte der Soziologie im deutschsprachigen Raum*, vol 1. (Wiesbaden: Springer), pp. 997–1007.

Forster, Rudolf, 1997a, *Psychiatriereformen zwischen Medikalisierung und Gemeindeorientierung: Eine kritische Bilanz* (Opladen: Westdeutscher Verlag).

Forster, Rudolf, 1997b, *Psychiatrische Macht und rechtliche Kontrolle: Internationale Entwicklungen und die Entstehung des österreichischen Unterbringungsgesetzes* (Vienna: Döcker).

Forster, Rudolf, Franz Leitner and Jürgen M. Pelikan, 1975, *Untersuchung der Probleme des Krankenpflegepersonals Österreichs: Endbericht: Psychiatrische Versorgung und menschliche Bedürfnisse – Abteilungsanalysen in einem Psychiatrischen Großkrankenhaus*, part 5 (Vienna: Institute for Advanced Studies).

Forster, Rudolf and Jürgen M. Pelikan, 1978, *Patientenversorgung und Personalhandeln im Kontext einer psychiatrischen Sonderanstalt: Eine organisationssoziologische Untersuchung im Psychiatrischen Krankenhaus der Gemeinde Wien 'Baumgartner Höhe'*, vols 1–2 (Vienna: Institute for Advanced Studies).

Forster, Rudolf and Jürgen M. Pelikan, 1980, 'Menschliche Bedürfnisse und totale Institution – am Beispiel eines psychiatrischen Großkrankenhauses', in Kurt Heinrich and Ulrich Müller (eds), *Psychiatrische Soziologie: Ein Beitrag zur sozialen Psychiatrie? 3. Düsseldorfer Symposium am 14. April 1978* (Weinheim: Beltz), pp. 169–91.

Forster, Rudolf and Jürgen M. Pelikan, 1990, 'Psychiatriereform und Sozialwissenschaften: Einleitende Überlegungen', in Rudolf Forster and Jürgen M. Pelikan (eds), *Psychiatriereform und Sozialwissenschaften: Erfahrungsberichte aus Österreich* (Vienna: Facultas), pp. 1–18.

Fritsch, Sibylle and Gerhard Mayer, 1978, 'Die Herren vom Steinhof', *profil* (12 December 1978), pp. 42–4.

Gabriel, Eberhard, 2007, *100 Jahre Gesundheitsstandort Baumgartner Höhe: Von den Heil- und Pflegeanstalten am Steinhof zum Otto-Wagner-Spital* (Vienna: Facultas Verlag).

Gesellschaft für Demokratische Psychiatrie Wien, 1979, *Dokumentation der Demokratischen Psychiatrie Wien* (Vienna: Gesellschaft für Demokratische Psychiatrie).

Goffman, Erving, 1973, *Asyle: Über die soziale Situation psychiatrischer Patienten und anderer Insassen* (Frankfurt: Suhrkamp).

Heinrich, Kurt and Ulrich Müller (eds), 1980, *Psychiatrische Soziologie: Ein Beitrag zur sozialen Psychiatrie? 3. Düsseldorfer Symposium am 14. April 1978* (Weinheim: Beltz).

Hemprich, Rolf Dieter and Karl Peter Kisker, 1968, 'Die "Herren der Klinik" und die Patienten: Erfahrungen aus der teilnehmend versteckten Beobachtung einer psychiatrischen Station', *Nervenarzt*, 39:10, 433–44.

Hettlage, Robert and Karl Lenz, 1991, 'Erving Goffman – ein unbekannter Bekannter', in Robert Hettlage and Karl Lenz (eds), *Erving Goffman – ein soziologischer Klassiker der zweiten Generation* (Bern: Paul Haupt), pp. 7–21.

Irschik, Sandra, 2017, 'Es tobt der Wahnsinn! Verdeckte Recherchen in Psychiatrien im Nachrichtenmagazin "profil" der 1970er-Jahre im Spiegel der Österreichischen Psychiatriereform'. Diploma thesis, University of Vienna.

Ittelson, William H., Harold M. Proshansky, Leanne G. Rivlin and Gary H. Winkel, 1977, *Einführung in die Umweltpsychologie* (Stuttgart: Klett-Cotta).

Kardorff, Ernst von, 1985, 'Zwei Diskurse über die Ordnung des Sozialen – Zum Verhältnis von Eigenrationalisierung und Verwissenschaftlichung am Beispiel von Psychiatrie und Soziologie', in Wolfgang Bonß and Heinz Hartmann (eds), *Entzauberte Wissenschaft: Zur Relativität und Geltung soziologischer Forschung* (Göttingen: Otto Schwartz & Co.), pp. 229–53.

Kardorff, Ernst von, 1991, 'Goffmans Anregungen für soziologische Handlungsfelder', in Robert Hettlage and Karl Lenz (eds), *Erving Goffman – ein soziologischer Klassiker der zweiten Generation* (Bern: Paul Haupt), pp. 327–54.

Katschnig, Heinz, Ingo Grumiller and Rainer Strobl, 1975a, *Daten zur stationären psychiatrischen Versorgung der österreichischen Bevölkerung: Eine Untersuchung über die Inzidenz in den psychiatrischen Universitätskliniken und Krankenhäusern Österreichs*, part 1 (Vienna: Österreichisches Bundesinstitut für Gesundheitswesen).

Katschnig, Heinz, Ingo Grumiller and Rainer Strobl, 1975b, *Daten zur stationären psychiatrischen Versorgung der österreichischen Bevölkerung: Eine Untersuchung über die Prävalenz in den psychiatrischen Krankenhäusern Österreichs*, part 2 (Vienna: Österreichisches Bundesinstitut für Gesundheitswesen).

Knorr, Karin, Hans Georg Zilian, Max Haller and Viktor Manhart, 1974, *Zur Situation der sozialwissenschaftlichen Forschung in Österreich. Endbericht; Teil 1: Ziel und Durchführung der Studie; Teil 2: Ressourcen und Aktivitäten der Sozialwissenschaften in Österreich* (Vienna: Institute for Advanced Studies).

Knorr, Karin, Hans Georg Zilian, Max Haller, Viktor Manhart, 1975, *Zur Situation der sozialwissenschaftlichen Forschung in Österreich: Endbericht: Der Produktions- und Verwertungszusammenhang sozialwissenschaftlicher Forschung*, part 4, vol. 1 (Vienna: Institute for Advanced Studies).

Kronen Zeitung, 1978, 'Die "Häfenbrüder" sind besser dran', 1978, *Kronen Zeitung* (20 June).

Ledebur, Sophie, 2015, *Das Wissen der Anstaltspsychiatrie in der Moderne: Zur Geschichte der Heil- und Pflegeanstalten Am Steinhof in Wien* (Vienna: Böhlau).

Leitner, Sebastian, 1978, 'Am Steinhof: Das Geständnis', *Kurier* (21 June).

Lepsius, Rainer, 1973, 'Stellungnahme der Deutschen Gesellschaft für Soziologie zur Institutionalisierung der "Medizinischen Soziologie"', *Kölner Zeitschrift für Soziologie und Sozialpsychologie*, 25:2, 954–5.

Mayer, Gerhard, 1978, 'Gepflegter Irrsinn', *profil* (12 December), pp. 44–7.

Meissner, Isabella, 1976, 'Wir leben wie in Watte', *profil* (27 January), pp. 26–7.

Mühlich-von Staden, Christine, Eike Wolff and Wolfgang Mühlich, 1982, *Ein Bett ist keine Wohnung: Bedürfnisse und Wünsche psychiatrischer Langzeitpatienten* (Rehburg-Loccum: Psychiatrie Verlag).

Naschold, Frieder, 1975, *Systemanalyse des Gesundheitswesens in Österreich: Eine Studie über Entstehung und Bewältigung von Krankheit im entwickelten Kapitalismus*, vol. 4 (Vienna: Institute for Advanced Studies).

Neues Volksblatt, 1978, 'Wien: Skandalöse Zustände an Psychiatrischem Krankenhaus', *Neues Volksblatt* (20 June).

Neun, Oliver, 2018, 'Geschichte des Verhältnisses zwischen Soziologie und Öffentlichkeit in der deutschsprachigen Nachkriegssoziologie', in Stephan Moebius and Andrea Ploder (eds), *Handbuch Geschichte der deutschsprachigen Soziologie: Geschichte der Soziologie im deutschsprachigen Raum*, vol. 1 (Wiesbaden: Springer), pp. 503–29.

P., Eva, 1977, 'In der Scheiße. Erzählungen aus dem Steinhof', *Forum* (August/September), pp. 50–1.

Pelikan, Jürgen, 1983, 'Patienten im Psychiatrischen Krankenhaus gesehen vom Standpunkt der Sozialwissenschaft', in Presse- und Informationsdienst der Stadt Wien (ed.), *Patienten im Psychiatrischen Krankenhaus: Verhandlungen des 8. Steinhof-Symposions* (Vienna: Vorwärts).

Pelikan, Jürgen M. and Fritz Leitner, 1974, *Untersuchung der Probleme des Krankenpflegepersonals Österreichs: Endbericht: Selektion und Sozialisation in der Krankenpflegeausbildung: Analysen einer Fragebogenerhebung in öesterreichischen Krankenpflegeschulen*, part 1, vol. 1 (Vienna: Institute for Advanced Studies).

Presse- und Informationsdienst der Stadt Wien (ed.), 1979, *Psychiatrische und psychosoziale Versorgung in Wien: Zielplan*, vol. 2 (Vienna: Vorwärts).

Presse- und Informationsdienst der Stadt Wien (ed.), 1983, *Patienten im psychiatrischen Krankenhaus: Verhandlungen des 8. Steinhof-Symposiums* (Vienna: Vorwärts).

Rehor, Thomas, 2019, 'Gegen das Sterben vor der Zeit: Die Gesundheitspolitik in der Ara Kreisky 1970–1983'. Thesis, University of Vienna.

Reimann, Helga, 1973, 'Die Entwicklung der Psychiatrischen Soziologie', *Kölner Zeitschrift für Soziologie und Sozialpsychologie*, 25:2, 240–56.

Schäfer, Gustav, 2016, 'Finanzströme spiegeln die Gesellschaft wider – finanzielle und personelle Ressourcen der Psychiatrie in Wien zwischen 1946 und 1970', *Virus: Zeitschrift zur Sozialgeschichte der Medizin*, 14, 335–42.

Schwarz, H., 1980, 'Umweltpsychologische Untersuchungen über den Einfluss der räumlichen Umgebung auf das Verhalten stationärer psychiatrischer Patienten'. Thesis, University of Munich.

Schwarz, Walter J., 1978, 'Reform in der Schlangengrube', *Kurier* (20 June).

Schwediauer, Karl, 1981, 'Die soziale Situation von Geisteskranken in einer psychiatrischen Großanstalt: Teilnehmende Beobachtung im Psychiatrischen Krankenhaus der Stadt Wien Baumgartner Höhe'. Masters thesis, Vienna.

Schwediauer, Karl, 1984, *Alltag in Steinhof: Leben in einer psychiatrischen Großanstalt* (Vienna: Böhlau).

Scull, Andrew, 1980, *Die Anstalten öffnen?: Decarceration der Irren und Häftlinge* (Frankfurt: Campus).

Volksstimme, 1978, 'Menschenwürdig – vielleicht in 5 Jahren', *Volksstimme* (20 June).

Weiss, Hans, 1976, 'Das Tagebuch eines Irrenwärters', *profil* (25 May), pp. 30–5.

10

Writing patients: group psychotherapy and reform efforts in 1970s GDR university psychiatry

Henriette Voelker

In 1974, a psychotherapy patient at the Charité psychiatric hospital in East Berlin wrote to his therapists: 'I am not fully occupied, i.e., the activity does not satisfy me. However, I use my free time for conversations and pleasant talks with my fellow patients. In general, I do not like the laxity. The daily schedule is carried out much too casually. Many things would have to be organised more tightly.'[1] Another patient reported: 'Afternoon: Club afternoon (organised by us, worked out because there was a lot of laughter). Lots of good-looking therapists in the afternoon in the corridor! It's great that they showed themselves from a very natural side (no need for a supervisor's facial expression).'[2]

These excerpts are taken from medical records, in which patients documented their stay in a psychotherapeutic ward themselves. In the evening, these patients were expected to note what concerned them during the day. They handed over their writings via a postbox next to the therapists' office by the following day. The therapists read and stored the reports. Sometimes the addressees changed, suggesting monthly reading shifts. The writing practice was part of the therapeutic concept of what was termed dynamic group psychotherapy, which was introduced at the psychiatric hospital of the Charité in the early 1970s. The reports' therapeutic aim was to encourage patients' self-reflection and understanding of transference phenomena in the group. This therapeutic method was developed especially for the treatment of neurotic disorders and was one of the main methods for inpatient psychotherapeutic treatment in the German Democratic Republic (GDR) from the 1970s.[3]

The daily reports as material artefacts of this practice were bundled in the medical records and are preserved in the Historical Psychiatric Archive of the Charité (HPAC). Their scope ranges from a sentence to several pages a day. Some bundles had only a few, others up to several hundred pages. One hundred and forty-eight such medical records from this group psychotherapeutic ward have been analysed, covering a time span from the introduction of the method in 1974 to the end of the current archival holdings in 1978.[4] The sources allow patient voices to come to the fore and are a rare finding in patient history, which, since Porter's call, has sustainedly faced a source problem inherent to psychiatry (Porter, 1985). Usually, psychiatrists wrote about their patients, but in the case of the present practice the relationship was reversed – even if the patients wrote the reports for the psychiatrists and the reports were read with a medical eye. The particularity of this practice lies in the fact that patients were its main actors and took over a task that otherwise lay in the psychiatrists' sphere of competence.

From a praxeological perspective, daily reporting had a variety of diagnostic, therapeutic, social and political-ideological implications that are worth exploring. The quotes above suggest changes in the traditional hierarchy of the therapist–patient relationships in such departments. Here, the reports will serve to examine reformist efforts, namely the introduction of the 'therapeutic community' concept, and their limitations in the context of group psychotherapy in a psychiatric university hospital in the GDR.[5] It should be mentioned that the East Berlin university clinic was the most prestigious medical institution in the German Democratic Republic, but it was not among the leading places for the development of psychiatric reforms (see, for example, Steinberg, 2014). The chapter will discuss the ambivalent effects of daily reporting as a writing practice and the reciprocal effects it had on local reform efforts. The daily reports will exemplify that even rather mundane psychiatric practices could have contradictory impacts on the implementation of larger structural agendas.

Daily reporting was a reflexive practice, as the patients as authors referred to themselves when writing. Yet the practice as such reflected on the social fabric and therapeutic space of the ward in two other ways. As a primary effect, it could trigger a conscious moment of reflection on the therapists' own actions in terms of evaluation and thereby impact on the social setting. Here, the analysed material offers only limited insights: while the patients wrote daily, the therapists only rarely documented their reactions to the writing in the medical files and did not publish about this practice either. Moreover, underlining and annotations in the sources can be assigned to the group of therapists but rarely to individuals, so that the therapists appear as a rather amorphous group. The focus of the present analysis will thus lie on the secondary reflexive effects of the writing practice. The chapter takes as a premise that practices can reverberate on the social fabric of the institution in a manner which did not correspond to or could even counteract the original motivation to act. Secondary effects of the present writing practice could thus be unintended repercussions for the therapist–patient relationships.

Group psychotherapy, therapeutic communities and psychiatric reforms in the GDR

The dissemination of psychotherapeutic approaches was among the reformist demands to improve psychiatric care in the GDR in the 1960s and 1970s. The first psychotherapeutic wards had been established in university hospitals in the 1950s, for example in Leipzig and East Berlin. Increasingly, from the 1970s, specialised departments for psychotherapy were introduced in several psychiatric district hospitals as well. According to an inventory from 1990, there were 35 such psychotherapeutic departments or institutions with about 760 beds at the end of the GDR (Dührssen *et al.*, 1990: 155). Considerable differences in material and personnel conditions as well as in the number of beds must be assumed. Due to the slow improvement in outpatient care structures, such facilities took over a significant share of all psychotherapeutic treatments provided. From the 1970s, there was a trend towards group psychotherapies in the GDR, which has been described for capitalist countries (Elberfeld, 2019), but also for other socialist countries such as Yugoslavia (Savelli, 2018). A variety of these facilities used the dynamic group psychotherapy developed by Kurt Höck (1920–2008) at the House of Health, the GDR's largest polyclinic.[6] In 1964, he established an associated hospital for neurotic disorders in East Berlin for inpatient group psychotherapy. On Höck's initiative, a training programme was set up. Consequently, a substantial number of therapists adapted the method and thereby established psychodynamic approaches in their facilities. Among them was Helmut Kulawik (1941–93), head of the psychotherapy department at the Charité since 1973.[7]

Höck developed the method from the 1960s. The term 'dynamic' ambiguously stands for group dynamics and psychodynamic therapy. As a student of Harald Schultz-Hencke (1892–1953), Höck was strongly influenced by his 'neopsychoanalysis', which had turned away from traditional Freudianism. However, psychoanalysis had been taboo since the Pavlov campaign of the mid-1950s, and the term 'psychodynamic' also served to cover this theoretical backdrop.

According to Höck, psychodynamic processes would improve the integration and harmony of the patients' personalities (Höck and König, 1976). The knowledge that others might have similar fates would relieve and liberate them from isolation. The therapeutic group allowed one to test and correct one's own behaviour. Moreover, participants could simultaneously project affects onto different group members. Dynamic group psychotherapy was based on the theory of group dynamics and foresaw five phases of group interaction: warm-up, dependency, activation, toppling process and work phase. Therapists were to provoke these by reserved behaviour. Serving as a projection screen for patients' expectations, they should not encourage, confirm, or provide any psychoeducation, dictate topics, or guide the group. The frustration of such expectations should enforce interaction among the patients. Uncertainty about authority and emotionality should arise. Eventually, a new ranking structure and a field of tension would emerge as a foundation for the therapeutic process. A central element of this method was to deny authoritarian guidance and support empowerment – which in turn, could lead to pressures of expectation and adaptation. Because the toppling process could be interpreted as a metaphor for the overthrow of the socialist social system, the therapeutic concept gave rise to debates about its political implications among psychotherapists after reunification (Leuenberger, 2001).

At the behest of the therapists, patients submitted handwritten reports on non-uniform paper. As this routine was part of dynamic group psychotherapy, it was also practised in the hospital for neurotic disorders of the House of Health (Hess, 2011b) and in an unknown number of other inpatient and outpatient institutions, such as a Magdeburg polyclinic (Weise, 2011). According to all the evidence so far, this writing practice was not subject to research in the GDR.[8] Höck's colleague, Czech clinical psychologist Stanislav Kratochvíl (born 1932), described a similar technique, with the term 'diary', in a therapeutic community for neurosis therapy in Kroměříž, Ceskoslovenská socialistická republika (CSSR). He highlighted a therapeutic and an administrative function, which can be assumed for the Charité as well: 'The function of the diary is to inventory one's own thoughts and at the same time everyday communication between the patient and the staff who reads through the diaries during the morning shift' (Kratochvíl, 1976: 225).

When dynamic group psychotherapy was introduced at the Charité in 1974, voices were raised in the GDR calling for social psychiatric reforms based on the concept of the 'therapeutic community' according to British social psychiatrist Maxwell Jones (1907–90). The first reform agenda, called the Rodewisch Proposition (1963), is considered to be the epitome of social psychiatric reform attempts in the GDR and has received wide scholarly attention (e.g. Schmiedebach *et al.*, 2000; Hanrath, 2002; Hennings, 2015). Nevertheless, it is associated with the notion that the reforms of the 1960s 'got stuck' (see Richter, 2001). Material, financial and personnel shortages, inhibitions from the professional society and university psychiatry, as well as the political unwillingness of crucial officials of the Socialist Unity Party to implement the reforms, hindered their progress (Kumbier and Haack, 2018: 247). In the 1970s, reform-oriented psychiatrists ventured a new attempt. A 'turn to the inside' (Hanrath, 2002: 438–47; Balz and Klöppel, 2015) marked the developments, which culminated in a second reform agenda, called the Brandenburg Proposition (1974). It no longer sought to expand outpatient, community-based care structures. Instead, the new agenda aimed at turning large asylums, which were seen as places of safekeeping and social seclusion, into institutions with a therapeutic agenda. In the same respect, the internal order should be restructured and traditional hierarchies flattened by the installation of therapeutic communities.

How these therapeutic communities should be put into practice remained a matter of negotiation: Jones's concept was ideologically controversial and should be adapted to socialism – not least to demarcate it from the West German anti-psychiatric movement (Thom, 1976). Although the relationship between political interference and self-censorship could not yet be further elaborated, it can be stated that professional and political discussions resulted in an adaptation of the Brandenburg Proposition to 'socio-political goals and their principles of collective education' (Kumbier and Haack, 2017: 434).[9] In 1976, an adjusted version was published (Schirmer *et al.*, 1976). This agenda no longer criticised societal conditions but held the psychiatric institutions themselves responsible for deficiencies. A debate had been ignited around the compatibility of the concept with socialism and the understanding of authority and democracy in socialist societies.[10] Yet the demands to transform mental hospitals into therapeutic institutions remained. It is still an open question how these endeavours influenced the large psychiatric hospitals and how the practical implementation consequently differed from Jones's concept.

The psychotherapeutic hospital for neurotic disorders in East Berlin, founded by Kurt Höck in 1964, was later referred to as a therapeutic community (Hess, 2011b: 373). Two years after the opening, Höck hosted an international symposium on dynamic group psychotherapy in East Berlin. It was a rare opportunity for East German therapists to get in touch with Western colleagues after the construction of the wall. With his contribution to this conference, Maxwell Jones popularised the therapeutic community among group psychotherapists in the GDR (Jones, 1967).

At the 1966 symposium, he complained that neither 'organic and descriptive psychiatrists' nor the 'psychoanalytic school' had 'so far given sufficient attention to the world of patients in the asylum or hospital' (Jones, 1967: 187). A vague concept of social psychiatry would be sufficient for the sake of its flexibility, but it demanded that psychiatry 'devotes increasing attention to the patient's social environment' (Jones, 1967: 189). In this sense, Jones sought to maximise patient involvement, give patients the role of therapists and use the authority of the therapeutic staff only when needed. This 'patient accountability' was not only to concern the organisation of ward life. For example, staff and patients were to decide together on dismissals or transfers to other wards. This should counteract the lack of trust and build self-esteem and independence. The 'mainstay for any therapeutic community' should be 'daily ward or community meetings with all patients and all staff ... followed by a staff meeting of 30 to 60 minutes ... where the interactions between staff and patients can be discussed during community meetings'. These meetings should be similar to the working mechanisms of group treatment, and thus be conducive to the therapeutic process: 'The manifest and latent content, the unconsciousness and the ego-defence are gradually understood in a similar way to small groups' (Jones, 1967: 191). Subsequently, Höck emphasised for psychotherapeutic departments: 'the structure, the workflow, the entire atmosphere of the clinic differs substantially from the usual hospital environment' (Höck and König, 1976: 154). Psychotherapists from the GDR, Poland and CSSR further developed the combination of group psychotherapy and therapeutic communities during the 1970s (Geyer, 2011a: 248). Moreover, in 1978, the curriculum for the newly introduced medical specialisation in psychotherapy included references to the therapeutic community (Akademie für Ärztliche Fortbildung, 1978: 201–6). Professional discussions on this combination were continued at the second international symposium on group psychotherapy in 1982 (Hess, 2011a: 277). Eventually, psychotherapists from other institutions and psychotherapeutic orientations also retrospectively stated that, since the 1970s, they had increasingly applied the basic principles of the therapeutic community – even though some faced considerable resistance from other staff members (Maaz, 2011; Misselwitz, 2011).

Even though the concepts could function without one another, structural overlaps between the therapeutic community and dynamic group psychotherapy seem to consist in the rejection of authoritarian guidance and the empowerment of patients, accompanied by a participatory ward life. The patient's position in the hospital setting and the therapeutic process should be enhanced. It appears that in addition to the Brandenburg Proposition, group psychotherapy contributed to the dissemination of the basic ideas of the therapeutic community. In the case of the Charité, an employee publicly referred to the psychotherapy department of the university hospital as a 'therapeutic community' on GDR television.[11] The following examples will help to assess the extent to which the implementation corresponded with Jones's visions.

Ward life through the lens of daily reports

Dynamic group psychotherapy was developed exclusively for certain forms of neurotic disorders. During the period of study, this diagnosis was an exclusion criterion for psychotherapeutic treatment at the Charité. Moreover, quantitative evaluation of the sample of psychotherapy patients at the Charité by social structure reveals additional admission criteria. The files document the stay of adults, who were predominantly between 25 and 50 years old, as one aim of the therapy was reintegration into employment. In the socialist society, the social imperative to work endorsed this tendency. In principle, the treatment was open to all genders and in the sample, seventy-four patients each were registered as male and female. Typically, the patients spent two to three months in the ward – in rare cases up to half a year. Longer stays did not occur, as the length of therapy was inherently limited. The Charité was partly involved in local healthcare structures but could accept patients from other parts of the GDR who were deemed suitable. About half of the patients were resident in East Berlin, while the remaining people came from other districts of the GDR. Typically, the patients were referred to the Charité after unsuccessful treatment attempts elsewhere.

Pre-treatment with medication was particularly frequent, mainly with the newly emerged benzodiazepines or barbiturates. Sometimes the patients had learned autogenic training in earlier outpatient treatment, an autosuggestive relaxation method developed by German psychiatrist J. H. Schultz (1884–1970).[12] Only a small minority had previously been treated with other psychotherapeutic measures. Often, patients had been suffering from their symptoms for years and additionally accepted long waiting times for inpatient treatment in Berlin.

The therapists at the Charité had to select their patients based on a small number of beds. The sample shows a significant accumulation of people with a high level of education or academic training and of people whose profession involved textual work. One possible explanation would be that therapists expected better treatment results from patients with high therapeutic motivation and strong reflexive abilities. A more precise analysis proves difficult, as the reasons for admission were rarely made explicit and no records of rejected patients were archived. During reunification, a social psychiatrist from Leipzig criticised that admission to psychotherapy had been reserved for socially privileged patients (Weise, 1990: 291). This criticism of social inequality in the provision of mental healthcare connects to a discourse that had been going on since the first half of the twentieth century. Even though the sample includes counter-examples, the preponderance of people with elevated social status and education can hardly be denied. It is conceivable that the requirements of self-reflective writing reinforced therapists to favour patients with higher levels of education and conversely to exclude others, given the limited number of psychotherapy beds.

Shortly after admission, the patients began to write. Often, the bundles of writing began with a schematic breakdown into therapeutic and non-therapeutic activities. As the group discussions proceeded, social matters on the ward, as well as reflections on one's own challenges and those of others, became prevalent. In the following, some excerpts will help to approach the organisation of the daily routine in the ward.

One began with a list, which gives insight into the therapeutic spectrum: 'Morning: Psychodrama, playing table tennis, shopping done. Afternoon: Taking a stroll around town with my visitors. Evening: Handicrafts and reading.'[13] Shortly afterwards this patient added: 'I went swimming early in the morning. (I very much missed the sporting activities during my home leave.) In the morning I wanted to buy tablecloths for the common room of ward 5, which I unfortunately did not succeed in despite many efforts. Since the music therapy was cancelled, I could occupy myself with handicrafts until the club afternoon.'[14]

Sport was one of the core activities during the patients' stays. Most took part in groups for so-called foot, swing and cardio gymnastics. The standard programme included ball sports such as volleyball, badminton and table tennis, some swam or went bowling. Physical activity had been anchored in the psychotherapy department by former hospital director Karl Leonhard as part of his individual therapy in the late 1950s. He believed this would provide patients with distraction, conditioning and an understanding of their own physical capacities. On the downside, patients could find themselves confronted with the expectation that they had to appear sporty. Another continuity was the ideal of permanent occupation – for example, with handicrafts. Walks or department store visits could function as confrontation techniques. The occasional work therapy placement had also persisted since Leonhard's tenure. For instance, patients worked on an hourly basis in the archives, on the children's ward or at the reception of the polyclinic. Psychopharmaceuticals were continuously rejected on this ward in the 1970s, which an analysis of the respective medical records confirms. In terms of the group therapeutic programme, the patients listed autogenic training, music therapy, psychodrama, communicative movement therapy,[15] creative therapy and group discussions. Most of these methods were newly introduced in the 1970s and their experimental status becomes apparent for instance in patients' statements about organisational difficulties. Furthermore, the daily reports give insight into different evaluations of therapy components. One patient criticised a lack of effectiveness: 'The psychodrama disappointed me. Maybe I just expected more or too much of it, but I had the impression that not even the central person for whom all the plays were performed could be given helpful hints.'[16] Some evaluations seemed more positive: 'The communicative movement therapy was a bit unusual for me and the others, but I enjoyed it very much. The miracle [Wunder] that we created together in the creative therapy would not be very well received, but we laughed heartily, and I think we have certainly come a bit closer again.'[17]

As in the following case, it can be observed from some medical histories that the therapists evaluated the success of the therapy measures with the help of the daily reports: '3 March, cf. daily report from the weekend! Important insights adequately processed in the group discussion. Although influences of childhood were already pointed out by me in the individual discussion – by far no such resonance there!'[18]

Moreover, the daily reports often partially or completely replaced the medical histories. Even if this observation can hardly be quantified, it can be stated that patients took over the therapists' role in the documentation to a certain degree. As a result, there are only a few entries by therapists on the patients' writings. It is noticeable that they mainly commented on positive evaluations by patients. One patient observed the positive effect of music therapy in which music was listened to together: 'Supported by Händel in the music therapy and what I felt was a relaxed and constructive collaboration in the psychodrama, my optimism lasted throughout the day.'[19] Through such descriptions, the therapists perceived and documented how the therapies affected their patients: 'In music therapy, pat. regains "upper water": through the music (in the "react[ive] Music therapy") he felt encouraged, cf. the daily report.'[20]

Besides these evaluative functions, the daily reports were intended to have a therapeutic effect. Often, the reports were explicitly mentioned in a therapy plan at the end of the anamnesis.[21] The therapeutic effect of writing was, among other aspects, to foster self-reflection and help uncover unconscious conflicts. Some patients actively reflected on the therapeutic effects of writing. A woman highlighted the functionality of daily reports as an inventory: 'Writing a report means thinking about yourself and the day that has passed. I do nothing more than think about myself. Capturing thoughts and writing them down means bringing order to things.'[22]

In the following example, a patient purposefully developed the writing so that she could use it as an immediate reflection on the different therapies during the day:

> I think I have found a better method, or any method at all, to cope with my problem. I continuously write down insights, experiences, and situations throughout the day. The written form is for me, next to psychodrama and discussion groups, the most important method of dealing with my problem consciously, namely in that way and not as a daily report, which I usually only wrote in the evening.[23]

Most of the daily reports dealt with the authors themselves. When referring to others, the reports could illustrate certain expectations regarding their therapeutic motivation – on the part of the therapists, but also on the part of fellow patients: 'In my opinion, the group discussion "exposed" [another patient]. Now, I have the impression that she shuns all activity and personal responsibility, sees the guilt in others and feels sorry for herself (pouts to the point of inner defiance). At the moment, I see no will for change in her.'[24]

Patients were exposed to a variety of expectations and pressures on their behaviour and emotional lives. It was a fundamental part of the therapeutic concept of dynamic group psychotherapy to stand up to authority and imposed expectations. It repeatedly becomes clear, though, that such revolt was only wanted within a quite narrow therapeutic framework. Scepticism about the therapy, low motivation or refusal to write could be seen as problematic behaviour. For example, one patient did not want to write honestly about her feelings. She wrote on the top of an otherwise blank A4 page in small letters and thereby underlined her statement with the material appearance of the report: 'I ask you to spare me the daily reports. Firstly, I am not able to rationalise my thoughts and experiences so that I can write them down; secondly, you would spare me a probable lie.'[25]

She wrote several more reports expressing her aversion. Less than two weeks later, she was discharged from the clinic and took up her professional occupation again. In cases like this, no evidence of coercive disciplinary measures was found as a reaction to the reports or the general refusal, but there were indications that therapists repeatedly asked patients to write or to engage more in therapy. Patients' judgements about their fellow patients, like the one above, indicate possible social consequences in terms of social interaction on the ward. These, in turn, are scarcely constructible from the files.

It seems conceivable that close cohabitation may have increased the pressure to adapt one's own behaviour. The patients lived together in narrow rooms with four to six beds. The still image of a public TV documentary below shows that, at least for external presentation, value was placed on an appealing room design with pictures, plants and bedside lamps. However, the patients only had a small bedside table for their personal belongings. In addition, the beds were placed close together and hardly allowed for any privacy (see Figure 10.1).

Self-organised group activities dominated the patients' spare time. During 'colourful patient afternoons', they were supposed to practice lectures or music-making in front of others. Dance events and joint singing were a mostly popular pastime. Moreover, the patients were asked to put together a cultural programme, which could include visits to museums, theatres or sights. For instance, one report was entitled 'Weekend plan – ward 5', and gave an account of two visits to the cinema, one to the opera, one to a museum as well as an excursion to an outer Berlin district within three days.[26] The emphasis therapists seem to have placed on cultural activities provides some insight into normative ideas about the behaviour of patients. To some extent it may even reflect the impact of ideological ideals of an all-round educated socialist personality – even if this mission was rejected in Höcks's conceptual writings (Höck and König, 1976).

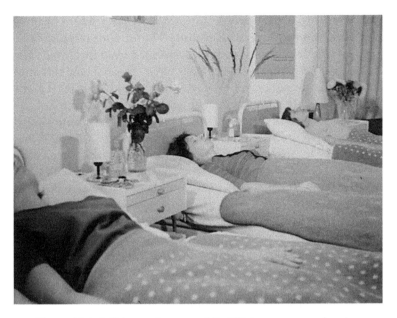

Figure 10.1 Still image from a public TV documentary, showing autogenic training in a patients' dormitory at the psychotherapy department of the Charité. Source: DRA, DRAB-H, 004167, 'Neurosen – Krank durch Überforderung?', DEFA, 9 March 1976.

While many patients enjoyed such excursions, some writers perceived collective ventures as a burden. Given the abundance of group activities, they addressed the pressure of expectation to integrate into the patient collective. Some notes from therapists clearly confirm such pressure, as in the case of the following entry in a medical record: 'Pat. shirks going to the cinema with the group.'[27] Under this impression, many dealt with tensions between privacy and group life in their reports:

> Three of us … were at the State Opera. Like the last time I went to the opera, my eyes fell shut with tiredness. I was not receptive at all. Both times I had gone with them so as not to isolate myself. Since I never sleep well anyway, and since I don't know beforehand whether I will be able to take a nap, I am even more tired the following day in such cases, which does not exactly improve my mood. Therefore, I consider this involuntary 'subordination' as pointless. The price I had to pay again is too high.[28]

Later, the same person added: 'I miss a quiet place where I can be
alone from time to time, undisturbed.'[29] In the same respect others
justified themselves when they had separated from the group. The
therapeutic benefits expected from group treatment could turn into
the opposite for patients if they craved privacy. In this regard, the
pressure to adapt was occasionally perceived to be coercive.

The two wards of the psychotherapeutic department were located
in a side wing of the psychiatric department of the Charité,[30] and
thus spatially separated from other psychiatric and neurological
wards. Consequently, the authors were mainly in contact with other
psychotherapy patients. The patients of both wards were involved
in the organisation of everyday life. As they were partly self-sufficient,
patients cleaned their rooms, went shopping, prepared meals and
did the dishes in kitchen duties. How community should be organised
could be perceived as a political question. This participatory concept
could be interpreted as a sign of democratisation, but some evolving
conflicts point towards frictional notions of social and societal
organisation in a broader sense among patients:

> By the way, [a fellow patient] wanted to suggest to the patient council
> to shift the breakfast from 7.30 to 7 o'clock (which would have
> spoken for him). But he did not do it. ... regarding the discussion
> about the kitchen duties, I was disappointed by the dishonesty in the
> patient council. The fact is: a) the patients of ward 4 sometimes start
> breakfast at 7.20 a.m. and are therefore finished sooner; b) the patients
> of ward 5 sometimes get the bucket trolley too late (because they do
> not get up in time), which may increase the time difference between
> the two wards; c) the claim that all patients always come to breakfast
> on time is untrue.
>
> I wish this complex matter to be completely clarified. My question
> is: Am I the victim of a primary neurotic maldevelopment? Are these
> conflicts typical for certain neuroses or is this specifically my problem?
> Does an already emerging anti-authoritarian society of egoists cast
> its shadow here? And if so, is it better for me to 'float with this
> current'?[31]

Until his release, he remained critical of the form of organisation:
'My thoughts and feelings circle around the discharge. I don't like
the dawdling that has occurred in the hospital. It is time to lead an
"orderly life" again.'[32]

As in the case of therapies, the patients could raise criticism also in relation to self-organised ward life, but it often remains vague as to what extent it was heard. Moreover, this patient implied a political dimension by suggesting that the community in the ward deviated too much from societal standards of the authoritarian ruled GDR, perhaps also approaching Western models too closely. His statement shows how differently patients reacted to the efforts to reorganise ward life. Among therapists and patients alike, the status of authority in the context of reform attempts and dynamic group psychotherapy seems to have been controversial.

In isolated cases, the patients' political attitudes are recognisable from their daily reports, but political debates seemingly rarely took place. To prevent betrayals, therapists of the same methods in other institutions asked their patients to focus on the here and now in group sessions and to leave political issues aside. It is likely that the same policy was followed at the Charité. From the patients' point of view, too, surveillance by state security had to be feared and presumably prefiltered their writings.

In addition, the author above referred to committees that resembled political bodies and were designed to enable patients to participate in organisational issues, represent their interests and resolve conflicts. A so-called 'patient council' was held once a week. It was composed of elected representatives from the patient dormitories and had an elected chairperson. The 'general assembly', in turn, was attended by all patients.[33] The combination of therapeutic components seems to have been non-negotiable, but when it came to cohabitation issues, patients could raise topics of concern and contribute to their solution. Details on these gatherings were rarely included in the reports. It still becomes apparent that not all patients were satisfied with these solutions or the way they were found.

The institution aimed to guarantee orderly social interaction and the course of therapy by a set of house rules. The precise wording has not been preserved. From the medical records it appears that curfews in the evening with open doors during the rest of the day and a ban on taking medication were central. In case of violations, the therapists issued admonishments or implied disciplinary measures. When a patient took medication on her own and lost consciousness, the medical history read:

Determination:

1) Pat. gave up all medication in the presence of Dr. ... + nurse ... (Dormutil, Caffeine, Gelonida, Titretta Supp, Obridan, Regulax).
2) Pat. informs the chairman of the pat. council until the departmental meeting.
3) Urine check on Friday.[34]

On the one hand, this is an example of how such patient committees could be incorporated in the execution of disciplinary measures. The patients' council was supposed to have a monitoring function here and the case should be negotiated in the patients' assembly. In this way, the patients were urged to control and discipline one another. On the other hand, the patient's reaction shows how strongly such social pressure could affect those concerned: 'Tomorrow, I will be lined up against the wall in the patients' assembly to be shot. I don't think I can endure it.'[35]

In the case of repetition, therapists threatened exclusion from psychotherapy, seemingly without consulting the other patients. Disciplinary measures which had not been jointly agreed upon with the patient community were also used in other conflicts. When a patient did not agree to her transfer to another dormitory, an argument arose. The medical history read: 'A short time later, the patient demonstratively wanted to leave the ward. Consultation with Dr. Seidel: no exeat!'[36]

This note emphasises that the therapists were still able to take away patients' freedoms as a disciplinary means, even though the ward was organised as a therapeutic community. In this example, the patient's protest was not perceived as legitimate criticism, but was instead interpreted as a negative behavioural trait. The following complaint emphasises that the hierarchy between the clinical professional groups and patients persisted and provided further potential for conflict: 'Again, I was "kicked out" by nurse ... Her harassing manner causes me to need more instead of less time, to her disadvantage. It is unacceptable that she wants to close the ward before 4 p.m. while I treat my nail fungus ..., especially since Dr. ... did not give us a time limit in response to our explicit question (witnesses: [two fellow patients]).'[37]

Despite these conflicts and the continued hierarchical positioning of therapists and patients, the latter often used the daily reports to give strong voice to their opinions. Due to the nature of the sources, it is hardly possible to assess the weight of their statements for conflict resolution. How such disputes were dealt with is rarely documented. In this respect, the daily reports served as a medium for complaints, not as a space for resolution. Where therapists attached importance to the patients' problems, solutions were sought through direct verbal exchange or in one of the patient committees.

At the same time, however, it should be emphasised that the liberties granted to the patients were high compared to other departments of the psychiatric hospital of the Charité and that, overall, the patients' statements in this regard were mostly positive. Patients were allowed to receive visitors or leave the hospital grounds during the day – for example, to meet family or acquaintances in East Berlin. In so-called 'stress test leaves' on weekends, the treated were to keep up or re-establish a connection to their social environment. It seems that this strategy also had to compensate for inadequate outpatient aftercare in other districts of the GDR (see, for example, Rose, 2005: 137–8). Patients who lived close by could continue their treatment as day patients. Yet patients had to ask for permission for weekend leaves and longer time out in the evening and the decision was made by the institution. Open doors can be seen as an expression of reformist efforts, even though institutionally imposed rules were still enforced hierarchically, and violations were sanctioned. To conclude, the following observation of a patient highlights pronounced differences to other psychiatric wards: 'Since I was here on the ward, my reservations about the inner thought-and-rumour-knot "mental hospital" had pretty much faded into the background. Now it's all back again. Not on our ward, but we are close to other departments where there is more going on between nursing staff and patients than the absent doctor could dream of.'[38] The patient was able to overcome her reservations about a psychiatric clinic in the setting of the psychotherapy. She did not specify her experience of visiting other wards. However, they made a strong negative impression on her and made her draw a contrast between the psychiatric and psychotherapeutic wards. Despite all the ambivalences, the psychotherapeutic ward seemed more advanced to this patient in a reformist sense.

The lens of the daily reports allowed for some spotlights on the group psychotherapy ward of the psychiatric hospital of the Charité in the mid-1970s. This perspective revealed attempts to reorganise social ward life. The establishment of a therapeutic community in a psychiatric hospital in the GDR required renegotiation of the status of authority and participatory decision-making on psychotherapeutic wards. The therapeutic community, as envisaged in Jones's model, was generated by the subordination of clinical hierarchy to consensus-oriented decision-making based on democratically controlled bodies. At the same time, however, some patients' complaints demonstrate that concessions were made to maintaining institutional authority, which could not and should not be overcome by the emancipation process envisaged by the group psychotherapy. In view of the debates on the Brandenburg Proposition, this may also suggest adaptations to the authoritarian societal system.[39]

Moreover, the concept had to be adapted to personnel and material circumstances. As the Charité was a university hospital, it can be assumed that the latter were exceptionally good compared to other institutions in the GDR (Janssen, 2012). In the present case, hierarchical structures eroded, but were not dissolved to the extent envisaged by Jones. Moreover, the reformist efforts were tied to the department and hardly transferred to non-psychotherapeutic psychiatric spaces, as broad implementation according to the Brandenburg Proposition would have required. This kind of 'islandisation' can also be observed in other attempts to establish therapeutic communities in sociotherapy wards (Falk and Hauer, 2007: 248). Among others, such attempts and the reservation of other professionals are known from Brandenburg-Görden and Berlin-Buch (Eichhorn and Busch, 1979; Späte and Otto, 2011).

Ambivalent effects of daily reporting as a practice

Unlike what Kratochvíl's explanations might suggest, the daily reports were no 'diaries', as the patients directly addressed their therapists. Thus, it was a hybrid form of writing that combined self-analysis and interpersonal communication. The fact that both were demanded simultaneously appeared to some patients as an intrusion into a private process – they refused. Others responded with technical descriptions of daily routines, while for those with a trusting relationship to the therapists, daily reports could become an appreciated means of expression and a helpful, if not central, therapeutic tool. Based on these different perceptions, our focus turns to the various implications that the practice had for social life on the ward.

Writing at first appears as a reformist practice and blended into the general therapeutic concept. The daily reports materially reflect a diversified psychotherapeutic spectrum. Due to its self-reflexive nature, the practice had a therapeutic effect itself, as several patients made use of it to uncover their unconscious mental conflicts. Moreover, the daily reports offered an additional means of communication. In this way, they promoted the flow of information and stand for an enhancement of the patient perspective in the therapists' perception. This means of communication had the potential to foster participatory organisation of the ward as well. Requests for private consultations were frequent and allowed for exchange in addition to the group sessions, when accepted. In some cases, therapists sought individual talks because of patients' writings, especially concerning suicide risks. Furthermore, the daily reports strengthened patients' voices in the documentation about themselves. Storing the daily reports in the patient records filed a 'second voice' next to the institutional one and enhanced the patients' subjective perception of their stay in the hospital. In this respect, patients even took over the responsibilities of therapists, when their reports replaced the journal in the medical files.

In addition, the patients' daily reports offered a means of evaluation for their treatment. Reading offered the therapists a moment of conscious reflection on their patients' assessments of the therapeutic effects and critiques. Thus, the reception was conductive to therapeutic ambitions, but the effect on their individual reformist endeavours can only be estimated. What can be substantiated, for the most part, are confirmatory perceptions of positive therapeutic or organisational effects. From the present sources, the impact criticism had on the therapists remains largely an open question. It is especially difficult to deduce whether protest was seen as therapeutic progress in terms of critique towards authorities, or whether the therapists took it into consideration as such, and either dismissed or ignored it, or adapted their behaviour or the respective circumstances. Still, the reports allowed patients to address the staff with questions, comments and sometimes sharp criticism concerning psychotherapy and everyday organisation. The writing practice thus strengthened the patients' capacity for action – a concern that the therapeutic community pursued as well.

However, this scope remained in distinct dependence on the therapists as representatives of the institution. This circumstance hints at some downsides that run counter to reformist ideas. First and foremost, the practice performed a hierarchy between therapists and patients in a way, which opposed the erosion of traditional hospital structures. Writing only took place in one direction, as therapists did not write back, but continuously requested the patients to write. Instead, they accumulated knowledge from each individual's written communication. In turn, the patients faced a certain kind of social control, as they did not know what their fellows wrote, and could not respond to it, even if it concerned them. It remained up to the therapists to decide when they considered the concerns important enough to respond. The hierarchical distribution of roles between therapists and patients remained and ultimately the writing practice repulsed attempts at its erosion.

Additionally, patients' testimonies were not free from institutional constraints. Their writing was subject to expectations in terms of commitment and therapy motivation, as well as assimilation into the group and predetermined hospital structures. There was pressure to appear sporty, hardworking and willing to reintegrate into work life. These values were considered therapeutically beneficial, but they also depict – whether intended or not – societal ideals of socialism in the therapeutic context. It seems reasonable to assume that patients were subject to these structures and that their statements were shaped accordingly. Personal testimonies are widely considered 'impressively unfree' and it seems conceivable that, in this case too, the patients made repressive mechanisms of the institution operative through writing (Osten, 2010: 8). Meanwhile, frequency, tone and the extent of criticism in some reports suggest a relative openness and seem to challenge the structural determinacy of patient perspectives to some extent. After all, this dilemma depicts one of the therapy itself: it aimed at emancipation from authoritarian structures, but ultimately remained bound to the institutional and societal context.

Apart from this, it seems plausible that the writing practice indirectly affected the choice of patients among those with neurosis diagnoses. The small number of psychotherapy beds were noticeably more likely to be given to people with a higher school education _ademic qualification. As an integral part of therapy, this _ence may have intensified the notion that higher education was necessary for psychotherapy. In the final account, this observation remains an assumption, as the sample also contains a few examples to the contrary. Finally, daily reporting may have hampered the transfer of the therapeutic concept to other psychiatric wards and institutions. Staff capacities might have been a limiting factor, as reading and processing the reports required time and a close supervisory relationship. Perhaps the practice contributed in small part to the fact that this psychotherapy remained out of reach for most psychiatric patients. Instead, the psychotherapy of neurotic disorders was further differentiated and bridges to the rest of psychiatry remained scarce.

The polyphony of patient opinions shows that the examined reform attempts were still in the making. They were subject to ideological and social negotiation not only on the part of therapists, but also of several patients. A similarly ambiguous picture emerges when looking at the implications of daily reporting as a practice. In an almost contradictory way, it strengthened the voices of patients in everyday life and in the medical documentation, while limiting them to an inferior role in the institutional system. Daily reporting can be seen as an expression of reformist endeavours, as it facilitated the expression of criticism and placed attention on patients' perceptions. If one considers secondary reflections of the practice on the social fabric, a more ambivalent picture emerges: daily reporting upheld the performance of hierarchy and thus eventually limited attempts at its erosion. Finally, the practice may serve as an allegory for the challenges of psychiatric reform projects in the context of socialist society.

Notes

1 Historisches Psychiatriearchiv der Charité [Historical Psychiatric Archive of the Charité] (henceforth HPAC), Berlin, 557/74M, Daily report from 6 January 1974.
2 HPAC, 449/74M, Daily report from 11 December 1974.
3 For a broad compilation of contemporary testimonies on the development of psychotherapy see Geyer (2011b).

4 The quotations of patients' speech in this article are used to express the polyphony of patient opinions and voices. To protect the patients' identities, this article does not include names or information on living conditions and renounces coherent case histories. From 1978, other patients from the second psychotherapeutic department with an individual therapy focus wrote as well. These twenty-six files were supplementarily included in the analysis. At the time of the research, the medical records of the 1980s had not yet been transferred from the clinic to the Historical Psychiatric Archives. These files will first be made accessible to researchers in 2022.

5 The concept of a 'therapeutic community' is also significant for Chapters 1, 2 and 5.

6 See Malich, 2019 for an outline of Höck's career.

7 The psychotherapy department was founded by Karl Leonhard (1904–88) in 1959 in order to put his Individual Therapy for Neuroses into practice.

8 Interviews with two psychotherapists working in the GDR revealed that the interviewees were not aware of any research based on the daily reports or on their use in therapy. Moreover, volumes from the 1970s and 1980s of the only psychiatric journal in the GDR, 'Psychiatrie, Neurologie und medizinische Psychologie', were examined.

9 The criticism of medical historian and philosopher Achim Thom had a decisive influence on the reformulation. He considered the psychodynamic understanding of illness and the individual psychological view of groups to be incompatible with Marxist ideas of society and the individual. Under socialism, a 'therapeutic community' could only be a 'rehabilitation collective' with an educational mission in the sense of forming socialist personalities, Kumbier and Haack (2018), referring to Thom (1974).

10 For example, disciplinary aspects of therapies were rejected in the first version, but in 1976 they were considered necessary, as was the maintenance of institutional authority (Kumbier and Haack, 2017: 439).

11 Deutsches Rundfunkarchiv [German broadcasting archive] (henceforth DRA), Potsdam, DRAB-H, 004167, 'Neurosen – Krank durch Überforderung?', DEFA, 9 March 1976.

12 Suggestive methods were widespread in the GDR as well as in other Eastern bloc countries, cf. Marks, 2018.

13 HPAC, 577/74F, Daily report from 12 December 1974.

14 HPAC, 577/74F, Daily report from 9 January 1975.

15 A group and self-awareness method developed at the Leipzig University Psychiatric Clinic (Kohler and Wilda-Kiesel, 1972)

16 HPAC, 319/78F, Daily report from 21 June 1978.

17 HPAC, 502/78F, Daily report from 14 September 1978.

ɪtry in the medical history from 3 March

from 16 August 1978.

entry in the medical history from 16

76M.

om 28 June 1977.

ɔm 9 June 1977.

rom 14 September 1976.

⎯, ͻͻᴑ/ʔ4ꜰ, Daily report from 4 November 1974.
26 HPAC, 477/77F, Daily report from 2 October 1977.
27 HPAC, 514/78M, Therapist's entry in the medical history from 2 February 1979.
28 HPAC, 557/74M, Daily report from 30 January 1975.
29 HPAC, 557/74M, Daily report from 13 March 1975.
30 Dynamic group psychotherapy and individual therapy respectively were practised there, but there were interferences in terms of therapeutic components. Prospective patients were distributed according to diagnoses.
31 HPAC, 557/74M, Daily report from 18 April 1975.
32 HPAC, 557/74M, Daily report from 8 and 9 May 1975.
33 On the general assembly as therapeutic practice see Chapter 2.
34 HPAC, 121/77F, Therapist's entry in the medical history from 16 March 1977.
35 HPAC, 121/77F, Daily report from 16 March 1977.
36 HPAC, 414/78F, Therapist's entry in the medical history from 3 October 1978.
37 HPAC, 557/74M, Daily report from 15 and 16 May 1975.
38 HPAC, 420/76F, Daily report from 11 August 1976.
39 Nevertheless, some therapeutic communities in the United States were criticised by European practitioners for maintaining authoritarian patterns and the leadership of a charismatic leader (Ottenberg 1982: 171). In this respect, the gradient in authority may not be explained by the East–West divide alone.

References

Akademie für Ärztliche Fortbildung (ed.), 1978, *Weiterbildung zum Facharzt* (Berlin: Ministerium für Gesundheitswesen der DDR).

Balz, Viola and Ulrike Klöppel, 2015, 'Wendung nach Innen: Sozialpsychiatrie, Gesundheitspolitik und Psychopharmaka in der Deutschen Demokratischen Republik, 1960–1989', *Vierteljahreshefte für Zeitgeschichte*, 63:4, 539–67.

Dührssen, Annemarie, Jürgen Körner, Gerd Rudolf, An[...]
    Elke Schultz-Dierbach, Dieter Kallinke, Michael Wirs[...]
    Müller-Küppers, Hellmuth Kleinsorge, Ulrich Rüger, Han[...]
    Rudolf Faber, Rudolf Haarstrick, Heinz Schepank, Eibe-R[...]
    Reinhard Leidtke, Hans-Werner Künsebeck, Hellmuth Freyberge[...]
    Holm-Hadulla and Michael Lukas Moeller, 1990, 'Die Psychothe[...]
    zum Ende des 20. Jahrhunderts im deutschsprachigen Bereich: E[...]
    Übersicht', *Zeitschrift für psychosomatische Medizin und Psychoanalyse,*
    36:2, 101–85.
Eichhorn, Hans and K.-T. Busch, 1979, 'Erfahrung über die Einrichtung
    einer therapeutischen Gemeinschaft für Psychotherapie im Bereich eines
    großstädtischen Klinikums', in Heinz A. F. Schulze and W. Poppe (eds),
    Konzeptionen und Modelle der langfristigen Betreuung in der Nerven-
    heilkunde: Ergebnisse des Kongresses der Gesellschaft für Psychiatrie
    und Neurologie der DDR vom 20.-22. Oktober 1977 mit 62 Beiträgen
    (Leipzig: S. Hirzel Verlag), pp. 143–4.
Elberfeld, Jens, 2019, 'Das Ich und das Wir: Gruppentherapie zwischen
    Sozialisierung der Psyche, Gemeinschaftserfahrung und Regierungstechnik',
    Mittelweg 36, 6:1, 137–59.
Falk, Beatrice and Friedrich Hauer, 2007, *Brandenburg-Görden: Geschichte*
    eines psychiatrischen Krankenhauses (Berlin: be.bra wissenschaft).
Geyer, Michael, 2011a, 'Ostdeutsche Psychotherapiechronik 1970–1979',
    in Michael Geyer (ed.), *Psychotherapie in Ostdeutschland: Geschichte*
    und Geschichten 1945–1995 (Göttingen: Vandenhoeck & Ruprecht),
    pp. 245–56.
Geyer, Michael (ed.), 2011b, *Psychotherapie in Ostdeutschland: Geschichte*
    und Geschichten 1945–1995 (Göttingen: Vandenhoeck & Ruprecht).
Hanrath, Sabine, 2002, *Zwischen 'Euthanasie' und Psychiatriereform:*
    Anstaltspsychiatrie in Westfalen und Brandenburg: Ein deutsch-deutscher
    Vergleich (1945–1964) (Paderborn: Schöningh).
Hennings, Lena, 2015, 'Die Entstehungsgeschichte der Rodewischer Thesen
    im Kontext von Psychiatrie, Sozialhygiene und Rehabilitationsmedizin
    der DDR'. Dissertation, Universität zu Lübeck.
Hess, Helga, 2011a, 'Die Gründung der Sektion Dynamische Gruppenpsycho-
    therapie und die Ausbildung in Gruppenselbsterfahrung', in Michael Geyer
    (ed.), *Psychotherapie in Ostdeutschland: Geschichte und Geschichten*
    1945–1995 (Göttingen: Vandenhoeck & Ruprecht), pp. 276–86.
Hess, Helga, 2011b, 'Die Herausbildung eines Institutes für Psychotherapie
    und Neurosenforschung (IfPN) mit Integration der Ambulanz, Klinik und
    Forschung', in Michael Geyer (ed.), *Psychotherapie in Ostdeutschland:*
    Geschichte und Geschichten 1945–1995 (Göttingen: Vandenhoeck &
    Ruprecht), pp. 372–3.

Höck, Kurt and Werner König, 1976, *Neurosenlehre und Psychotherapie* (Jena: VEB Gustav Fischer Verlag).

Janssen, Wiebke, 2012, 'Medizinische Hochschulbauten als Prestigeobjekt der SED: Das Klinikum Halle-Kröllwitz', *Deutschland Archiv*, 45:4, 703–12.

Jones, Maxwell, 1967, 'Traditionelle Psychiatrie, Sozialpsychiatrie und die therapeutische Gemeinschaft', in Kurt Höck (ed.), *Gruppenpsychotherapie in Klinik und Praxis: Ergänzter Bericht des Internationalen Symposions über Gruppenpsychotherapie in Berlin vom 20. bis 22.01.1966* (Jena: Gustav Fischer Verlag), pp. 187–95.

Kohler, Christa and Anita Wilda-Kiesel, 1972, *Bewegungstherapie für funktionelle Störungen und Neurosen* (Leipzig: Barth).

Kratochvíl, Stanislav, 1976, 'Organisation und Erfahrung einer therapeutischen Gemeinschaft für Neurosentherapie', in Kurt Höck and Karl Seidel (eds), *Psychotherapie und Gesellschaft* (Berlin: VEB Deutscher Verlag der Wissenschaften), pp. 217–42.

Kumbier, Ekkehardt and Kathleen Haack, 2017, 'Psychiatrie in der DDR zwischen Aufbruch und Stagnation: Die Brandenburger Thesen zur "Therapeutischen Gemeinschaft" (1974/76)', *Psychiatrische Praxis*, 44:8, 434–45.

Kumbier, Ekkehardt and Kathleen Haack, 2018, 'Die Psychiatrie in der DDR zwischen Aufbruch und Stagnation: Die Brandenburger Thesen zur "Therapeutischen Gemeinschaft" (1974/1976)', in Ekkehardt Kumbier and Holger Steinberg (eds), *Psychiatrie in der DDR: Beiträge zur Geschichte* (Berlin: be.bra wissenschaft), pp. 247–60.

Leuenberger, Christine, 2001, 'Socialist psychotherapy and its dissidents', *Journal of the History of Behavioral Studies*, 37:3, 261–73.

Maaz, Hans-Joachim, 2011, 'Die Klinik für Psychotherapie und Psychosomatik im Diakoniewerk Halle: Ein Freiraum zur Integration von Methoden der Humanistischen Psychologie', in Michael Geyer (ed.), *Psychotherapie in Ostdeutschland: Geschichte und Geschichten 1945–1995* (Göttingen: Vandenhoeck & Ruprecht), pp. 565–8.

Malich, Lisa, 2019, 'Kurt Höck oder der verordnete Aufstand des neurotischen Körpers', in Alexa Geisthövel and Bettina Hitzer (eds), *Auf der Suche nach einer anderen Medizin: Psychosomatik im 20. Jahrhundert* (Berlin: Suhrkamp), pp. 300–12.

Marks, Sarah, 2018, 'Suggestion, persuasion and work: Psychotherapies in communist Europe', *European Journal of Psychotherapy and Counselling*, 20:1, 10–24.

Misselwitz, Irene, 2011, 'Aufbau der Psychotherapie in der Klinik für Psychiatrie und Neurologie der Universität Jena', in Michael Geyer (ed.), *Psychotherapie in Ostdeutschland: Geschichte und Geschichten 1945–1995* (Göttingen: Vandenhoeck & Ruprecht), pp. 568–71.

Osten, Philipp (ed.), 2010, *Patientendokumente: Krankheit in Selbstzeugnissen* (Stuttgart: Franz Steiner Verlag).

Ottenberg, Donald J., 1982, 'Therapeutic community and the danger of the cult phenomenon', *Marriage & Family Review*, 4:3–4, 151–73.

Porter, Roy, 1985, 'The patient's view: Doing medical history from below', *Theory and Society*, 14:2, 175–98.

Richter, Eva A., 2001, 'Psychiatrie in der DDR: Stecken geblieben – Ansätze vor 38 Jahren', *Deutsches Ärzteblatt*, 98:6, 307–8.

Rose, Wolfgang, 2005, *Anstaltspsychiatrie in der DDR: Die brandenburgischen Kliniken zwischen 1945 und 1990* (Berlin: be.bra wissenschaft).

Savelli, Mat, 2018, '"Peace and happiness await us". Psychotherapy in Yugoslavia, 1945–85', *History of the Human Sciences*, 31:4, 38–57.

Schirmer, Siegfried, Karl Müller and Helmut F. Späte, 1976, 'Brandenburger Thesen zur therapeutischen Gemeinschaft', *Psychiatrie, Neurologie und medizinische Psychologie*, 28:1, 21–6.

Schmiedebach, Heinz-Peter, Thomas Beddies, Jörg Schulz and Stefan Priebe, 2000, 'Offene Fürsorge – Rodewischer Thesen – Psychiatrie-Enquete: Drei Reformansätze im Vergleich', *Psychiatrische Praxis*, 27:3, 138–43.

Späte, Helmut F. and Klaus-Rüdiger Otto, 2011, *Irre irren nicht* (Leipzig: Ille & Riemer).

Steinberg, Holger, 2014, 'Karl Leonhard hat "kein Interesse!" – Hintergründe über das Rodewischer Symposium aus neu aufgetauchten Quellen', *Psychiatrische Praxis*, 41:2, 71–5.

Thom, Achim, 1974, 'Auf dem Weg zu einer Psychiatrie der sozialistischen Gesellschaft', *Psychiatrie, Neurologie und medizinische Psychologie*, 26:10, 578–87.

Thom, Achim, 1976, 'Bedeutsame Differenzierungen der sozialpsychiatrischen Bewegung in der kapitalistischen Gesellschaft: Teil II', *Psychiatrie, Neurologie und medizinische Psychologie*, 28:2, 99–105.

Weise, Gerlinde, 2011, 'Ambulante psychotherapeutische Komplextherapie am Modell einer Magdeburger poliklinischen Einrichtung: Zur Entstehungsgeschichte und Struktur der ambulanten psychotherapeutischen Behandlungsform im Rahmen der Organisation der Polikliniken', in Michael Geyer (ed.), *Psychotherapie in Ostdeutschland: Geschichte und Geschichten 1945–1995* (Göttingen: Vandenhoeck & Ruprecht), pp. 402–5.

Weise, Klaus, 1990, 'Psychotherapie in der Psychiatrie', in Achim Thom (ed.), *Psychiatrie im Wandel: Erfahrungen und Perspektiven in Ost und West* (Bonn: Psychiatrie Verlag), pp. 288–307.

Osten, Philipp (ed.), 2010, *Patientendokumente: Krankheit in Selbstzeugnissen* (Stuttgart: Franz Steiner Verlag).

Ottenberg, Donald J., 1982, 'Therapeutic community and the danger of the cult phenomenon', *Marriage & Family Review*, 4:3–4, 151–73.

Porter, Roy, 1985, 'The patient's view: Doing medical history from below', *Theory and Society*, 14:2, 175–98.

Richter, Eva A., 2001, 'Psychiatrie in der DDR: Stecken geblieben – Ansätze vor 38 Jahren', *Deutsches Ärzteblatt*, 98:6, 307–8.

Rose, Wolfgang, 2005, *Anstaltspsychiatrie in der DDR: Die brandenburgischen Kliniken zwischen 1945 und 1990* (Berlin: be.bra wissenschaft).

Savelli, Mat, 2018, '"Peace and happiness await us". Psychotherapy in Yugoslavia, 1945–85', *History of the Human Sciences*, 31:4, 38–57.

Schirmer, Siegfried, Karl Müller and Helmut F. Späte, 1976, 'Brandenburger Thesen zur therapeutischen Gemeinschaft', *Psychiatrie, Neurologie und medizinische Psychologie*, 28:1, 21–6.

Schmiedebach, Heinz-Peter, Thomas Beddies, Jörg Schulz and Stefan Priebe, 2000, 'Offene Fürsorge – Rodewischer Thesen – Psychiatrie-Enquete: Drei Reformansätze im Vergleich', *Psychiatrische Praxis*, 27:3, 138–43.

Späte, Helmut F. and Klaus-Rüdiger Otto, 2011, *Irre irren nicht* (Leipzig: Ille & Riemer).

Steinberg, Holger, 2014, 'Karl Leonhard hat "kein Interesse!" – Hintergründe über das Rodewischer Symposium aus neu aufgetauchten Quellen', *Psychiatrische Praxis*, 41:2, 71–5.

Thom, Achim, 1974, 'Auf dem Weg zu einer Psychiatrie der sozialistischen Gesellschaft', *Psychiatrie, Neurologie und medizinische Psychologie*, 26:10, 578–87.

Thom, Achim, 1976, 'Bedeutsame Differenzierungen der sozialpsychiatrischen Bewegung in der kapitalistischen Gesellschaft: Teil II', *Psychiatrie, Neurologie und medizinische Psychologie*, 28:2, 99–105.

Weise, Gerlinde, 2011, 'Ambulante psychotherapeutische Komplextherapie am Modell einer Magdeburger poliklinischen Einrichtung: Zur Entstehungsgeschichte und Struktur der ambulanten psychotherapeutischen Behandlungsform im Rahmen der Organisation der Polikliniken', in Michael Geyer (ed.), *Psychotherapie in Ostdeutschland: Geschichte und Geschichten 1945–1995* (Göttingen: Vandenhoeck & Ruprecht), pp. 402–5.

Weise, Klaus, 1990, 'Psychotherapie in der Psychiatrie', in Achim Thom (ed.), *Psychiatrie im Wandel: Erfahrungen und Perspektiven in Ost und West* (Bonn: Psychiatrie Verlag), pp. 288–307.

Höck, Kurt and Werner König, 1976, *Neurosenlehre und Psychotherapie* (Jena: VEB Gustav Fischer Verlag).

Janssen, Wiebke, 2012, 'Medizinische Hochschulbauten als Prestigeobjekt der SED: Das Klinikum Halle-Kröllwitz', *Deutschland Archiv*, 45:4, 703–12.

Jones, Maxwell, 1967, 'Traditionelle Psychiatrie, Sozialpsychiatrie und die therapeutische Gemeinschaft', in Kurt Höck (ed.), *Gruppenpsychotherapie in Klinik und Praxis: Ergänzter Bericht des Internationalen Symposions über Gruppenpsychotherapie in Berlin vom 20. bis 22.01.1966* (Jena: Gustav Fischer Verlag), pp. 187–95.

Kohler, Christa and Anita Wilda-Kiesel, 1972, *Bewegungstherapie für funktionelle Störungen und Neurosen* (Leipzig: Barth).

Kratochvíl, Stanislav, 1976, 'Organisation und Erfahrung einer therapeutischen Gemeinschaft für Neurosentherapie', in Kurt Höck and Karl Seidel (eds), *Psychotherapie und Gesellschaft* (Berlin: VEB Deutscher Verlag der Wissenschaften), pp. 217–42.

Kumbier, Ekkehardt and Kathleen Haack, 2017, 'Psychiatrie in der DDR zwischen Aufbruch und Stagnation: Die Brandenburger Thesen zur "Therapeutischen Gemeinschaft" (1974/76)', *Psychiatrische Praxis*, 44:8, 434–45.

Kumbier, Ekkehardt and Kathleen Haack, 2018, 'Die Psychiatrie in der DDR zwischen Aufbruch und Stagnation: Die Brandenburger Thesen zur "Therapeutischen Gemeinschaft" (1974/1976)', in Ekkehardt Kumbier and Holger Steinberg (eds), *Psychiatrie in der DDR: Beiträge zur Geschichte* (Berlin: be.bra wissenschaft), pp. 247–60.

Leuenberger, Christine, 2001, 'Socialist psychotherapy and its dissidents', *Journal of the History of Behavioral Studies*, 37:3, 261–73.

Maaz, Hans-Joachim, 2011, 'Die Klinik für Psychotherapie und Psychosomatik im Diakoniewerk Halle: Ein Freiraum zur Integration von Methoden der Humanistischen Psychologie', in Michael Geyer (ed.), *Psychotherapie in Ostdeutschland: Geschichte und Geschichten 1945–1995* (Göttingen: Vandenhoeck & Ruprecht), pp. 565–8.

Malich, Lisa, 2019, 'Kurt Höck oder der verordnete Aufstand des neurotischen Körpers', in Alexa Geisthövel and Bettina Hitzer (eds), *Auf der Suche nach einer anderen Medizin: Psychosomatik im 20. Jahrhundert* (Berlin: Suhrkamp), pp. 300–12.

Marks, Sarah, 2018, 'Suggestion, persuasion and work: Psychotherapies in communist Europe', *European Journal of Psychotherapy and Counselling*, 20:1, 10–24.

Misselwitz, Irene, 2011, 'Aufbau der Psychotherapie in der Klinik für Psychiatrie und Neurologie der Universität Jena', in Michael Geyer (ed.), *Psychotherapie in Ostdeutschland: Geschichte und Geschichten 1945–1995* (Göttingen: Vandenhoeck & Ruprecht), pp. 568–71.

18 HPAC, 14/75M, Therapist's entry in the medical history from 3 March 1975.
19 HPAC, 339/78M, Daily report from 16 August 1978.
20 HPAC, 339/78M, Therapist's entry in the medical history from 16 August 1978.
21 E.g. in the case of HPAC, 499/76M.
22 HPAC, 179/77F, Daily report from 28 June 1977.
23 HPAC, 228/77F, Daily report from 9 June 1977.
24 HPAC, 391/76M, Daily report from 14 September 1976.
25 HPAC, 356/74F, Daily report from 4 November 1974.
26 HPAC, 477/77F, Daily report from 2 October 1977.
27 HPAC, 514/78M, Therapist's entry in the medical history from 2 February 1979.
28 HPAC, 557/74M, Daily report from 30 January 1975.
29 HPAC, 557/74M, Daily report from 13 March 1975.
30 Dynamic group psychotherapy and individual therapy respectively were practised there, but there were interferences in terms of therapeutic components. Prospective patients were distributed according to diagnoses.
31 HPAC, 557/74M, Daily report from 18 April 1975.
32 HPAC, 557/74M, Daily report from 8 and 9 May 1975.
33 On the general assembly as therapeutic practice see Chapter 2.
34 HPAC, 121/77F, Therapist's entry in the medical history from 16 March 1977.
35 HPAC, 121/77F, Daily report from 16 March 1977.
36 HPAC, 414/78F, Therapist's entry in the medical history from 3 October 1978.
37 HPAC, 557/74M, Daily report from 15 and 16 May 1975.
38 HPAC, 420/76F, Daily report from 11 August 1976.
39 Nevertheless, some therapeutic communities in the United States were criticised by European practitioners for maintaining authoritarian patterns and the leadership of a charismatic leader (Ottenberg 1982: 171). In this respect, the gradient in authority may not be explained by the East–West divide alone.

References

Akademie für Ärztliche Fortbildung (ed.), 1978, *Weiterbildung zum Facharzt* (Berlin: Ministerium für Gesundheitswesen der DDR).
Balz, Viola and Ulrike Klöppel, 2015, 'Wendung nach Innen: Sozialpsychiatrie, Gesundheitspolitik und Psychopharmaka in der Deutschen Demokratischen Republik, 1960–1989', *Vierteljahreshefte für Zeitgeschichte*, 63:4, 539–67.

Dührssen, Annemarie, Jürgen Körner, Gerd Rudolf, Annelise Heigl-Evers, Elke Schultz-Dierbach, Dieter Kallinke, Michael Wirsching, Manfred Müller-Küppers, Hellmuth Kleinsorge, Ulrich Rüger, Hans Kind, Franz Rudolf Faber, Rudolf Haarstrick, Heinz Schepank, Eibe-Rudolf Rey, Reinhard Leidtke, Hans-Werner Künsebeck, Hellmuth Freyberger, Rainer Holm-Hadulla and Michael Lukas Moeller, 1990, 'Die Psychotherapie zum Ende des 20. Jahrhunderts im deutschsprachigen Bereich: Eine Übersicht', *Zeitschrift für psychosomatische Medizin und Psychoanalyse*, 36:2, 101–85.

Eichhorn, Hans and K.-T. Busch, 1979, 'Erfahrung über die Einrichtung einer therapeutischen Gemeinschaft für Psychotherapie im Bereich eines großstädtischen Klinikums', in Heinz A. F. Schulze and W. Poppe (eds), *Konzeptionen und Modelle der langfristigen Betreuung in der Nervenheilkunde: Ergebnisse des Kongresses der Gesellschaft für Psychiatrie und Neurologie der DDR vom 20.-22. Oktober 1977 mit 62 Beiträgen* (Leipzig: S. Hirzel Verlag), pp. 143–4.

Elberfeld, Jens, 2019, 'Das Ich und das Wir: Gruppentherapie zwischen Sozialisierung der Psyche, Gemeinschaftserfahrung und Regierungstechnik', *Mittelweg 36*, 6:1, 137–59.

Falk, Beatrice and Friedrich Hauer, 2007, *Brandenburg-Görden: Geschichte eines psychiatrischen Krankenhauses* (Berlin: be.bra wissenschaft).

Geyer, Michael, 2011a, 'Ostdeutsche Psychotherapiechronik 1970–1979', in Michael Geyer (ed.), *Psychotherapie in Ostdeutschland: Geschichte und Geschichten 1945–1995* (Göttingen: Vandenhoeck & Ruprecht), pp. 245–56.

Geyer, Michael (ed.), 2011b, *Psychotherapie in Ostdeutschland: Geschichte und Geschichten 1945–1995* (Göttingen: Vandenhoeck & Ruprecht).

Hanrath, Sabine, 2002, *Zwischen 'Euthanasie' und Psychiatriereform: Anstaltspsychiatrie in Westfalen und Brandenburg: Ein deutsch-deutscher Vergleich (1945–1964)* (Paderborn: Schöningh).

Hennings, Lena, 2015, 'Die Entstehungsgeschichte der Rodewischer Thesen im Kontext von Psychiatrie, Sozialhygiene und Rehabilitationsmedizin der DDR'. Dissertation, Universität zu Lübeck.

Hess, Helga, 2011a, 'Die Gründung der Sektion Dynamische Gruppenpsychotherapie und die Ausbildung in Gruppenselbsterfahrung', in Michael Geyer (ed.), *Psychotherapie in Ostdeutschland: Geschichte und Geschichten 1945–1995* (Göttingen: Vandenhoeck & Ruprecht), pp. 276–86.

Hess, Helga, 2011b, 'Die Herausbildung eines Institutes für Psychotherapie und Neurosenforschung (IfPN) mit Integration der Ambulanz, Klinik und Forschung', in Michael Geyer (ed.), *Psychotherapie in Ostdeutschland: Geschichte und Geschichten 1945–1995* (Göttingen: Vandenhoeck & Ruprecht), pp. 372–3.

IV

Crossing institutional boundaries

11

Neuroleptics outside psychiatry: sedating deviant youth in the 1960s and 1970s in Belgium's juvenile institutions

Benoît Majerus and David Niget

Histories of neuroleptics

The introduction of neuroleptics into psychiatry in the 1950s has been and continues to be described as a revolution on several levels. Firstly, the new drugs are said to have made psychiatric hospitals more manageable, with patients becoming less agitated and less noisy. Second, they are said to have definitively brought psychiatry into the therapeutic age, bridging the gap with other medical disciplines. With the gradual adoption of double-blind protocols to test them, neuroleptics seemed to endow psychiatry with a universally recognised degree of scientificity, and because their development was based on an understanding of molecular action in the brain, they hinted at new hypotheses regarding the causes of, and eventual cure for, mental illness. Finally, neuroleptics were described as having paved the way for psychotherapy within psychiatric hospitals and were even said to have contributed to the deinstitutionalisation that took place in various Western countries beginning in the 1960s.[1]

This narrative, which was endorsed by psychiatrists, nurses and patients (as well as by pharmaceutical companies), has long been called into question, and in recent years has undergone several revisions that paint a more nuanced picture. The introduction of neuroleptics is, first of all, part of a longer history of drugs in psychiatry and of psychiatric biology, which had given rise to therapeutic hopes as early as the inter-war period (e.g. shock therapy, brain surgery, etc.) (Missa, 2006; Snelders *et al.*, 2006). A revisionist historiography has also shown that the definition of chlorpromazine as an antipsychotic drug took several years and that in psychiatric hospitals its introduction did not prevent the use of other drugs and therapeutic interventions. In addition to their therapeutic function, it became clear that neuroleptics, like other biological therapies, also had strong disciplinary potential. By paying more attention to discordant contemporary voices and by taking a more refined approach to the different actors in the story, a complex and multi-layered history has emerged (Majerus, 2019). Finally, the reality of psychiatric deinstitutionalisation and the factors that made it possible have given rise to a particularly lively historiography (Kritsotaki *et al.*, 2016; Guillemainet *al.*, 2018). The fact that the story of deinstitutionalisation has been told for many countries – even if, at present, only for countries in the West – has helped to further refine the narrative.

The historiography of neuroleptics is therefore particularly rich, and their use is certainly one of the best-studied phenomena in the history of twentieth-century psychiatry. However, as with other subjects, Greg Eghigian's call ten years ago to 'look for psychiatric work outside the asylum' has hardly been heeded with respect to the history of psychiatric medication (Eghigian, 2011: 209). The present work seeks to address this lack by examining the practices at one youth guidance institution in Belgium, emphasising three elements. Firstly, this chapter highlights the mobility of drugs – i.e. their ability to 'travel' across institutional barriers, unlike other therapies such as electroshock or insulin treatment, which are much less fluid. While the concept of 'drug trajectories' (Gaudillière, 2005) provides the starting point for this chapter, it of course raises questions about the mobility of practices. Historians often remain trapped by those who produce the sources they consult; by following an object – in this case a drug – they can leave the walls of psychiatry and discover new spaces (Ankele and Majerus, 2020). Secondly, we show how impoverishing it is to look at psychiatric institutions in isolation, since the various institutions of social deviance are linked through inmates, staff, objects and other elements – although their respective historiographies have often remained separate. Finally, we seek to deepen the debate around the therapeutic and/or disciplinary functions of these psychotropic drugs.[2]

Biological psychiatry: an opportunity for child and youth psychiatry?

In order to sketch the prescriptive framework of the local practices at this Belgian institution, we consulted three relevant academic journals: *Sauvegarde de l'enfance* (1950–80), created in 1945 by French regional child protection associations, *Revue de Droit Pénal et de Criminologie* (1954–68), the leading journal for penal sciences in Belgium, and *Revue de neuropsychiatrie infantile et d'hygiène mentale de l'enfance* (RNIHME), created in 1953 by French-speaking psychiatrists, including Georges Heuyer, an international leading figure in child psychiatry.

Biological psychiatry was almost completely absent from the first two publications,[3] but in the RNIHME the situation was completely different. First of all, the journal illustrates a recent trend in the historiography on psychotropic drugs, which underscores to what extent the history of the latter must be understood within the broader field of early twentieth-century psychiatric biology: the child psychiatrists publishing in the RNIHME welcomed the entire arsenal of biological treatments. Shock therapies were considered 'feasible with children and adolescents' and electroshock was considered the 'easiest shock method to use with children' (Leroy, 1957). It is therefore not very surprising that psychotropic drugs were also seen as a therapy to be embraced. The vast majority of the articles that appeared in the RNIHME were enthusiastic about this new pharmacopoeia, which was described as 'a real revolution in psychiatry' (Brauner and Pringuet, 1963: 574). Support for the 'new' drugs was nearly unanimous. Most of the studies published in this journal dealt specifically with 'mentally deficient children' but the authors regularly used a broader framework: the most detailed study published in the 1960s covered a fairly heterogeneous population drawn from 'either the children's ward of the psychiatric hospital; or from an IMP [*Institut Médico-Pédagogique*]; or from a boarding school for children in the public assistance system; or from a delinquent's home' (Faure and Faure, 1960: 255). This endorsement was only slightly tempered by a warning of younger populations' high sensitivity to the new drugs. Thus, the above-mentioned study on the neuroleptic Levomepromazine underlined in its conclusion 'the extreme sensitivity of children to Nozinan [Levomepromazine]; the absolute necessity of giving very low doses' (Faure and Faure, 1960: 279). From the late 1960s onwards, advertisements for drugs became more common in the RHIME. Most of these advertisements, such as the 1967 ad for the neuroleptic Haloperidol shown below, did not highlight their use with younger patients. Only the tranquilliser Diazepam, in 1968, promoted its specific use in paediatrics.

These elements – the importance of biological psychiatry and the positive reception of psychotropic drugs – must nevertheless be carefully put into context. The name of the source – the *Revue de neuropsychiatrie infantile* – also indicates its limitations: neuropsychiatry was not the major current within the field of deviant youth studies, which was dominated by criminology and rehabilitation-focused approaches, as we can see from the titles of the two other journals – *Sauvegarde de l'enfance* and *Revue de Droit Pénal et de Criminologie*.

Saint-Servais: a particular place

In order to carry out this study, we looked at a specific type of institution that was born in the first half of the twentieth century in Western countries: medical-pedagogical observation centres/child guidance institutions, which were attached to the juvenile justice system.

In order to understand how and why psychiatric expertise entered the field of juvenile justice in Belgium and why it persisted in the 1960s and 1970s, it is important to look back at the new penal rationality that founded it. It may be recalled that the turn of the twentieth century was marked by the emergence of a new penal doctrine called 'social defence', influenced by the heightened importance of criminology. This reflected a paradigm shift from a liberal conception of the law, which focused on evaluating criminal facts and sanctioning them in proportion to their gravity, to a preventive conception linked to identifying and treating criminals. In this context, where the priority was on reducing the risk of further criminal behaviour, children and adolescents became legitimate and favoured targets of 'predictive' and socially efficient penal interventions (Niget, 2012). This new legislation was considered progressive at the time, favoured by experts and promoted by politicians such as the socialist Emile Vandervelde, the Belgian Minister of Justice (Wagnon, 2017).

The 1912 Belgian Child Protection Act, which established juvenile courts, was part of the new penal rationality. This law replaced the notion of 'discernment' (the ability to tell right from wrong) with that of the educability of the individual offender. The juvenile justice system thus had to determine whether a young offender was educable. The question then arose of mental deficiency, the prevalence of which was pointed out by many pedagogical experts at the beginning of the century (including the Belgian educationalist and psychologist, Jean-Ovide Decroly), particularly among working-class families. Thus, the new law mandated a preliminary study of young delinquents' environments and personalities, with input from a 'social inquiry' on the one hand, and a medical and psychological examination on the other. This examination, mandated by the juvenile court judge, was to be carried out in a 'child guidance' institution. Quantitative measurements of intelligence (IQ tests), along with a great number of psycho-technical tests imposed on the children, were therefore used to identify 'mildly retarded' individuals and to establish the boundary of the norm, below which intervention was necessary. In the aftermath of World War I, two Belgian state observation institutions, one for boys (Mol) and one for girls (Saint-Servais), successfully occupied the new formal space for experts created by the 1912 Child Protection Act. These two institutions were responsible for carrying out 'observations', but they were also reform schools. Despite the symbolic role of science in assessing juvenile delinquents, the inter-war years were still marked by a highly moral conception of deviance (De Koster and Niget, 2015). Similarly, the modalities used to treat 'incorrigible' youth within the reform schools remained predominantly disciplinary, even if experts pointed to problems of physiological or psychiatric origin (Massin, 2014).

The post-war period was one of institutional change in the area of child protection in Belgium. More generally, all over the Western world, children were subject to 'therapeutisation' by the sciences of the psyche, a process that gave birth to the concept of 'maladjusted children' (Heuyer, 1948). From 1947 onwards, the Saint-Servais staff were made up of professionals: trained social workers, both religious and non-religious, who acted as educators (case workers), a professional psychologist, a psychologist's assistant and a psychiatrist.

At the time, psychology enjoyed great legitimacy, and the discipline gained great influence over juvenile justice practices and procedures. In addition to psychometric tests, many so-called 'projective' tests (e.g. the Rorschach) were used to assess the emotional states of young people. Nevertheless, one can observe the persistence of a medical approach towards juvenile inmates, which increased with the appearance of antipsychotic, antidepressant and anxiolytic drugs in the 1950s. In 1958, a group of psychiatrists working with the juvenile justice administration decided there was a need to create 'relaxation sections' for 'difficult pupils'[4] at the institutions, where drug treatment would be the principal treatment.[5] Thus, in 1959, a Special Section was opened at Saint-Servais, where depressed and violent inmates were sent, away from the groups in the pavilion system. The juvenile reform system's swift adoption of the scientific discovery of psychiatric drugs marked the return to a disciplinary order and a very deterministic interpretation of behavioural disorders in terms of pathological corporeality, while post-war psychology had promoted a more comprehensive approach to deviance.

The Special Section on which our observations are based was in operation from September 1959 to June 1976.[6] It was a small section, with just five beds originally (later eight). A case worker explained in 1966: 'It would be reserved for more difficult cases, i.e. especially for nervous cases requiring a special diet. This experience would be halfway between the pavilions, which were suitable for most of the pupils and already well specialised, and the psychiatric clinics, where the most serious cases would continue to be sent' (Caprasse, 1966: 1). It should be noted that the use of antipsychotic and neuroleptic drugs was not restricted to the Special Section; they were used in the other pavilions, but in limited quantities. Any patient receiving heavy medication that required more supervision was referred to the Special Section.

While the average number of placements per year for the entire observation institution was 200 during the 1960s, there were generally between 60 and 80 stays in the Special Section per year. Given that a number of girls stayed there several times, it can be estimated that 25 per cent of inmates were placed in the Special Section each year. In the 1970s, general admissions to the institution dropped to an average of 160 per year, and the number of young women in the

Special Section decreased to about 30 stays per year (less than 20 per cent of pupils).[7]

This Special Section saw a number of young women coming from and returning to the pavilions after their stay in the section, but there were also cases of girls entering the institution directly in a condition considered problematic, requiring isolation, medication and 'thorough observation'.

The disciplinary dimension of the section was not hidden; as one case worker stated: 'one of the main aims of the section will be to relieve the pavilion of troublesome elements' (Caprasse, 1966: 2). Moreover, the staff testified to the difficulty of getting disciplinary cases to peacefully coexist in the section with truly pathological cases.

A heterogeneous pharmacopoeia

Within the specific environment of the Special Section at Saint-Servais, we must first note the high rate of young women receiving psychoactive medication:[8] 57 per cent were subject to it. There is a notable discrepancy between the commonality of this practice and its relative invisibility in the sources. Psychoactive drugs hardly appear in the inmates' individual files (see below), nor were they thematised in the annual reports, in which the psychiatrist on duty wrote a two-to-three-page subchapter every year without ever mentioning medication. Our quantitative results come from monthly synthetic tables summarising the situation in the Special Section.

Although only 65–100 women passed through the Special Section per year, making for a fairly small data set, it seems that the use of medication can be divided into three time periods. During the first four years (1959–62), the distribution rate of drugs was very high: on average, more than 75 per cent of the young women received them. In the second phase (1963–70), which lasted the next eight years, the rate fell below 45 per cent, before becoming very irregular during the last years for which we have data.

This significant use of psychoactive drugs was characterised by a large and varied pharmacopoeia. Over the fifteen years in question, we count roughly eighty different psychoactive drugs. Some were prescribed on a regular basis; twelve were prescribed more than twenty times in the timespan. This great variety seems to indicate, on the one hand, a lack of standardisation, and on the other hand, a certain openness to experimentation. This intertwining of knowledge, practices and resources can be analysed as a form of 'bricolage' in the sense of Michel de Certeau (Certeau, 1980). Some drugs, moreover, were used in the same year as they were put on the psychiatric market, such as Haloperidol (in 1959) and Haloanisone (in 1961), two antipsychotics manufactured by the Belgian industrialist Janssen, as well as Swiss drugs such as the antidepressant Tofranil (in 1959) – indicating great porosity between the psychiatric and youth protection sectors. This porosity was perhaps also linked to the fact that the psychiatrist in charge of Saint-Servais was Fernand Arnould, a close collaborator of Joseph Paquay, one of the main Belgian psychopharmacologists.[9]

Four main groups of drugs were used: barbiturates, antipsychotics, antidepressants and minor tranquillisers.[10] Barbiturates were by far the most commonly prescribed drugs: 62 per cent of young women on medication at Saint-Servais took them, almost always Luminal (which accounted for 95 per cent of the barbiturates administered). This 'old' drug was first marketed in the early 1910s by Bayer, initially as an anticonvulsant for epileptics. It was widely used in (Belgian) psychiatry beginning in the inter-war period, both in and outside of hospitals, but was also commonly prescribed by general practitioners as a sleeping pill (Vijselaar, 2010; Majerus, 2016; Massin, 2017). Luminal, probably the most widely used drug in psychiatry in the late 1940s, is one of the barbiturates that 'survived' the introduction of neuroleptics and continued to be used in psychiatry in the 1960s.[11] In the monthly listings, the word 'Luminal' is very often accompanied by the words 'in the evening' indicating its use as a sleeping pill, which was also its main use during those years in psychiatry, as a nursing sister recounts in her autobiography: 'It was regularly given to patients in the evening. It calmed the patients and gave them a regular sleep schedule.'[12] While barbiturates did survive the introduction of neuroleptics, they were less resistant to the rise of minor tranquillisers. Whereas through the end of the 1960s, 75 per cent of the girls on medication at the institution were on barbiturates, after that the rate rapidly declined to below 10 per cent. At the same time the percentage of girls on tranquillisers rose.

The second major group of drugs were antipsychotics (33 per cent of young women in the institution, 58 per cent of those on medication). These came on the market in the early 1950s. Chlorpromazine, the first neuroleptic, was initially used in surgery, obstetrics and psychiatry. In the second half of the 1950s, it was increasingly defined and sold as an antipsychotic. Antipsychotics were characterised by fairly significant side effects, not only for the patients but also for those who distributed them (skin reactions). As with antidepressants, but in contrast to barbiturates, a great variety of antipsychotic drugs were used in Saint-Servais: Haloperidol (56 per cent), Truxal (10 per cent), Prazine and Largactil (each 11 per cent) were among the four most widely distributed antipsychotics, the latter being very present in the early years and then gradually disappearing. The sources do not give any explicit clues as to the reasons for this change; one hypothesis could be the particularly significant side effects of antipsychotics, which would then have been replaced by minor tranquillisers once those came on the market. These side effects, particularly trembling, explain why anti-Parkinson's drugs such as Cogentin and Disipal are also found among the list of administered drugs. Antipsychotics were prescribed two or three times a day, with the first administration normally taking place in the morning. In general, drugs seem to have been administered on a regular basis, rarely as a one-shot intervention. The posology varied greatly. A closer examination of Haloperidol administration shows that a patient received on average twelve drops (the range was between five and thirty drops) and that this did not fundamentally change over the years.[13]

The third most commonly used group of drugs were antidepressants (24 per cent of young women at the institution, 43 per cent of those on medication). Antidepressants had been on the market since 1955 and were a very gendered drug – they seem to have been absent from the equivalent institution for young men.[14] The antidepressants prescribed were quite varied: Tofranil (35 per cent), as well as Catovit (15 per cent) and Pertranquil (13 per cent), without any major changes over the years. Antidepressants were mainly administered in the morning and at midday, almost never in the evening.

The fourth and last major group were minor tranquillisers/anxiolytics (15 per cent of young women, 27 per cent of women on medication). First appearing in 1955, this was undoubtedly the most commercially successful group of psychiatric drugs outside of psychiatric and other institutions (Tone, 2009). As with barbiturates, one drug dominated: Quaname represents 57 per cent of the anxiolytics prescribed at Saint-Servais. Valium, which was sold on the Belgium market from 1963 on, was the second-most used.

The last element to be highlighted is the combined administration of these psychoactive drugs. In fact, few women (12 per cent) were given only one drug. Half of them took two per day and the remaining 40 per cent took three or even up to seven different drugs per day. All combinations were represented, with the most common being barbiturates and antipsychotics (28 per cent of all young women on medication) and barbiturates and antidepressants (23 per cent), but 12 per cent received antipsychotics and antidepressants. Further research on similar institutions, as well as prisons and homes for the elderly, will be necessary to better contextualise these results.

Uses of psychoactive drugs

The Special Section was run by a multidisciplinary team of specialists divided along typical gender lines, with psychiatry being considered a formalised and therefore male science, while psychology was seen as a more subjective and hence female discipline.[15] Medical treatment was determined by the doctor-psychiatrist, Dr Fernand Arnould, and stays were also supervised by the psychologist, Mrs G. Goosens. The therapeutic methods used were mostly individual, in contrast to care in the pavilions, which was based on a group dynamic. These were mainly 'occupational therapy' (i.e. manual activities and housework), play, and psychotherapy with the psychiatrist, including interviews and drug treatments. These methods were similar to those used in psychiatric clinics, without going as far as 'heavy' treatments, as the psychiatrist explained in 1966: 'no sleep cure here, no electroshock, no insulin cure'. The length of stays varied greatly, from a few days to several weeks, with frequent return visits for some patients, sometimes spread over several years.

It should be noted that the girls in the population studied were under judicial investigation. They were detained in the establishment by court order, so as to best inform the decision of the juvenile judge who would monitor their observation. They most often came from working-class families,[16] in which, according to the experts, they had frequently suffered violence or at least educational neglect. Those in the Special Section were older than the average girl at the institution. The majority were between 16 and 20 years of age, and about 20 per cent were between 14 and 16 years of age, covering the period of adolescence. With regard to their social situation, they were often failing at school or, in the case of working girls, were professionally unstable. Among the 'factors' contributing to their deviance, investigations (police investigations as well as social investigations) very frequently pointed to problems linked to sexuality that was deemed inappropriate: 'early' sexuality, early pregnancy, prostitution or the like, having many partners, homosexuality, having significantly older sexual partners, having leisure activities linked to sexuality or running away for reasons thought to have to do with sexuality, and finally, incest – which only began to be named as a reason for deviance in the 1970s (Niget, 2011). This preponderance of sexuality in the aetiology of girls' deviance contributed to a representation of sexuality as pathological, with girls being judged incapable of controlling their 'sexual impulses'. This had pathological and psychological consequences, which the psychiatrist referred to in his 1967 report as a 'kind of nymphomania' and which seemed to him to be generalised among the girls. Several other pathologies were gradually named in the 1960s and 1970s. These included 'depression', along with what experts considered to be its marker, suicide attempts, which were thus scrupulously noted in patients' files. In 1966, the director of Saint-Servais noted an increase in suicide attempts beginning in 1964 (Caprasse, 1966: 71). In addition, drug use – hashish and LSD – was identified as a problem by the psychiatrist in his 1969 report and was quantified in the 1972 report, which stated that 62.5 per cent of inmates used drugs. The phenomenon was associated with 'hippie' culture, but in this case was considered not a form of political protest, but rather a manifestation of the anomic situation in which young people found themselves.[17] It is interesting to note that in spite of disapproval of the misuse of psychotropic substances among youth, the institution prescribed them large quantities of antipsychotic medications.

According to an assessment by the staff of Saint-Servais, about one-third of the pupils coming from all pavilions who entered the school had significant psychological or psychiatric problems, a phenomenon that would increase over the period under study.[18] However, the young people sent to the Special Section were not, from a psycho-pedagogical point of view, the most troubled: the reports and files show that they obtained better results on IQ tests than the average pupil at the institution.[19] This was in contrast to the image held by pupils in the other pavilions, who referred to the Special Section as 'the silly pavilion' (Caprasse, 1966: 68). However, the institution considered itself not a psychiatric institution but an educational one, which probably explains the relative rarity of strictly psychiatric comments in the archival material, whether in the aetiology of the causes behind a young person's placement in the institution, case analyses in individual files or the proposals for measures made to the judge.

In the monthly registers of the Special Section, which include individual case descriptions, there are few direct references to psychiatric diagnoses. If we focus on the two groups of drugs whose indications are clearly related to psychiatric diagnoses – antidepressants and antipsychotics – most used words to describe their behaviours give early suggestions of the behaviours that might lead to their administration.

While remaining cautious, it can be hypothesised that the two main families of drug treatments included here (antidepressants and antipsychotics) correspond more or less to the two main categories of causes for placement in the Special Section: namely, a depressive state on the one hand, and violent/undisciplined behaviour on the other.

When focusing on the most used words in the description for young women who were prescribed antidepressants,[20] it was, unsurprisingly, the term 'depressed' that was most frequently employed in relation to girls who were administered antidepressants, pointing to an institutional thematisation of depression as an emerging pathological form in the 1950s and 1960s. This can be associated with the reference to 'suicide attempts', which occurred relatively frequently. In 1966, a case worker noted that the proportion of depressed inmates had increased between 1963 and 1966, which for her corresponded to a morbid evolution in the mental health of young people. This phenomenon can be interpreted both as greater consideration of the issue of depression in educational and therapeutic practices, and as an effect of this new class of drugs, which required

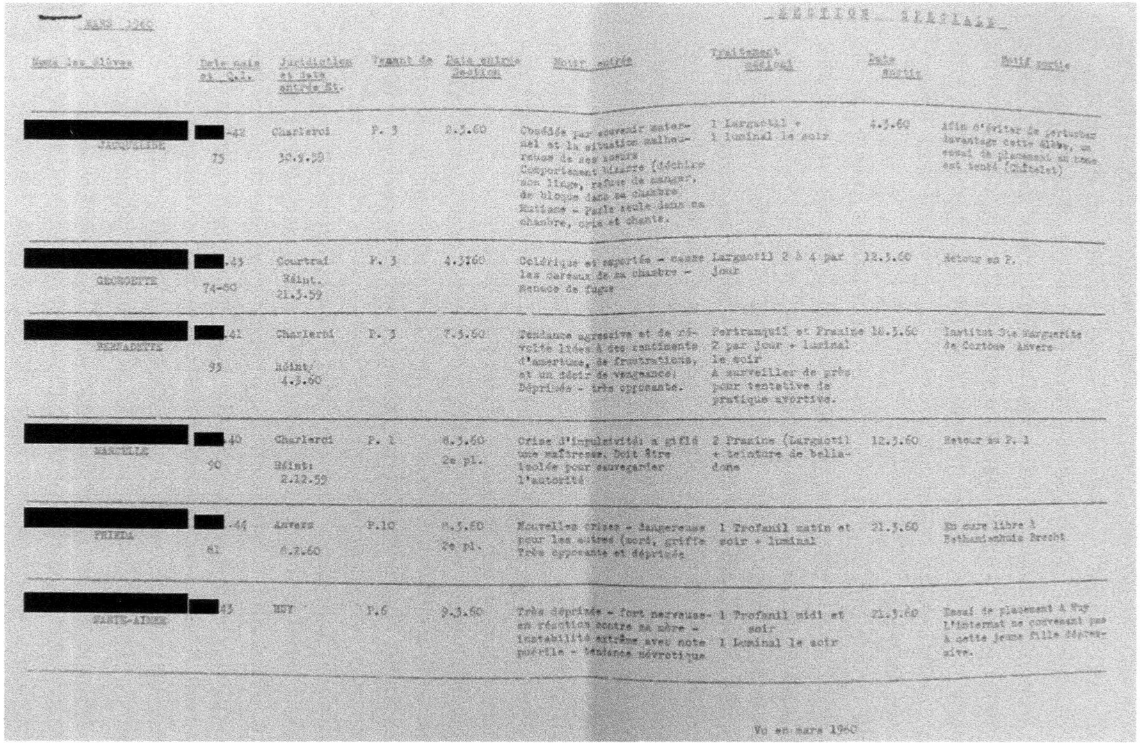

Figure 11.1 A sample of the monthly registers of the Special Section. AEB, Namur, EOESS, Call numbers 98–114 (1959–75).

a diagnosis of depression in order to be administered. Nevertheless, suicide was treated in a relatively varied manner: it was seen as a real risk for girls (who were therefore heavily medicated), but was also sometimes minimalised, with 'small attempts' reported more as a form of indiscipline than as a sign of suffering, and the terms 'pithiatism' or 'hysterical' used to describe situations where girls entered into suicidal crises judged to be 'exaggerated' and 'absurd' (i.e. not tangible).

The term 'group' is also very present in our corpus, pointing to the idea that the girls who were placed in Special Section were incapable of living among the pavilion groups (i.e., in the other sections of the institution): it was thought that 'group life' was harmful to them, given the vulnerability of their psyches. Another important aspect is that the staff were wary of the 'contagious' nature of depression within a group. For example, Anne-Laure,[21] who cried for hours, describing her suicidal thoughts, was said to need to be placed in the Special Section because she had caused a disturbance: 'several pupils start crying, show themselves depressed … [For some girls], the doses of drugs need to be increased, and some who were not taking them now ask for them' (Caprasse, 1966: 21).

Similarly, the term 'runaway' was also common among girls deemed 'depressed'. It indicated a desire for freedom expressed by the girls: for example, Henriette 'Did not return on her first weekend – upon return was very depressed and stubborn – does not accept any educational influence – remains and isolates herself in her only problem "need for freedom".'[22] Saint-Servais staff considered running away above all as a behavioural problem, a symptom of malaise. As a result, running away from the institution often justified drug treatment. There were frequent reports of 'mock runaways' – pupils pretending to run away to attract attention. Moreover, from 1968–69 onwards, running away was associated with the hippie movement and drug use, a factor that was seen to amplify the state of depression: Germaine was 'Returning from escape – very badly off physically – depressed – had new experiences (hippie groups, drugs, etc.).'[23]

Finally, despite the fact that depression was emphasised, the terms 'difficult', 'aggressive', 'refuses' and 'troublesome' indeed refer to behaviour deemed violent at the institution, from which we can conclude the relative porosity between the two main categories found in the institution's reports: the 'undisciplined' and the 'depressed'.

Administration of antipsychotics was linked to a state of opposition to or even violence against institutional discipline, as is shown by the terms 'difficult', 'aggressive', 'disruptive' and 'impulsive' among the reasons for sending girls to the Special Section and giving them antipsychotic drugs. The generic term used in the annual reports was 'caractérielles' (temperamental). This aggressiveness could be directed against 'the group', i.e. fellow inmates, but also against 'authority', i.e. the staff. It frequently took a rather violent turn, with many episodes of 'anger', the breaking of windowpanes, objects and furniture, and physical violence between girls or towards the staff (knife threats, beatings). The consequences of episodes included frequent running away and threats of suicide, as for Jeanne: 'Spectacular scenes, screams – attempts to run away – protests – hair pulling, etc… Threatened to throw herself out of the window – stood for a long time on the windowsill with a knife in her hand.'[24] In the clinical descriptions of these cases, the disciplinary issue seemed to take precedence; thus Janine was 'Sowing evil spirits in the group – undermining authority. Strong impulsivity with violent reactions – dangerous to self and others.'[25] Indeed, a number of girls interviewed about their time in the Special Section considered their stay 'punishment' rather than therapeutic treatment (Caprasse, 1966: 27).

The terms 'bizarre', 'nervous', and 'stubborn' refer to the perception of more marked pathological states, generally referred to as 'psychopathological cases', which the monthly situation reports attest to: Jacqueline was 'obsessed by maternal memory and the unfortunate situation of her sisters. Strange behaviour (tears her laundry, refuses to eat, locks herself in her room) mutism – talks alone in her room, shouts and sings';[26] Maryvonne had 'Hysterical tendencies – strange, even dangerous external behaviour – requires more individual observation.'[27] The proportion of inmates with a severe mental disorder increased during the period studied. Caregivers saw this as a deterioration in the mental health of the young people sent to the institution, but we can also interpret it as a progressive inclination to problematise juvenile deviance in more psychiatric terms, a turn that may have been encouraged by the very existence of the Special Section. In the 1960s, the director even considered creating a new section for these 'psychopathological' cases, but this did not happen. It should be pointed out that some girls deliberately engaged in erratic behaviour to protest against an institutional regime that they considered harsh and, in a way, grotesque. Acting foolishly may thus have been a form of resistance for the girls, ironically displaying public behaviour at odds with their private views. In the last years of the Special Section's operation, the annual reports mentioned the difficulty of caring for this population of 'neurotic' young people.[28]

From treatment to placement: the institutional trajectories of medicated youth

What were the institutional trajectories of girls placed on antipsychotic medication? Did they differ from those of the general population of girls in Saint-Servais? Was the therapeutic approach consistent with subsequent placement decisions? Analysis of the reasons why girls who were given medication left the Special Section yields several interesting insights. Firstly, the overwhelming majority were returned to the institution after their stay in the Special Section (43 per cent), either to the same pavilion or to another pavilion where the group and educational methods differed significantly (more or less autonomy given to the young people). Thus, many girls went back and forth between the Special Section, where they received heavy medication, and the living quarters, where the administration of medication was lighter.

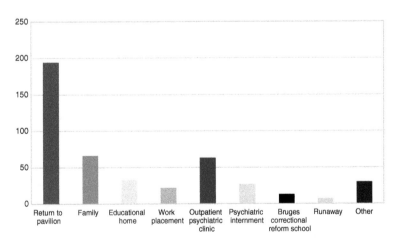

Figure 11.2 Reason for release from the Special Section, St Servais (1959–75).

Returning to the family home (15 per cent) was considered by staff and judges to be the preferred outcome for the girls, especially those who seemed vulnerable, depressed, and to whom the family could offer support – provided the family was not the cause of anxiety in the eyes of the Saint-Servais staff. Medical or psychological follow-up could then be recommended at home, in cooperation with the parents.

Placement in educational homes – small institutions with more flexible routines – was also an option (7 per cent), especially for girls who demonstrated a 'weariness' of institutional 'discipline' (a euphemism used to indicate that they were exhausted or hopeless), but who were not deemed dangerous or antisocial.

Work could also have been seen as a form of rehabilitation: 5 per cent of the girls were placed with employers in the nearby city of Namur, in 'semi-liberty', often working as domestic servants in upper-class houses or in shops or workshops in the city and returning to the institution in the evening.

The most significant form of outplacement for our study was in psychiatric institutions, which accounted for 20 per cent of all placements after a stay in the Special Section. Fourteen per cent of these placements were designated as 'free cures' in a psychiatric clinic or medical-pedagogical institute. Young people would attend these institutions during the day (ambulatory) and return home in the evening. The best known and most frequently recommended was Dr Titeca's clinic in Brussels. It should be noted that 'free' did not mean 'freedom': if girls did not comply, the children's judge could request that they be returned to Saint-Servais, which happened relatively often according to our records.

Aside from free cures, 6 per cent of the inmates were placed in residential psychiatric institutions. This sometimes also entailed legal internment that was equivalent to detention (a measure called 'col-location' in Belgium), which was used for psychiatric cases deemed serious and lasting. These institutions included the state asylum in Mons and the clinic in Braine l'Alleud, south of the Brussels conurbation. The famous Geel psychiatric colony was also favoured. Several girls were sent to the Beau Vallon psychiatric clinic, located a few hundred metres from the Saint-Servais reform school.

Finally, we note the persistence of a strictly disciplinary treatment for a few cases deemed problematic. Throughout the period under study, girls judged 'unmanageable' were regularly sent to the correctional institution of Bruges (3 per cent, or thirteen individual cases). This was a public institution specially dedicated to the treatment of unruly girls. The last resort there was the use of coercion and extreme surveillance, which led to institutional violence, as Veerle Massin has shown in her research (Massin, 2014). Being sent to this disciplinary institution could also be a prelude to psychiatric confinement, as this 1959 file shows: 'Strong oppositional tendencies: refusal to stand up, to work – which manifests itself in very violent aggression – is dangerous – was observed in 1954. Transferred to State Reform School of Bruges and from there collocated at the asylum in Mons.'[29]

Lastly, running away offered an alternative to institutional constraints for a certain number of young inmates (2 per cent) who refused placements that they considered arbitrary. Running away was considered an indication of a pathological condition by the experts at Saint-Servais, who used this to justify heavy medication upon the runaway's return to the institution. Overall, analysis of the institutional trajectories of the medicated young women shows that although they were more likely to be sent to psychiatric care institutions than anywhere else, the majority were not. This indicates that the main purpose of medication was to serve as a transitional therapy and possibly also to improve discipline.

Subjectivities: perception of antipsychotic treatments

In addition to the quantitative approach detailed above, we also took a closer look at individual young women's files. We studied the files of thirty-seven young women who received psychoactive medication: in just over half the files (twenty), medication was not mentioned at all, while in the other files it was most often only briefly referenced. These files nevertheless allow some additional glimpses of practices. The young women interned at Saint-Servais had the option of refusing medication. Margot, aged 17, was given heavy antipsychotics – Haloperidol in the morning and at noon – and antidepressants in the evening. At one point, she clashed with the educational team over a question of borrowing books and refused to eat or to take her medication. She was obliged to sign a form clearing the institution – 'I certify that I refused the following meals on Wednesday 23 March: snack, supper and medication' – but according to this document, her refusal had no other consequences.[30] Secondly, the same file indicates that the doctor gave some latitude in his prescriptions, and the drugs were clearly framed in terms of a behaviour control paradigm. On the one hand, the psychiatrist indicated that the ten drops of Haloperidol at lunchtime could be replaced by the weaker Truxal tablet once Margot started to work, probably to avoid the excessive drowsiness caused by Haloperidol. At the same time, he also wrote that 'in case of minor worsening, we could double the morning and evening dosages, adding about twenty drops of Prazine.'[31] The third element found in some of the files is that several young women had already taken psychotropic drugs before coming to Saint-Servais, either in other institutions or on an outpatient basis through a general practitioner's prescription – a sign of the ubiquity of psychoactive drugs in the 1960s.[32]

Conclusion

At the end of this exploratory study dealing with a new object in historiography, we would like to emphasise that the introduction of neuroleptics changed institutional practices in Saint-Servais significantly with the setting up of this Special Section, gradually transforming the problem of indiscipline, which was the primary reason for the introduction of drug treatments, into a question of pathology and care. The treatment of a significant proportion of inmates between 1959 and 1975 within the Special Section (20 to 25 per cent), as well as the massive use of neuroleptics and antidepressants within this section, is a significant fact in the history of the institution. It marks a moment in the history of youth welfare, when juvenile deviancy was seen as a behavioural problem, under the combined influence of the 'sciences of the psyche', psychology and psychiatry. This trend was transnational, as evidenced, among other sources, by work of the World Health Organization in the 1950s and 1960s (Bovet, 1951; Gibbens, 1961). Moreover, faced with increasing contestation of discipline within institutions, both by the young people themselves and by various staff members, the introduction of neuroleptics may have offered an alternative deemed less authoritarian, one based on the rationality of care rather than correction. It can also be argued that neuroleptics offered a way of updating or perpetuating coercive practices through science and therapy, which would soon be called into question by the social and political contestation of the sixty-eighters. It should also be considered that as physical punishment was increasingly prohibited in youth welfare institutions, therapeutic discipline offered an alternative that was regarded as more humane. This question remains to be discussed from our contemporary point of view as historians of youth welfare and psychiatry.

At the same time, the introduction of neuroleptics can be described as a 'non-event' since it was rarely mentioned in the archives other than as a formality. One possible hypothesis for this silence would be that psychiatry was not central to these youth welfare institutions. The dominant paradigm was that of education, not of care/cure. Although the introduction of neuroleptics did indeed change institutional practices, it did not change the regime of institutional discourse. The rationality of child guidance institutions was based mainly on an aetiology of deviances rooted in moral fault (due to the penal judicial origin of this rationality), and on the possibility of 're-education' through pedagogical techniques, reinforced after World War II by psychological techniques that centred on the person as a subject. From this perspective, psychiatry appeared to be peripheral, and even underscored a certain failure of the institution to rehabilitate young people, which explains why the treatment method for 'neurotic' inmates remained segregation, either in a special section or in correctional institutions (such as the one in Bruges) or in purely therapeutic institutions (psychiatric clinics).

Whatever the meaning of this silence, the cohabitation of two correctional regimes – the first based on deviance and its retribution, the second on behaviourism and a therapeutic approach – opened up a space after World War II for experimenting with multiple practices at the intersection of care and punishment.

The question of how young people perceived these psychiatric practices, particularly the use of medication, remains to be more precisely documented. It is possible that the use of medication profoundly changed the institutional experience of young people, but this remains to be verified through a meticulous search for youth voices in the individual case files.

Notes

1 See the many books by Edward Shorter, including Shorter, 1997. For a critical discussion of these apparent breaks with the past see Henckes, 2016.
2 The quantitative data used in this text are based on exhaustive encoding of the monthly entry and exit registers of the Special Section of Saint-Servais, from its opening in 1959 to its closure in 1975, which include 820 entries (some inmates appear several times). The encoded data are as follows: surname, first name, date of entry, reason for entry, medical treatment (name of medication, dosage and frequency of administration), date of exit, measures taken on exit (type and location of placement). A reproduction of the register is available in this article (see below). The qualitative data are based on examination of a sample of thirty-seven individual files randomly selected from among the files of girls who were treated with neuroleptics. Archives de l'Etat en Belgique (hereafter AEB), Namur, Etablissement d'Observation de l'Etat de Saint-Servais (hereafter EOESS), Record number BE-A0525.444, Call number 98–114, Monthly registers of the Special Section (1959–75).
3 One of the only articles in these two journals that explicitly discussed the use of psychotropic drugs seemed to prefer shock therapy as it considered these new drugs dangerous (Aubin and Aubin, 1962).
4 The population at Saint-Servais was comprised of young women aged 12 to 20 who were legally mandated to be there and could not lawfully leave at will, yet the institution considered itself not a prison or psychiatric institution but rather a reform school. Therefore, in keeping with the source material, we refer to the young women who lived there as 'inmates', 'pupils', 'young women' and 'girls'. It may be noted that the term 'patient' is never used.
5 AEB, Beveren, RK/ROG Brugge, n°72, Minutes of a meeting of psychiatrists organised by the administration, 21 November 1958. Quoted by Veerle Massin (Massin, 2014).
6 The monthly reports and the annual report for 1976 attest to this, but no qualitative comments are made in the available documents regarding the reasons for this closure. However, it should be noted that, from 1973 onwards, the Special Section was no longer the subject of specific analysis in the annual reports (statistical tables). It should also be noted that in 1972, a 'pavilion 9' was opened, reserved for the 'most difficult cases', which may explain why the Special Section then lost part of its disciplinary function. AEB, Namur, EOESS, Call numbers 29–53, Annual reports (1931–89).

7 The model for juvenile deviance treatment then shifts from custodial institutions to the outplacement system.

8 AEB, Namur, EOESS, Call numbers 98–114, Monthly registers of the Special Section (1959–75).

9 Missa, 2010. Within this framework, Arnould co-published about ten scientific articles on antipsychotics between 1959 and 1965, for example, Paquay *et al.*, 1959.

10 We have adopted a categorisation used by Tone (2009) and others which mixes substance-oriented and effect-oriented categories, illustrating the blurred boundaries that characterise psychiatric drugs.

11 It continues to be used today as an anticonvulsant.

12 'On le donnait régulièrement aux malades le soir. Il calmait les malades et donnait un sommeil régulier' (De Cock, 1986: 58).

13 According to Benkert and Hippius (1976: 164–6), ten drops correspond to one milligram. The same book suggests three times 0.5 mg per day for Haloperidol as a standard dose.

14 At the Etablissement central d'observation pour garçons in Mol, the parallel institute for young men, the invoices for medication contain the names of antipsychotics but not antidepressants: AEB, Beveren, Etablissement central d'observation pour garçons à Mol, Call number 2381, Factuurboek 1958–59.

15 The ability of women to enter the field of child psychology in the twentieth century, in the name of maternalist arguments, nevertheless led to the undermining of this professional practice in the face of the medical and psychiatric disciplines, which were held by men and therefore considered more scientific (Hoogland Noon, 2004: 107–29).

16 This broad category needs to be refined, but this is not the purpose of this chapter.

17 See in particular the 1972 annual report, which provides an in-depth analysis of the 'causes' of youth deviance. AEB, Namur, EOESS, Call numbers 29–53, Annual reports (1931–1989).

18 For example, the 1972 report mentions a 'large percentage of pupils with insufficient nerve balance (29.5%)'. *Ibid.*

19 *Ibid.*; Caprasse, 1966: 7.

20 We have fully transcribed the 'entry patterns' for all women admitted, as recorded in the monthly summaries, and entered them into Voyant Tools which is an open-source, web-based application for performing text analysis. On Voyant Tools: Alhudithi, 2021.

21 First names have been changed to preserve anonymity.

22 'Pas rentrée lors de son premier W.E.- à son retour est très déprimée et butée – n'accepte guère l'influence éducative – reste et s'isole dans son unique problème "besoin de liberté".' AEB, Namur, EOESS, Call

numbers 98–114, Monthly registers of the Special Section, HJ, Entry 1970-08-01.

23 AEB, Namur, EOESS, Call numbers 98–114, Monthly registers of the Special Section, GD, Entry 1969-11-14.

24 AEB, Namur, EOESS, Call numbers 98–114, Monthly registers of the Special Section, JS, Entry 1960-01-04.

25 AEB, Namur, EOESS, Call numbers 98–114, Monthly registers of the Special Section, JL, Entry 1959-09-01.

26 AEB, Namur, EOESS, Call numbers 98–114, Monthly registers of the Special Section, JB, Entry 1960-03-02.

27 AEB, Namur, EOESS, Call numbers 98–114, Monthly registers of the Special Section, MS, Entry 1970-05-21.

28 AEB, Namur, EOESS, Call numbers 29–53, Annual reports (1931–89).

29 AEB, Namur, EOESS, Call numbers 98–114, Monthly registers of the Special Section (1959–75).

30 AEB, Namur, EOESS, Call numbers 570/1 to 862 for the observation files for minors, Observation file, A1012.

31 AEB, Namur, EOESS, Call numbers 570/1 to 862 for the observation files for minors, Observation file, A1108, Medical form (undated, unsigned).

32 An article published in 1962 by a child psychiatrist who treated children on an outpatient basis states that half of the children had already received medication before being treated by him (Lécuyer, 1963: 408).

References

Alhudithi, Ella, 2021, 'Review of voyant tools: See through your text', *Language Learning & Technology*, 25:3, 43–50.

Ankele, Monika and Benoît Majerus (eds), 2020, *Material Cultures of Psychiatry* (Bielefeld: Transcript).

Aubin, Henri and Bernard Aubin, 1962, 'Formule nouvelle d'assistance: Clinique neuro-psychiatrique infantile: Bilan d'une expérience de cinq ans', *Sauvegarde de l'enfance*, 17:8, 495–503.

Benkert, Otto and Hanns Hippius, 1976, *Psychiatrische Pharmakotherapie: Ein Grundriß für Ärzte und Patienten* (Berlin: Springer).

Bovet, Lucien, 1951, *Psychiatric Aspects of Juvenile Delinquency: A Study Prepared on Behalf of the World Health Organization as a Contribution to the United Nations Programme for the Prevention of Crime and Treatment of Offenders* (Geneva: World Health Organization).

Brauner, F. and G. Pringuet, 1963, 'Les traitements médicaux des enfants déficients mentaux', *Revue de neuropsychiatrie infantile*, 11:9–10, 571–82.

Caprasse, Claire, 1966, *La Section Spéciale dans le cadre de l'Etablissement d'Observation et d'Education de l'Etat, de Saint-Servais* (Brussels: Ministère de la Justice, Office de la protection de la jeunesse, Centre de formation et de perfectionnement des cadres).

Certeau, Michel de, 1980, *Arts de faire* (Paris: Union d'éditions).

De Cock, Françoise, 1986, *Plus d'un demi-siècle au service des malades mentaux* (Namur: n.p.).

De Koster, Margo and David Niget, 2015, 'Scientific expertise in child protection policies and juvenile justice practices in twentieth-century Belgium', in Joris Vandendriessche, Evert Peeters and Kaat Wils, *Scientists' Expertise as Performance: Between State and Society, 1860–1960* (London: Pickering & Chatto), pp. 161–72.

Eghigian, Greg, 2011, 'Deinstitutionalizing the history of contemporary psychiatry', *History of Psychiatry*, 22:2, 201–14.

Faure, H. and M. L. Faure, 1960, 'Le Nozinan en neuro-psychiatrie infantile', *Revue de neuropsychiatrie infantile et d'hygiène mentale de l'enfance*, 8:5–6, 254–86.

Gaudillière, Jean-Paul, 2005, 'Introduction: Drug trajectories', *Studies in History and Philosophy of Biological and Biomedical Sciences*, 36:4, 603–11.

Gibbens, Trevor Charles Noël, 1961, *Trends in Juvenile Delinquency* (Geneva: World Health Organization).

Guillemain, Hervé, Alexandre Klein and Marie-Claude Thifault (eds), 2018, *Fin de l'asile?: Histoire de la déshospitalisation psychiatrique dans l'espace francophone au XXe siècle* (Rennes: Presses universitaires de Rennes).

Henckes, Nicolas, 2016, 'Magic bullet in the head? Psychiatric revolutions and their aftermath', in Jeremy Greene, Flurin Condrau and Elizabeth Siegel Watkins (eds), *Therapeutic Revolutions: Pharmaceuticals and Social Change in the Twentieth Century* (Chicago, IL: University of Chicago Press), pp. 65–96.

Heuyer, Georges, 1948, *Aspect médical de l'Enfance inadaptée* (Paris: Ecole des Parents et des Educateurs).

Hoogland Noon, David, 2004, 'Situating gender and professional identity in American child study, 1880–1910', *History of Psychology*, 7:2, 107–29.

Kritsotaki, Despo, Vicky Long and Matthew Smith (eds), 2016, *Deinstitutionalisation and After: Post-War Psychiatry in the Western World* (London: Pickering & Chatto).

Lécuyer, Robert, 1963, 'De l'utilisation de la thioridazine comme traitement symptomatique de l'instabilité psychomotrice chez l'enfant (81 cas traités en ambulatoire)', *Revue de neuropsychiatrie infantile*, 11:7–8, 407–13.

Leroy, Robert, 1957, 'Thérapeutiques de choc en neuro psychiatrie infantile', *Revue de neuropsychiatrie infantile et d'hygiène mentale de l'enfance*, 5:11–12, 547–51.

Majerus, Benoît, 2016, 'Making sense of the "chemical revolution": Patients' voices on the introduction of neuroleptics in the 1950s', *Medical History*, 60:1, 54–66.

Majerus, Benoît, 2019, 'A chemical revolution as seen from below: The "discovery" of neuroleptics in the Paris of the 1950s', *Social History of Medicine*, 32:2, 395–413.

Massin, Veerle, 2014, '"La Discipline". Jeunes délinquantes enfermées, violence institutionnelle et réaction disciplinaire: Une dynamique (Belgique, 1920–1970)', *Crime, Histoire & Sociétés / Crime, History & Societies*, 18:1, 31–56.

Massin, Veerle, 2017, 'La consultation d'hygiène mentale, le patient et le psychiatre (Belgique, 1920–1940)', *Journal of Belgian History*, 48:4, 144–64.

Missa, Jean-Noël, 2006, *Naissance de la psychiatrie biologique: Histoire des traitements des maladies mentales au XXe siècle* (Paris: Presses universitaires de France).

Missa, Jean-Noël, 2010, 'Peut-on parler de militantisme psychopharmacologique chez les pionniers de la psychiatrie biologique (1952–1960)?', *Sud/Nord*, 25:1, 105–20.

Niget, David, 2011, 'Le genre du risque: Expertise médico-pédagogique et délinquance juvénile en Belgique au XXe siècle', *Histoire@Politique*, 14:2, 38–54.

Niget, David, 2012, 'L'enfance irrégulière et le gouvernement du risque', in David Niget and Martin Petitclerc (eds), *Pour une histoire du risque: Québec, France, Belgique* (Québec: Presses de l'Université du Québec), pp. 297–316.

Paquay, Joseph, Fernand Arnould and P. Burton, 1959, 'Le traitement par le Tofranil de la phase dépressive de la psychose maniaco-dépressive', *Acta Neurologica et Psychiatrica Belgica*, 59:8, 958–65.

Shorter, Edward, 1997, *A History of Psychiatry: From the Era of the Asylum to the Age of Prozac* (New York: John Wiley & Sons).

Snelders, Stephen, Charles Kaplan and Toine Pieters, 2006, 'On cannabis, chloral hydrate, and career cycles of psychotrophic drugs in medicine', *Bulletin of the History of Medicine*, 80:1, 95–114.

Tone, Andrea, 2009, *The Age of Anxiety: A History of America's Turbulent Affair with Tranquilizers* (New York: Basic Books).

Vijselaar, Joost, 2010, *Het gesticht: Enkele reis of retour* (Amsterdam: Uitgeverij Boom).

Wagnon, Sylvain, 2017, 'Entre libéralisme et progressisme: l'influence d'Adolphe Prins (1845–1919) dans la théorisation de la défense sociale et la construction de la protection de l'enfance en Belgique', *Criminocorpus*. https://doi.org/10.4000/criminocorpus.3410 (accessed 7 August 2023).

12

Psychiatric practices beyond psychiatry: the sexological administration of transgender life around 1980

Ketil Slagstad

A central component of psychiatric expertise is the preparation of expert opinions in non-therapeutic settings. An obvious example is the evaluative role of forensic psychiatrists in assessing criminal responsibility in the courtroom (Skålevåg, 2016). Evaluative psychiatric expertise has developed hand in hand with modern bureaucracy and modern legal systems. However, the psychiatrist has also provided more diffuse, albeit expansive, evaluative expertise in clinical decisions about non-psychiatric treatment. At the interface between society and administrative bureaucracy, between medicine and public opinion, psychiatric expertise has sought to secure public trust and safeguarded bureaucratic intervention *beyond* the therapeutic qualifications of the psychiatrist. This expertise is an example of the social practice of psychiatry solving practical problems with expert knowledge as a precondition and enabler of change (Geisthövel and Hess, 2017).

The topic of this chapter is the co-constitutive relationship between the psychiatrist and the administrative bureaucracy in the role not of healer but of evaluator. In Scandinavian welfare states, such as Norway, the psychiatrist has cared not only for the individual patient, but also safeguarded the interests of the public and administrative bureaucracy. Extensive public health systems, free healthcare and strong public trust in state institutions have made the psychiatrist a key element of the state, which is understood as the institutional tools for communities and populations to negotiate with each other

(Skinner, 2012: 85–6). At least that is the argument of this chapter, in which I examine the psychiatric practice of assessing trans patients for hormonal and surgical treatment in Norway in the 1970s and 1980s as an example of this restrictive, evaluative psychiatric gatekeeping practice.[1] The role of psychiatric expertise in trans healthcare, i.e. the administrative function of psychiatrists in decisions about non-psychiatric hormonal and surgical treatment, is an example of the historical significance of psychiatry's non-formalised evaluative expertise – of psychiatric practices beyond psychiatry.

The historical importance of the psychiatrist in making decisions about hormonal and surgical treatment for medical transitioning is not unique to Norway. In various national contexts, the psychiatrist has been a crucial element in deciding who should have access to treatment, from the United States (Edgerton, 1974) to France (Sekuler, 2018: 99–115), Germany (Klöppel, 2010: 547–84; Meyer, 2018), Denmark (Holm, 2017), Finland (Parhi, 2018) and Iran (Najmabadi, 2014: 15–37). The evaluative role of psychiatrists has also been highlighted in the international Standards of Care guidelines, first published by the Harry Benjamin International Gender Dysphoria Association in 1979. These stated that the patient needed the approval of two psychiatrists or psychologists for sex reassignment surgery (The Harry Benjamin International Gender Dysphoria Association, 1979).

The history of psychiatric expertise in administering the lives of trans people is a history of the welfare state in miniature. The Scandinavian welfare state was built by the mobilisation of science, social science and medicine (Slagstad, 1998; Schiøtz, 2003; Sejersted, 2011; Bauer, 2014; Lie, 2014). While historians of the welfare state and public healthcare system have often taken a top-down approach, focusing on the role of grand ideas, ideology and central public institutions such as the Directorate of Health (Nordby, 1989; Berg, 2009), less attention has been paid to the significance of mundane medical and psychiatric practices. Using selected findings from my research on the history of transgender medicine in Norway in the twentieth century, this chapter takes a bottom-up approach to the welfare state and bureaucracy by centring psychiatric practices: their work in evaluation and in the distribution of welfare state benefits, their implementation in practice and their manifold logics, which include the consequences of administering trans life.

The chapter begins with an overview of the unformalised practices of trans medicine in Norway in the 1950s and 1960s. This provides historical background for the discussions in the 1970s about the institutionalisation and streamlining of medical practices. In a situation with little clinical experience and scientific literature to support treatment decisions, and in a context of professional disagreements and criticism, psychiatrists and psychologists sought to secure the legitimacy of diagnostic and therapeutic practices by anchoring them in a formalised public health structure. Following scholars in science and technology studies, this chapter argues that experts had to incorporate the epistemologies and infrastructures already in place – sexological expertise and the Oslo Health Council – to make diagnostic and therapeutic guidelines into a standard. But the administration of trans life also modified these networks and infrastructures. As a way of knowing and practicing psychiatry, sexology mobilised a network of patients, concepts, objects and spatial arrangements in which 'sex change' itself became an important vehicle. Sexology and the formalised structure of the Oslo Health Council secured the evaluative expertise of psychiatry in the space between bureaucracy and medicine.

Negotiating trans care: a troubled past and a hopeful future

After the Health Act was passed in 1860, the health councils formed the backbone of the Norwegian public health system.[2] Inspired by the reorganisation of British health laws, the act responded to major societal challenges, most importantly the cholera epidemics. The councils consisted of elected officials and were directed by a state-employed physician, the *stadsfysikus*, the chief city physician in the cities and the *distriktslege*, the medical district officer in the counties and communes. This body cared for the health of the population and ensured that doctors had a leading political role in the country's health system (Schiøtz, 2003: 41–50, 235–71). The *stadsfysikus* and the *distriktslege* cooperated closely with the centralised health administration.

After World War II, a new Directorate of Health was established within the Ministry of Social Affairs. The directorate was a hybrid creature, functioning both as a professional administrative body making independent decisions in public health issues and as a policy-making body for the minister. The director general of health was throned at the top of the directorate, and with direct access to the minister was the most powerful person in the Norwegian health bureaucracy. Both Karl Evang, director general of health until 1972, and his successor Torbjørn Mork, who held the position until 1992, were physicians and specialists in epidemiology and public health. Both were members of the Labour Party and had been politically appointed to the post. The Directorate of Health and the health councils, with the Oslo Health Council as a prime example, became vehicles for implementing the health politics of the expanding welfare state, but also for creating new forms of medical expertise.

Hormone replacement therapy and sex reassignment surgery have been offered to trans people in Norway since the 1950s, albeit in a very restricted manner. In the early 1950s, the massive media spectacle surrounding the American Christine Jorgensen and her hormonal and surgical treatment in Copenhagen led many people to request the same treatment in Norway. As doctors were unsure whether such treatment was legally permissible, the issue was quickly taken to the highest level of the health bureaucracy. The authorities decided that such treatment should not be formalised in a public health facility or structure. Clinical decisions were left to experts, and in the following decades, a handful of interested physicians made decisions regarding treatment (Sandal, 2020). In Oslo, the capital, many trans feminine patients were assessed by a psychiatrist at Ullevål Hospital. The psychiatrist started hormone therapy before referring the patients to a plastic surgeon at Rikshospitalet, the national hospital. An endocrinologist at Aker Hospital, another Oslo hospital, together with a team of medical specialists, assessed most trans masculine patients and made decisions about androgen treatment and chest surgery.[3] Until the establishment of a specialised service for trans care at the Oslo Health Council, the routine for medical transition was unregulated and conducted in a non-standardised manner.

Sex reassignment was a marginal, albeit controversial, field of medicine. Among the harshest critics was the psychiatrist Johan Bremer, the chief physician of the women's department at Gaustad Hospital, the country's first state mental asylum. Psychiatry was too immature, he argued, too little was known about the nature of mental illness to let surgeons conduct 'irreversible procedures' on patients. 'You don't give small children sharp objects to play with. A psychiatry that is on the stage of development that probably corresponds to the toddler stage should not play around with knives and scissors', he said (Bremer, 1982: 95). To justify his position, Bremer invoked psychiatry's recent past: the psychopharmacological 'era' had left psychosurgery on the ash heap of history,[4] and it was probably 'only a matter of time' before 'sex change surgery' would end there too. In one patient, for example, a multidrug cocktail consisting of 50 mg of nialamide once a day (a monoamine oxidase inhibitor), 0.40 mg of meprobamate three times a day (a tranquilliser) and 50 mg of chlorpromazine four times a day (a high-dose neuroleptic) had made the patient's desire to transition 'disappear' (Bremer, 1961). The best a psychiatrist could offer was psychotherapeutic support – or to institute a multidrug psychotropic regime.

Some psychiatrists disagreed. Several case reports about attempts to change the patient's gender identity, whether through aversion therapy or psychoanalysis, had shown that these interventions were not only useless but also harmful. Some psychiatrists argued that it was their professional duty as physicians to help patients as best as they could, even when this required the use of hormones or surgery to treat what they considered to be a psychiatric condition. In a 1957 article in the main Scandinavian psychiatric journal, psychiatrist Per Anchersen argued that 'it would be unjustifiable not to do everything possible to help him to a satisfactory psychosocial adjustment', writing about so-called 'male transvestites', ignoring the patients' identities and preferred pronouns (Anchersen, 1957). The task of the psychiatrist was 'To help the transvestites, not to cure genuine transvestism', he wrote, referring to the older term for transsexuality.[5] But only a very selected group of patients should undergo hormonal and surgical treatment: 'Surgical treatment seems to be advisable only for a proportion of those who approach doctors with a desire for "sex change".'[6] Anchersen distinguished between transvestism as a fetish associated with sexual desire and genuine transvestism as permanent desire for change of sex, which included a 'disgust' towards the genitals. In addition, he selected patients for surgery based on physical appearance, stature and personality according to an idea about who would pass well in society after treatment (Slagstad, 2022a).

Trans healthcare in a queer time

These opposing professional positions shaped the backdrop of the clinical assessment of patients in the 1970s. The psychiatric examination of trans patients in the Oslo Health Council, which became the main institution for trans medicine in Norway, developed from sexology.[7] Sexology was an emerging 'thought style' in some circles of Scandinavian psychiatry in the 1970s and 1980s (Fleck, 1980), but in social medicine there was a much longer tradition of viewing health and disease through the lens of sexuality. For the Director General of Health Karl Evang, sexuality was an integral part of health (Nordby, 1989; Berg, 2002). However, information and education were not enough; society had to be fundamentally reorganised to create the fundament for 'new forms of human sex lives more suited to human nature than the present ones' (Evang *et al.*, 1932). When the Kinsey Reports were published in the 1940s and 1950s, a ground-breaking study of sexual behaviour in the United States, Evang praised them for providing empirical evidence of the dissonance between people's lives and laws, conventions and conservative morality (*Æsculap*, 1948: 99).

Internationally, the 1970s were big for sexology, and it increasingly became a scientific, professionalised and clinically applied field. The International Academy of Sex Research was founded in 1973, followed by the World Association for Sexology in 1978. Following the publication of a World Health Organization report (1975) on the training of health professionals in a plethora of aspects of human sexuality, psychiatrists increasingly recognised *sexual health* as a fundamental concept for human well-being: 'Sexual health is the integration of the somatic, emotional, intellectual, and social aspects of sexual being, in ways that are positively enriching and that enhance personality, communication, and love', the report stated (World Health Organization, 1975). During the same period, sexology also gained a firm foothold in European countries. In several European countries, sexology became a separate profession, with its own curricula for sexology training (although not necessarily officially recognised as a speciality), and sexologists published textbooks, organised conferences and founded professional organisations: the Nordic Association for Clinical Sexology (1978), the Norwegian Association for Clinical Sexology (1981), a Nordic journal of sexology

(1983) and the European Federation for Sexology (1988) (Langfeldt, 1981; Fugl-Meyer *et al.*, 1999).

To understand the role of sexology in the history of trans medicine in Scandinavia, it is necessary to shift the analytical focus from traditional professions to *expertise* broadly construed (Eyal, 2013). Sexology was not the expertise of *one* profession but was enacted by a network of professions, structures and objects. Moreover, sex reassignment legitimised sexology as a field of knowledge, for instance by creating transatlantic professional bonds between Scandinavia and the United States. The Norwegian psychologist Thore Langfeldt, the Danish psychiatrist Preben Hertoft, the American psychiatrist Richard Green and psychologist John Money were all sexologists and close friends working with trans patients.[8] Hertoft founded the Sexology Clinic at Rigshospitalet, the national hospital, in Copenhagen in 1986, and his textbook *Klinisk sexologi* (Clinical sexology), became a reference work in sexology and in the care for trans patients in Scandinavia (Graugaard and Schmidt, 2017).

Amid major societal changes such as student activism, the women's movement and lesbian and gay liberation, the Oslo Health Council became a laboratory for developing and experimenting with new ideas on sexology and social medicine on grand scale, not least in hammering out efficient responses to HIV/AIDS (Slagstad, 2020). Prejudices against homosexuals were firmly entrenched in society, and also among medical professionals. Sex between men had only been decriminalised in Norway in 1972 and homosexuality was still a psychiatric diagnosis.[9] This was the background for the establishment of a counselling service for homosexuals within the Oslo Health Council in 1977. The service was run by health professionals who themselves were lesbian and gay – general practitioners, nurses and social workers – and supervised by a group of psychiatrists and psychologists. Among their supervisors was Berthold Grünfeld. He was appointed to the country's first position in sexology in a new department of medical sexology in the council.[10] To Grünfeld, sexuality was 'a primitive force in life, a fundamental dimension. ... The more one tries to suppress it, the greater worry it becomes. Suppression dehumanises it, turns it into something dirty and frugal, something we are ashamed of. Unfortunately, our culture has far too much of this destructive attitude towards sexuality' (Grünfeld, 1979: 114). Grünfeld became a leading expert in transgender medicine in Norway, and when patients applied for hormonal and surgical treatment, they first had to convince the sexologists at the Oslo Health Council.[11]

Material preconditions for psychiatric expertise

The Oslo regime for sex reassignment was an attempt to safeguard professional decision-making in a situation where clinical knowledge and experience were sparse. None of the experts had any clinical experience with trans health. 'I don't know if I had heard the word "transsexualism" before. I was completely blank', one of the psychologists said.[12] The professionals were concerned that their interventions would harm the patients: 'I felt very strongly that I or we cared about the patients' situation, their feelings, their integrity, that bad things should not be made worse, that nothing should be started without a proper foundation.'[13] To support decisions, the clinicians wanted to formalise the assessment in a separate institution or clinic. If they had the support and security of an institutional framework, it would take some of the responsibility off their shoulders.

However, the Director General of Health Torbjørn Mork opposed the formalisation or institutionalisation of transgender medicine. The moment a clinic was established, more people would seek treatment, he argued. This was also an efficient strategy to keep thorny legal issues such as marriage rights and the change of name, personal identification number and legal gender at a bay.[14] Moreover, it kept medical transition out of the media spotlight. The health authorities generally tried to avoid public attention to sensitive and potentially controversial issues such as artificial insemination (Bjørvik, 2018: 76–7). In articles about transsexuality and sex reassignment published in the 1950s and 1960s, the *Journal of the Norwegian Medical Association* would often print a note in italics above the title: 'May not be mentioned in the daily press.' The medical practice was to remain secret and restricted.

Doctors and health authorities restricted medical transition to avoid public attention, circumvent legal issues and safeguard clinical decisions. Gatekeeping practices of trans medicine were not restricted to clinical practice but also included psychiatric-bureaucratic efforts to limit the dissemination of knowledge about treatment procedures and the refusal to institutionalise treatment. The authorities decided that this area of psychiatry and medicine would be better handled by dedicated, independent doctors with a personal interest in the topic. And it was precisely this professionally independent but state-sanctioned position of providing expert opinions on issues of public importance on behalf of the bureaucracy that shaped the evaluative role of psychiatry.

Since the authorities refused to establish a specialised clinic, professionals looked for other ways to protect the credibility and legitimacy of clinical decisions. The healthcare workers met several times with the authorities and experts from abroad, and this process created the basis of formalised guidelines for sex reassignment. The guidelines stabilised a therapeutic system and secured the credibility of professional expertise, but they also changed the therapeutic system and institutional context. The guidelines streamlined the medical administration of trans patients by entrusting various professions with specific diagnostic and therapeutic tasks and setting the path for diagnostic and therapeutic practice. A new structure for trans health was established. This is what Stefan Timmermans and Marc Berg poetically described in another context as the crystallisation of an existing and changed world (Timmermans and Berg, 1997). And the existing world that secured the legitimacy of sexology was cast in concrete.

The Oslo Health Council was originally located in a school building from 1869, but this was demolished in 1969 and replaced by a new building. In the new building, all the different departments of the Oslo Health Council were brought under one roof, from the department of epidemic diseases, housing hygiene, venereal diseases and food hygiene to school healthcare and the department for mother and child. During the 1970s, eight new departments were added, in general practice medicine, community nursing, physiotherapy and medical genetics, as well as a support service for families with disabled children. As early as 1958, a large social-psychiatric department for outpatient services was added, dedicated to prophylactic and acute psychiatric care and follow-up of patients discharged from the mental hospitals. By the mid-1970s, the council coordinated the psychiatric services for the entire Oslo population (Borg, 1983), and by 1984 the council employed more than 1,200 full-time staff (Mellbye, 1987; Smith and Siem, 2020). Ironically, the counselling service for homosexuals, where trans patients were assessed, was part of the Department for Mother and Child. But even though some of the clients and the professionals found this somewhat amusing, it also provided institutional credibility.

The brutalist building in natural concrete from 1969, with a building cost of 29 million kroner, was designed by Erling Viksjø and Inge A. Dahl (Figure 12.1). By this time, Viksjø had already established himself as one of the country's most sought-after architects. Ten years earlier, he had designed the high-rise government building in the city centre, just a stone's throw from the health council. It quickly became a prominent symbol of the social-democratic welfare state. Because of the location of the new health council, the architects gave the building a stringent triangular shape, and the architectural design, floor plan and choice of materials were evidence of a hyper-modern unified vision of architecture, science and medicine: a small laboratory was set up in the basement, each room was equipped with a sink, and the more than 1,000 windows were made of solid aluminium (Figure 12.2) (Dahl and Viksjø, 1969). In many ways, the two brutalist edifices in sandblasted natural concrete and con-glomerate concrete – the government buildings and the Oslo Health Council – materialised a new muscular post-war policy and an ambitious modernist political programme. For politicians and doctors alike, the architecture of the new health council embodied a bright medical future, an expansive public healthcare system and the importance of medicine, science and psychiatry for the welfare state. In this programme, sexology now found its rightful place. In theory, sexology stood for gender equality and sexual liberation, a future 'reform psychiatry' that fit perfectly with ideals of a modern welfare state. The modernist, 'social-democratic' architecture and infrastruc-ture of the Oslo Health Council legitimised sexological expertise in the eyes of the government and the public, which in turn secured the evaluative role and authority of the psychiatrist in trans issues. The new Oslo Health Council brought trans medicine under one roof, and the concrete cast concretised the role of sexology in trans medicine, psychiatry and the public healthcare system in general.

Making a psychiatric expert opinion

The professionals sought to protect the integrity of the treatment regime by anchoring it in the public health body but also in the

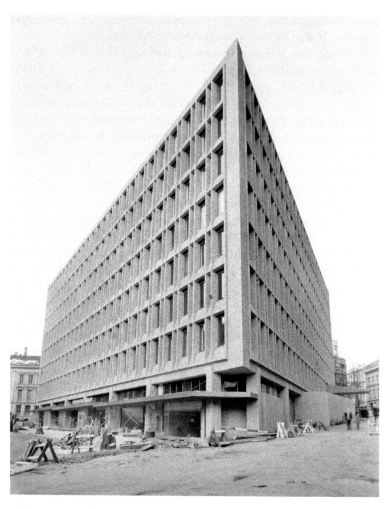

Figure 12.1 The Oslo Health Council anno 1969. The location posed
several problems for the architects. The triangular shape was 'not
particularly well-suited for an office building', the architects stated, and
it had caused a range of technical and constructional problems.
However, 'the client saw a central location as the best solution'.
Photo by Leif Ørnelund. With permission from the Oslo Museum,
Creative Commons 3.0. http://www.oslobilder.no/OMU/
OB.%C3%9869/0319. Image available under a Creative Commons
(CC BY-NC-ND 4.0) licence, https://creativecommons.org/licenses/
by-nc-nd/4.0/.

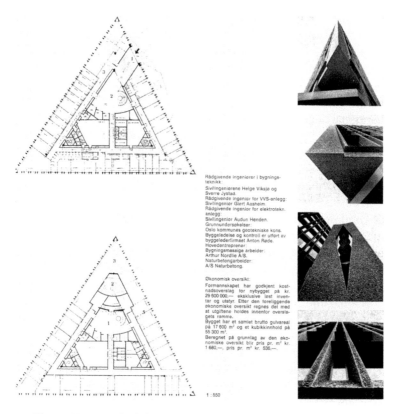

Figure 12.2 On the left, the architectural plan of the Oslo Health Council. The building had a triangular shape, and all offices were aligned along the outer walls. Stairs, elevators and facilities such as kitchenettes, toilets and locker rooms were placed in the core of the building. Separate windows in every office ensured bright working conditions for the health staff. On the right, details of the building and the entrance sculpture designed by Ramon Isern. Byggekunst, 1969. With permission from Arkitektur N and Tone Viksjø. Image available under a Creative Commons (CC BY-NC-ND 4.0) licence, https://creativecommons.org/licenses/by-nc-nd/4.0/.

clinical approach to the individual patient. Diagnostic and therapeutic decisions were made by a team of experts that included psychiatrists, psychologists, endocrinologists, social workers and plastic surgeons. From the beginning, the patient was examined by 'every potential clinician' and all decisions were based on the views of 'all the aforementioned specialists'.[15] The team-based multidisciplinary approach ensured that each patient was thoroughly assessed from a range of biological, psychological and social viewpoints. A general practitioner or surgeon conducted a clinical examination to examine every aspect of the patient's 'somatic sex' to exclude 'genetic, hormonal or genital incongruence'. A psychiatrist carefully scrutinised the 'sexological state' of the patient, including sexual fantasies, self-perception, experience of femininity and masculinity, 'gender role behaviour' and sexual practice. A psychologist or psychiatrist examined the patient's personality using clinical interviews and testing instruments to decide whether concomitant psychiatric symptoms or conditions were primary or secondary to transsexuality. Finally, the social worker scrutinised the work situation and facilitated social transition in the workplace, even by arranging for occupational rehabilitation or, if needed, the relocation to a new job.

Broadly seen, the expert opinion on whether a patient was given hormonal and surgical treatment was shaped against two premises. There could be no contraindications and the patient had to fulfil the criteria of transsexuality. Contraindications ranged from age and social issues to physical characteristics and psychiatric illness. The professionals argued that the younger the patient, the better the prognosis; ideally, the patient should be in their twenties or early thirties. The barrier to access treatment was much higher if the patient had children or was married. The patient should preferably have a stable job and secure income, as well as social and psychological support among family, friends and colleagues. 'To exaggerate a bit', Hanna said in an interview, 'if everyone had said they wanted a husband, two children, a family car, a villa and a dog, they would've been very happy.'[16] She went through the diagnostic assessment in the early 1980s.

'Unsuitable body type' was another contraindication that primarily prevented access to treatment for tall trans women or patients with a sturdy body type. 'One of the criteria for sex change, which was very strict, was that one had to be able to pass as the other gender [*kjønn*]', one of the doctors recalled. 'So tall men didn't get treatment and people who had big shoes. I remember very well how this criterion of being able to pass was talked about. Talk about cultural production of masculinity and femininity and what is right and wrong and normal and abnormal. It's very strange to think about today, I think.'[17]

'Psychotic traits' posed a firm contraindication to medical therapy, but the psychiatrists and psychologists did not relate psychotic symptoms to stigma or minority stress. In rare cases, the Oslo guideline stated, 'the desire for sex change' was part of a psychotic illness. Depression, on the other hand, could be the result of 'having waited for treatment for a long time and experienced many negative reactions along the way'.[18] Therefore, major depression was not a firm contraindication to treatment. The different approach to psychosis and depression established a hierarchy of contraindication. Psychosis became a separate disease entity unrelated to minority stress, while the professionals saw depression in relation to psychological and societal factors such as stigma. Professionals realised trans health was inextricably linked to the negative health effects of marginalisation, stigmatisation and ostracism. The different approach to patients with psychotic and depressive symptoms probably reflected a much longer tradition in psychiatry of distinguishing between severe and milder forms of mental illness, and of psychiatrists automatically attributing lower self-knowledge to people with psychosis and impaired decision-making capacity.

The second obligatory passage point was that the patient had to be diagnosed as a transsexual and not as a transvestite or homosexual. The diagnostic criteria for transsexuality corresponded to those of the ICD-9, published in 1978: the patients had to have the experience of 'belonging to the opposite sex' since childhood and 'feelings of disgust' towards their 'own biological sex', as well as the desire to be recognised as the 'opposite sex' and a wish for hormonal and surgical therapy to align the body with their gender identity.[19] An important objective of psychiatric expertise therefore was to probe the 'consistency' of the gender identity and the psychosexual development including 'sexual fantasies, self-image, experience of masculinity/femininity, gender role behaviour and sexual behaviour.'[20] The diagnostic reasoning was based on the idea that transsexuality had to be separated from so-called effeminate homosexuality. For trans women to pass through the diagnostic system, for example, they had to convince the professionals that they were only sexually interested in heterosexual men.

The unsolvable paradox of the restrictive Oslo model was that the medical treatment that would have made it easier for patients to fulfil the stereotypical gender conceptions of transsexuality was withheld until the very end. 'They were very afraid that people would regret it', Hanna said. 'If you were a heterosexual woman like me, everything was okay, but if you were a lesbian woman, it was not okay, then they would not operate on you.'[21] At first, the professionals concluded that she was an effeminate homosexual man since she also dated gay men. But at that time, Hanna did not really care much if the men she went on dates with were gay or straight, and besides, it was much easier for a trans woman to meet men in Oslo's gay scene. 'I tried to explain to Grünfeld all the things I tried to do that night without him [her date] trying to feel me up down there, which turned into a big mess, poor guy, but Grünfeld then decided to believe I was a gay man', Hanna said. 'But when I told him that I had gone out with straight guys, gone to the cinema and had a glass of wine, he asked me why it had stopped there. And I said: 'Look, I have not yet had genital surgery, and I don't have breasts either.'[22]

One of the doctors confirmed Hanna's experience: 'At that time, I think nobody believed that transgender people, or "sex change clients", as we used to say, could be anything but heterosexual. It was part of the definition that if they wanted to become the opposite sex, then they wanted a partner of the same sex as they were born. It was almost a requirement.'[23] The health professionals feared that trans patients requested medical treatment as a 'cheap solution' to self-repressed homosexuality:

> Back then it was much harder to be gay, and if you could disguise it with surgery, hormones, clothes, and social role, that was more attractive to some people. We thought we knew quite a lot about sexual orientation, so with some of the people we talked to, we concluded: he is gay, do not pursue this project, sex change is not the solution for this. But at the same time, there was a lack of understanding that transgender people could have a non-heterosexual orientation. At that time, sexual orientation was very binary, you were either homosexual or not. Any form of fluidity, which has become much more apparent the last ten years, did not exist in people's minds.[24]

According to the experts' self-understanding, sexology was about approaching human sexuality in sex-positive, health-promoting, depathologising and non-normative ways. However, the Oslo model also reflected ingrained scepticism about the medicalisation of social and sexual issues. In sexology, transgender was not considered a minority condition or included in the human variation they otherwise advocated. The sexological legacy of sex, gender and sexuality, and how these concepts related to one another, became a barrier to accessing medical treatment for trans patients (see Gill-Peterson, 2018). Trans patients were subjected to a medical regime of psychiatric-sexological inspection and adjustment, and sexology became a tool for psychiatrists, psychologists and other sexologists to administer trans life. However, there would have been no sexology without the patients who willingly, but most often unwillingly, shared stories with the professionals and who had to surrender their bodies and identities to psychiatric, medical and sexological inspection, examination and administration. Ultimately, sexology became a gatekeeping model in trans medicine, a way of organising trans-specific healthcare which has faced much criticism (Stone, 1991; Spade, 2006; Alm, 2018; Horncastle, 2018; Ashley, 2019; Shuster, 2021).

Paradoxically, Grünfeld was aware of the hierarchical problems and unequal distribution of power in the system he overlooked: the paternalism of the doctors making these decisions often remained unconscious, he wrote, 'disguised as so-called medical reasoning' (Grünfeld, 1987: 203). In the end, very few patients succeeded in receiving treatment and most people were left to fend for themselves. There were simply few other ways of accessing hormones and surgery for trans patients within the public healthcare system.[25]

The manifold practices of psychiatric expertise

This chapter has attempted to extend a historical analysis of the psychiatric-bureaucratic administration of trans life beyond anachronism or moral indignation over the actions of individual actors. This would overlook the systemic role of psychiatric expertise in the welfare state in negotiating and resolving problems between the public and the bureaucracy. The psychiatric expert opinion was an attempt at providing an answer to a practical question – who should be allowed to change sex? – in a situation where the major goal of medicine and bureaucracy was to restrict and limit this type of care to a minimum. The preparation of psychiatric expert opinions was not limited to the clinical encounter between the individual patient and psychiatrist or the evaluation of contraindications, aetiological reasonings or nosological demarcation. Psychiatric expertise was one building block in a comprehensive social fabric that also included medical publication culture and the health bureaucracy. Expert opinions gained their legitimacy and authority by tying together patients and health professionals, concepts and objects, paper and concrete, institutional and spatial arrangements. This included the old public health institution of the Oslo Health Council with its new architectural design, and it included the flowering field of sexology with its organisations, publication channels, conferences, textbooks and curricula.

Standardisation processes are central to modern medicine, scholars in science and technology have noted (Bowker and Star, 1999). However, standards cannot be seamlessly teleported to any social context. For standards to work, they must recruit and become embedded in pre-existing institutional and material relations and practices. Protocols and standards are 'technoscientific scripts which crystallize multiple trajectories', the scripts enable and modify pre-existing infrastructures (Timmermans and Berg, 1997). Sexology as reform psychiatry mobilised old institutions and structures while fostering new spatial, material and architectural arrangements.[26] As psychiatrists and sexologists developed diagnostic routines and treatment protocols for trans patients, they worked hard to embed these practices into the pre-existing Oslo Health Council and the counselling service for homosexual patients, expanding, transforming and modifying the infrastructure already in place. Faced with the 'new' issue of sex change, the professionals tried to secure expert authority and legitimacy by anchoring decisions in an interdisciplinary team. Trans care enabled new ways of doing psychiatry. This reform built on an old epistemological framework of sex and sexuality and their interrelations, and the old framework hindered a subversive and inclusive potential in sexology from being applied to the new field of trans health. This legacy continues to reverberate in the present. In the early 2000s, a new gender identity clinic was established at Rikshospitalet under psychiatric control. Yet people who transgress binary norms of gender are still excluded from treatment (Jentoft, 2019; Slagstad, 2022b).

The Oslo story of sexological expertise on trans issues is an example of psychiatric expertise as social practice. Sexology, as a form of psychiatric expertise, prepared, mediated and solved problems between the bureaucracy and the public. The sexological administration of trans patients was a response to the 'new' issue of medical transition which secured the evaluative role of psychiatry in the welfare state. Sexology became the fundament for a new diagnostic and therapeutic programme and standard of trans medicine that changed the existing world of psychiatry.

Funding

The research for this chapter was funded by the Norwegian Research Council (Grant No. 283370) and the research project Biomedicalization from the Inside Out (BIO).

Notes

1 One could argue that it is anachronistic to use 'trans' for a time when the term was not in use. However, I do not use it as an identity category but as an analytical category to avoid reproducing the pathologising terms of hegemonical actors (i.e. doctors).

2 The health councils (helserådene) were originally known as health commissions (*sunnhetskommisjoner*).

3 For the regulation of sex reassignment in the Scandinavian medico-judiciary system, see Alm, 2018; Hartline, 2020; Honkasalo, 2020; Alm, 2021.

4 For more on psychosurgery see the contribution by Florent Serina in Chapter 6.

5 Magnus Hirschfeld had already coined the term *Transvestitismus* in 1910. In Denmark and Norway, 'genuine transvestism' was in use in the 1950s and 1960s. In Sweden, 'transsexualism' was in use from the 1960s – see Wålinder, 1967. 'Transsexualism' gradually replaced 'genuine transvestism' in 1970s Norway. American doctors and psychiatrists mostly referred to 'transsexuality' or 'transsexualism' (Benjamin, 1953; Benjamin, 1966).

6 The National Archives of Norway, Oslo, RA/S-1286/D/Dc/L0611, Sosialdepartementet, Helsedirektoratet, Kontoret for psykiatri, H4, Dc,

Box 611, Folder Transseksualitet, Per Anchersen to the Directorate of Health, 31 July 1974.

7 For the role of social medicine see Slagstad, 2021.

8 Thore Langfeldt, interview with Ketil Slagstad, Oslo, 29 January 2020.

9 In 1977, the Norwegian Psychiatric Association recommended its members avoid using the diagnosis.

10 Oslo City Archives, Oslo (hereafter OCA), Oslo helseråd, Box 122, Homofile – transseksualitet, Hans Døvik, 'Rådgivningstjenesten for homofile – egen seksjon for medisinsk sexologi', 3 July 1979.

11 Berthold Grünfeld was born in Bratislava to Jewish parents, but was brought to Norway by the Nansen Relief before World War II.

12 Bodil Solberg, interview with Ketil Slagstad, Oslo, 20 January 2020.

13 *Ibid.*

14 OCA, Oslo helseråd, Box 122, Homofile – transseksualitet, Torbjørn Mork to Stadsfysikus in Oslo, Fredrik Mellbye, 'Transseksualitet', 16 February 1979.

15 OCA, Oslo helseråd, Box 122, Homofile – transseksualitet, Report, 'Utredning om transseksualitet', December 1979, p. 5.

16 Hanna, interview with Ketil Slagstad, 13 November 2019. 'Hanna' is a pseudonym.

17 Kirsti Malterud, interview with Ketil Slagstad, 24 October 2019. At the time, Kirsti Malterud worked as a general practitioner. She later became a professor in general practice with a research focus on qualitative methods and women's health.

18 OCA, Oslo helseråd, Box 122, Homofile – transseksualitet, Report, 'Utredning om transseksualitet', December 1979, p. 5.

19 *Ibid.*, p. 6.

20 *Ibid.*

21 Hanna interview.

22 *Ibid.*

23 Malterud interview.

24 *Ibid.*

25 It was not possible to find out what happened to those patients who were denied treatment.

26 See also Chapters 4 and 9.

References

Æsculap, 1948, '8. oktober: Kinsey-rapporten', *Æsculap*, 28:8, 89–100.

Alm, Erika, 2018, 'What constitutes an in/significant organ? The vicissitudes of juridical and medical decision-making regarding genital surgery for intersex and trans people in Sweden', in Gabriele Griffin and Malin Jordal (eds), *Body, Migration, Re/Constructive Surgeries* (London: Routledge), pp. 225–40.

Alm, Erika, 2021, 'A state affair? Notions of the state in discourses on trans rights in Sweden', in Erika Alm, Linda Berg, Mikela Lundahl Hero, Anna Johansson, Pia Laskar, Lena Martinsson, Diana Mulinari and Cathrin Wasshede (eds), *Pluralistic Struggles in Gender, Sexuality and Coloniality: Challenging Swedish Exceptionalism* (Cham: Springer International Publishing), pp. 209–37.

Anchersen, Per, 1957, 'Problems of transvestism', *Acta Psychiatrica et Neurologica Scandinavica*, 31:106, 249–56.

Ashley, Florence, 2019, 'Gatekeeping hormone replacement therapy for transgender patients is dehumanising', *Journal of Medical Ethics*, 45:7, 480–2.

Bauer, Susanne, 2014, 'From administrative infrastructure to biomedical resource: Danish population registries, the "Scandinavian laboratory," and the "epidemiologist's dream"', *Science in Context*, 27:2, 187–213.

Benjamin, Harry, 1953, 'Transvestism and transsexualism', *International Journal of Sexology*, 7:1, 12–14.

Benjamin, Harry, 1966, *The Transsexual Phenomenon* (New York: Julian Press).

Berg, Ole, 2009, *Spesialisering og profesjonalisering: En beretning om den sivile norske helseforvaltnings utvikling fra 1809 til 2009: Del 1: 1809–1983 – Den gamle helseforvaltning* (Oslo: Statens helsetilsyn).

Berg, Siv Frøydis, 2002, *Den unge Karl Evang og utvidelsen av helsebegrepet* (Oslo: Solum Forlag).

Bjørvik, Eira, 2018, 'Conceiving Infertility: Infertility Treatment and Assisted Reproductive Technologies in 20th Century Norway'. PhD dissertation, University of Oslo.

Borg, Egil (ed.), 1983, *Psykiatrisk poliklinikk i sentrum: Oslo Helseråds avdeling for psykiatri 25 år* (Oslo: Universitetsforlaget).

Bowker, Geoffrey C. and Susan Leigh Star, 1999, *Sorting Things Out: Classification and its Consequences* (Cambridge, MA: MIT Press).

Bremer, Johan, 1961, 'Mutilerende behandling av transseksualisme?', *Tidsskrift for Den Norske Lægeforening*, 68:13–14, 921–3.

Bremer, Johan, 1982, *Veier og villspor i psykiatrien* (Oslo: Tanum-Norli).

Dahl, Inge A. and Erling Viksjø, 1969, 'Oslo Helseråd', *Byggekunst*, 51:6, 232–3.

Edgerton, Milton T., 1974, 'The surgical treatment of male transsexuals', *Clinics in Plastic Surgery*, 1:2, 285–323.

Evang, Karl, Otto Galtung Hansen and Carl Viggo Lange, 1932, 'Vårt program', *Populært Tidsskrift for Seksuell Oplysning*, 1:1, 3–7.

Eyal, Gil, 2013, 'For a sociology of expertise: The social origins of the autism epidemic', *American Journal of Sociology*, 118:4, 863–907.

Fleck, Ludwik, 1980, *Entstehung und Entwicklung einer wissenschaftlichen Tatsache* (Frankfurt: Suhrkamp).

Fugl-Meyer, Kerstin, Elsa Almås, Espen Esther Pirelli Benestad and Osmo Kontula, 1999, 'Nordic sexology education and authorisation', *Scandinavian Journal of Sexology*, 4:1, 61–8.

Geisthövel, Alexa and Volker Hess, 2017, 'Handelndes Wissen: Die Praxis des Gutachtens', in Alexa Geisthövel and Volker Hess (eds), *Medizinisches Gutachten: Geschichte einer neuzeitlichen Praxis* (Göttingen: Wallstein Verlag), pp. 9–39.

Gill-Peterson, J., 2018, *Histories of the Transgender Child* (Minneapolis, MN: University of Minnesota Press).

Graugaard, Christian and Gunter Schmidt, 2017, 'Preben Hertoft (1928–2017)', *Archives of Sexual Behavior*, 46:6, 1551–4.

Grünfeld, Berthold, 1979, *Vårt seksuelle liv* (Oslo: Gyldendal).

Grünfeld, Berthold, 1987, 'Seksualitet som helseproblem', in Harald Siem, Kåre Berg and Berthold Grünfeld (eds), *Samfunnsmedisin i praksis: Oslo Helseråd i 80-årene* (Oslo: Universitetsforlaget), pp. 200–6.

'Hanna', 2019, Interview by Ketil Slagstad, Oslo, 13 November.

hartline, france rose, 2020, 'Exploring the (cis)gender imaginary in the Nordic region', *Journal of Gender Studies*, 1:23, 67–87.

Holm, M. [now Sølve M. Holm], 2017, 'Fleshing Out the Self: Reimagining Intersexed and Trans Embodied Lives Through (Auto)biographical Accounts of the Past'. PhD dissertation, Linköping University.

Honkasalo, Julian, 2020, 'In the shadow of eugenics: Transgender sterilisation legislation and the struggle for self-determination', in Ruth Pearce, Igi Moon, Kat Gupta and Deborah Lynn Steinberg (eds), *The Emergence of Trans: Culture, Politics and Everyday Lives* (Abingdon: Routledge), pp. 17–33.

Horncastle, J., 2018, 'Busting out: Happenstance surgery, clinic effects, and the poetics of genderqueer subjectivity', *TSQ: Transgender Studies Quarterly*, 5:2, 251–67.

Jentoft, Elian E., 2019, 'Through the Needle's Eye: A Qualitative Study of the Experiences of Adolescents with Gender Incongruence and their Families Seeking Gender Affirming Healthcare in Norway'. Master's thesis, University of Oslo.

Klöppel, Ulrike, 2010, *XX0XY ungelöst: Hermaphroditismus, Sex und Gender in der deutschen Medizin: Eine historische Studie zu Intersexualität* (Bielefeld: Transcript Verlag).

Langfeldt, Thore, 1981, 'Klinisk sexologi i Norden', *Tidsskrift for Norsk Psykologforening*, 18:12, 652–3.

Langfeldt, Thore, 2020, Interview by Ketil Slagstad, Oslo, 29 January.

Lie, Anne Kveim, 2014, 'Producing standards, producing the Nordic region: Antibiotic susceptibility testing, from 1950–1970', *Science in Context*, 27:2, 215–48.

Malterud, Kirsti, 2019, Interview by Ketil Slagstad, Bergen/Berlin, 24 October.

Mellbye, Fredrik, 1987, 'Embetet som stadsfyskikus i Oslo', in Harald Siem, Kåre Berg and Berthold Grünfeld (eds), *Samfunnsmedisin i praksis: Oslo Helseråd i 80-årene* (Oslo: Universitetsforlaget), pp. 22–7.

Meyer, Sabine (ed.), 2018, *Auf nach Casablanca?: Lebensrealitäten transgeschlechtlicher Menschen zwischen 1945 und 1980* (Berlin: Senatsverwaltung für Justiz, Verbraucherschutz und Antidiskriminierung and Landesstelle für Gleichbehandlung – gegen Diskriminierung (LADS)).

Najmabadi, Afsaneh, 2014, *Professing Selves: Transsexuality and Same-Sex Desire in Contemporary Iran* (Durham, NC: Duke University Press).

Nordby, Trond, 1989, *Karl Evang: en biografi* (Oslo: Aschehoug).

Parhi, Katariina, 2018, 'Boyish mannerisms and womanly coquetry: Patients with the diagnosis of Transvestitismus in the Helsinki Psychiatric Clinic in Finland, 1954–68', *Medical History*, 62:1, 50–66.

Sandal, Sigrid, 2020, '"Transvestittbehandlingsspørsmålet"', *Historisk tidsskrift*, 99:4, 316–31.

Schiøtz, Aina, 2003, *Folkets helse – landets styrke, 1850–2003* (Oslo: Universitetsforlaget).

Sejersted, Francis, 2011, *The Age of Social Democracy: Norway and Sweden in the Twentieth Century* (Princeton, NJ: Princeton University Press).

Sekuler, Todd, 2018, 'Un/Certain Care: From a Diagnostic to a Somatechnic Regime of Care for Medical Transition in Public Hospitals in France'. PhD dissertation, Humboldt-Universität zu Berlin.

shuster, stef m., 2021, *Trans Medicine: The Emergence and Practice of Treating* (New York: New York University Press).

Skålevåg, Svein Atle, 2016, *Utilregnelighet: En historie om rett og medisin* (Oslo: Pax forlag).

Skinner, Quentin, 2012, *Die drei Körper des Staates* (Göttingen: Wallstein Verlag).

Slagstad, Ketil, 2020, 'The amphibious nature of AIDS activism: Medical professionals and gay and lesbian communities in Norway, 1975–1987', *Medical History*, 64:3, 401–35.

Slagstad, Ketil, 2021, 'Society as cause and cure: The norms of transgender social medicine', *Culture, Medicine, and Psychiatry*, 45:3, 456–78.

Slagstad, Ketil, 2022a, 'Bureaucratizing medicine: Creating a gender identity clinic in the welfare state', *Isis*, 113:3, 469–90.

Slagstad, Ketil, 2022b, 'On the Boundaries of Care: The Ephemerality of Transgender Medicine in the Welfare State, Scandinavia 1951–2001'. PhD dissertation, University of Oslo.

Slagstad, Rune, 1998, *De nasjonale strateger* (Oslo: Pax forlag).

Smith, Anders and Harald Siem, 2020, 'Offentlig folkehelsearbeid i Oslo: et tilbakeblikk', *Michael*, 17:1, 528–35.

Solberg, Bodil, 2020, Interview by Ketil Slagstad, Oslo, 20 January.

Spade, Dean, 2006, 'Mutilating gender', in Susan Stryker and Stephen Whittle (eds), *The Transgender Studies Reader* (New York: Routledge), pp. 315–32.

Stone, Sandy, 1991, 'The empire strikes back: A posttransexual manifesto', in Julia Epstein and Kristina Straub (eds), *Body Guards: The Cultural Politics of Gender Ambiguity* (New York: Routledge), pp. 280–304.

The Harry Benjamin International Gender Dysphoria Association, 1979, *Standards of Care: The Hormonal and Surgical Sex Reassignment of Gender Dysphoric Persons* (Galveston, TX: n.p.).

Timmermans, Stefan and Marc Berg, 1997, 'Standardization in action: Achieving local universality through medical protocols', *Social Studies of Science*, 27:2, 273–305.

Wålinder, Jan, 1967, *Transsexualism: A Study of Forty-Three Cases* (Göteborg: Akademiförlaget).

World Health Organization, 1975, *Education and Treatment in Human Sexuality: The Training of Health Professionals* (Geneva: World Health Organization).

Index